A Hound Dog in Anderson
and other Essays on Medicine and Life

Charles S. Bryan, M.D., MACP

Forward by W. Curtis Worthington, M.D.

The South Carolina Medical Association
Columbia, South Carolina
2008

ISBN 978-1-60530-563-9

Printed in Columbia, South Carolina,
for the Phrontistery Press
by Wentworth Printing Corporation

For Donna

Contents

Forward   xi
Preface   xiii

Personalities and Reflections   1

Joseph Ioor Waring — An Appreciation   3
Bill's Lesion   8
Fond Memories of Emmett   12
Real Medicine   15
Eulogy Written in a Country Churchyard   20
"I've Been There"   24
Games Played with Balls   28
Flight 463   31
Doctor Weston   33
Nothing Could be Finer   36
Live as Though Seen   41
Pew Thoughts While Listening to Pachelbel's
    Cannon in D   45
The English Lesson   48
A Hound Dog in Anderson   51
Thoughts on *The Doctor*   54
E. Carwile Leroy (1933-2002): *Lacrimae Rerum*   58
His Blood Runneth Orange   60
"I'm not a Missionary"   64

The Profession of Medicine   69

Professional Responsibility   71
On the Verge of a New Golden Age?   75
William Osler and Medical Societies   79
Of Ideals and Heroes   84
What is Professionalism and can it be Measured?   88
Sacred Trust   91

A Very Short History of the Medical Profession,
    as Told to Patch Adams   94
What is a Doctor? Reflections on the Physician
    Charter on Professionalism   100
Advancing Medical Professionalism. I. Our
    Public Image   105
Advancing Medical Professoinalism. II. One Size
    Does Not Fit All   109
Advancing Medical Professionalism. III. Bearding the
    Evils of Specialization   115
Advancing Medical Professionalism. IV. Why Higher
    Professionalism Hurts   119
Advancing Medical Professionalism. V. The Social
    Contract, and Why Tort Reform is Essential   124
Advancing Medical Professionalism. VI.
    Summing Up   130
"I Like Science and I Want to Help People" —
    Introductory Remarks on Professionalism to
    Freshman Medical Students   133

The Virtues in Medicine   147

The Limits of Altruism   149
To Care and Not to Care   151
"Reverence for Life" — A Unifying Field for Ethical
    Decision Making?   155
Peace and Good Will   157
High Tech, High Touch   161
The V-Word and the Four C's   164
First Among the C's   167
The Duties of Patients: A Distant Mirror   172
Y2K.4. Virtues and Values   175
Medicine and the Seven Basic Virtues. I. Introduction   183
Medicine and the Seven Basic Virtues. II. Prudence
    (Practical Wisdom)   186
Medicine and the Seven Basic Virtues. III. Justice   192
Medicine and the Seven Basic Virtues. IV.
    Temperance   197

Medicine and the Seven Basic Virtues. V. Courage 204
Medicine and the Seven Basic Virtues. VI. Faith 208
Medicine and the Seven Basic Virtues. VII. Hope 212
Medicine and the Seven Basic Virtues. VIII. Love 216
Medicine and the Seven Basic Virtues. IX. Summing
   Up 220

Medical Education 227

Personality and Medical Students 229
Bedside Body Language 233
Found: A Point on the Compass 235
Should Philosophy be Required in the Premedical
   Curriculum? 237
Preparation for Medical School: What Have we
   Learned, and What Can we do Differently? 239
Second Schools: Second Thoughts 243
Comprehensive Health/Lifestyle Education in the
   Secondary Schools ... An Idea Whose Time
   has Come? 247
Whither Academic Health Centers? 249
Just Thinking 253
Reflections on the SMA-1 (A.K.A., the Medical History) 258
Physical Diagnosis and the Technological Imperative 264

Public Health and the HIV/AIDS Epidemic 269

Immunization against Swine Influenza: A Major
   Challenge for South Carolina Physicians 271
Physicians and the Environment 273
AIDS in South Carolina 275
AIDS Policies 280
Ethics and AIDS—One Year Later 282
Beliefs, Attitudes, and Health Promotion 285
HIV, Surgeons, and ... All of Us 289
Fort Host 297
"The Rights of the Child" Revisited 306

The Politics of Medicine   309

Physicians' Assistants   311
The New Nurse and Territorial Rights   314
Handgun Control   316
The CT Scan and the Technological Imperative   318
"Wellness" — New Catchword or Novel Concept?   320
Chiropractic Legislation: Two Broken Records   326
The New Economics of Health Care Delivery:
    A Time for Ideas and Input   331
Diagnosis Related Groups (DRGs): Implications
    and Uncertainties   335
Medical Education and DRGs   338
Of Cost Containment and Cat-Bellers   341
Black Physicians, South Carolina Medicine,
    and the SCMA   344
Appropriate Health Policy: A Larger View   348
When Democrats Last in the Dooryard Bloom'd   351
"The Character and Usefulness of This Calling":
    Thoughts on the Coming Sesquicentennial   354
Of Hegel and Health Care Financing   357
Rightsizing the Healthcare Workforce   359
Race and Health Care   364
Y2K.7. Myth, Magic, and Muggles: Harry Potter
    and the Future of Medicine   368
Health Care Reform: The Case for
    Communitarianism   371

Medical Journalism   377

The Case Report as Medical Scholarship   379
The Journal — Expectations   383

Bibliography: Editorials, 1976-2007   387

Index   399

Forward

This unusual and interesting collection of editorials was written by Dr. Charles S. Bryan during his thirty-one-year tenure as editor of *The Journal of the South Carolina Medical Association*. It was a period that saw many changes in medicine and society and these editorials reflect in a remarkably insightful way the consequences of many of these changes. They also demonstrate the author's grasp of lessons from history and philosophy as they may be applied to the numerous problems attendant upon scientific advances that sometimes boggle the mind of even the reasonably well-educated. They are for the most part not "editorials" at all in the usual sense, but rather short essays on a variety of topics of contemporary, historical, or philosophical import.

The book is divided into seven sections. The first, *Personalities and Reflections*, consists of eighteen pieces on events, personal incidents, biographical sketches, eulogies, and other reflections on life and a life in medicine.

The Profession of Medicine is devoted to medical professionalism, its virtues and vices. It begins with professional responsibility followed by six items on advancing medical professionalism, and ends with the text of a lecture energized from the previous considerations of the topic, given to freshman medical students.

Virtues in Medicine defines for the reader, among other considerations, the four classical virtues from Plato—prudence, justice, temperance, and courage—and the three theological virtues from the Apostle Paul: faith, hope, and love. The author gives a final analysis of this section by beginning and ending it with his actions in a particular case of his own. He also leads his readers into a discussion of how virtues relate to character, including some easy-to-understand charts, and concludes that "character represents the cumulative effect of making choices in tough situations. And the task of building character is never complete."

Medical Education addresses at length the questions of who should be admitted to medical school and who, when all is said and done, would become the most effective physicians. In recent years there have been numerous experiments such as modifications of admissions policies, early introduction of patient contact, rotations with doctors in the field, and changes of emphasis in the curriculum. All of these are examined to a greater or lesser extent in this section. The definition of academic health centers also comes under scrutiny. One muses on a quatrain from *Omar Kyam*:

> Myself when young did eagerly frequent
> Doctor and Saint, and heard great argument
> About it and About: but ever more
> Came out by the same door as in I went.

Public Health and the HIV/AIDS Epidemic is devoted primarily to HIV/AIDS including the beginning of the epidemic and its course in South Carolina. It is a primer on the topic for almost anyone who is interested and the author has been a central figure in understanding the ramifications of the disease.

The Politics of Medicine defies simple categorization. The essays—from physician's assistants through the new economics of health care delivery, to health care reform and the case for "communitarianism," all refer to segments of the health care community in a real or presumed need for change.

This book encompasses a significant portion of the professional life of a talented writer and sensitive physician. His writings project an air of enthusiasm and excitement as well as authority and significance. His dedication to medicine in its broadest sense is apparent throughout.

W. Curtis Worthington, M.D.
Director, The Waring Historical Library
Professor of the Health Sciences
Formerly Academic Dean
The Medical University of South Carolina
Charleston, South Carolina

Preface

Three motives explain this collection of editorials from *The Journal of the South Carolina Medical Association*. First, and atop Abraham Maslow's hierarchy of needs, is the desire to capture more than three decades of medical history in South Carolina. Over time I've written about many and perhaps most of the medical issues-of-the-day, largely because, as I sometimes say only partly in jest, monthly deadlines have denied me the luxury of letting many of my thoughts to go unpublished (as they perhaps should).

My second motive is to make accessible a body of writing that might someday be difficult to obtain as the major medical libraries, already pressed for space, shed their aging journals to make room for computers and the like. Changes in the SCMA's organizational structure (in 1984 a group of organizational consultants recommended that the journal editor no longer be an *ex-officio* member of the leadership group) and in my own research interests (which after 1992, when I became chair of the Department of Medicine at the University of South Carolina School of Medicine, focused less on infectious diseases and more on the history and philosophy of medicine) resulted in my editorials being less concerned with medical politics and more concerned with such abstractions as idealism, professionalism, and the virtues. Ideas that have been presented and published in various national forums were often developed first and/or more fully in *The Journal*, and hence this collection may hold some interest for the future researcher.

My third motive is to share these editorials with various friends around the United States, Canada, and abroad, and especially my many friends in the American Osler Society, an organization devoted to the continued relevance of the humanities to medicine. I'd also like to share them with the younger physicians in South Carolina as a way of encouraging them to take up what I've called "the ideal of idealism." Over time much of my writing has taken the form of gratuitous prescriptive advice. I'm a firm believer in setting and pursuing lofty goals, including such quixotic aspirations as the unity of the medical profession, and I'd consider this book successful if even one or two younger colleagues take up this banner and hold it higher than I've managed to do. This motive includes, of course, the vainglorious "struggle to singularize ourselves, to survive in some way in the memory of others and of posterity," to quote the Spanish philosopher Miguel de Unamuno. Hence, the desire to give these 92 editorials (out of 300 written for *The Journal* between 1976 and 2007) longer shelf-lives than might otherwise be the case.

I'd like to thank the presidents and other leaders of the SCMA for the privilege of serving so many years as editor of their journal. (At the time of this writing, and since the retirement of Dr. John Thomison from *Tennessee Medicine*, I'm probably the longest-tenured medical journal editor in the United States.) And I'd like to express my deep gratitude to the previous managing editors, all of whom became good friends: Joy Drennen, Audria Belton, Dana Kickey Yow, and Jeannette Mangels. I've enjoyed a close working relationship with the Waring Historical Library at the Medical University of South Carolina, Charleston, and would like to thank Dr. W. Curtis Worthington, Jr., its longtime director, and its previous curators, Anne Donato, Elizabeth (Betty) Newsom, and Jane Brown, who provided so many cover illustrations through the years. I thank Everose Alexander for transcribing many of these editorials, and I thank the current managing editors, Brandolyn Harper and Katherine Crosby, for their continued support. I thank Sanchia Mitchell, my longtime secretary, for her patience and also for her proofreading. I am especially grateful to Robert Ariail, the world class cartoonist whose cover illustration captures the moment of the title story ("A Hound Dog in Anderson"). Finally, I thank my wife, Donna, for her support of these and other projects through the years.

Charles S. Bryan, M.D., MACP

Columbia, South Carolina
December 2007

Personalities
and Reflections

Joseph Ioor Waring—An Appreciation

J SC Med Assoc 1978; 74: 105-106

To have many friends; to serve ably in one's profession and to teach others; to have one's avocation blossom into a second career; to become the acknowledged authority in one's field of interest; to receive just recognition during one's lifetime; to maintain one's perspective and sense of humor through it all; to live, in good health, well beyond the threescore year and ten; and to die at home after a full day's activities and with plans for the morrow—all these are things greatly to be prized. While we mourn the loss of Dr. Waring—for his family, for medicine, and for ourselves—we marvel at all he accomplished.

His death brought forth many recollections from those who knew him well. He was a prince of a man—genteel, friendly, witty, and patient. Many recall that his pace was invariably relaxed and unhurried. He must have possessed an exceptional ability to budget and organize his time and to set clear priorities. Some recall that he sometimes turned aside suggestions that he should seek high offices. He worked long and hard behind the scenes for causes of his choosing. Recognition came to him; he did not seek it.

He was an encourager. Dr. Neill W. Macaulay, for example, recalls that it was Dr. Waring who suggested that he create a permanent museum from his vast collection of historical items related to dentistry, and continued to promote the idea. When the Macaulay Museum of Dental History was finally dedicated, Dr. Waring's remarks were quite brief. Dr. Macaulay remembers that he tried to get his long-time friend to make a major address, but that Dr. Waring deferred to others. He simply accepted the collection on behalf of the Medical University of South Carolina. Such modesty was apparently characteristic of the man.

There are numerous South Carolina physicians more qualified to eulogize Dr. Waring than the present editor of *The Journal*. I offer one for reasons he would have appreciated. Shortly before is death, he told me: "The problem with being editor of *The Journal*

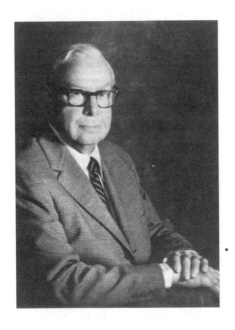

Joseph Ioor Waring
(1897-1977)

was meeting that deadline every month."

As a freshman medical student in Baltimore, I first heard of Dr. Waring and his reputation from an impeccable source: Dr. Owsei Temkin, then the dean of American medical historians. I had approached Dr. Temkin about the possibility of a summer research project. Upon learning that I came from South Carolina, he immediately began telling me about Joe Waring, the Charleston pediatrician who had made significant contributions to the field, and who was also much remembered by members of the American Association for the History of Medicine for the hospitality he had shown them at Old Town Plantation. Years later I first met Dr. Waring at the dedication of the Macaulay Museum of Medical History. When I complimented him on his writings, he referred to them as "mere cataloging." One knew otherwise.

When Dr. Edward E. Kimbrough resigned as editor, effective January 1977, he was made editor emeritus and Dr. Waring's name was deleted from our masthead. *The Journal* and the South Carolina Medical Association evidently meant a great deal to him, for Dr. Waring wrote us a charming letter in which he politely wondered how one could be "de-merited" from an "emeritus" position. The Council quickly created for him a new position, that of *senior* editor emeritus, and he was back on the masthead. The role of medical history in *The Journal* was of mutual concern. On the one hand, there was a long tradition of historical articles, including many of Dr. Waring's, and I was personally interested in this tradition and had been made a member of the Committee on Historical Medicine. On the other hand, our readership survey indicated a low priority for such articles. We corresponded, and he kindly invited me to visit him at the Waring Historical Library.

That visit, two months before his death, was most memorable. One can only envy his life-long friends, who surely treasure many such memories. He began by expressing concern as to where I had managed to park my car on the busy Medical University campus. I told him I'd left it in a place of doubtful legality, whereupon he immediately made it right. He and his assistant, Anne Donato, prepared a special placard for the windshield to the effect that I was a guest of the Waring Historical Library. Feeling thus secure, I joined Dr. Waring at his desk.

Eighty years of age, Dr. Waring was spry and alert. His desk seemed at first glance to be in cluttered disarray. Closer inspection disclosed the hallmarks of a busy, disciplined scholar: the scattered piles of books and journals possessed an order, and the numerous place marks indicating that a project was well underway. Dr. Waring explained that he was compiling a bibliography of medical history in South Carolina. He was clearly preparing a path for others to follow.

He conducted my tour of the library with obvious pleasure. He radiated pride in the collections, although he spoke of the need for additional funding. We browsed through some rare books. Dr. Waring was far from pedantic. His sense of humor made one feel immediately at ease. We paused for a few moments over William Hunter's illustrations of the gravid uterus, made two centuries ago. I reflected silently upon how the clinically relevant portion of the detail Hunter had drawn from cadavers can now be obtained noninvasively in the living patient by diagnostic ultrasound, a method introduced since Dr. Waring retired from clinical practice. But the users of newer technology can only be enriched by learning of the problems of their predecessors. The previous evening, I had gone over Temkin's essay "The usefulness of medical history for medicine." The value of such a place such as the Waring Historical Library on a medical school campus is great, if often intangible.

Dr. Waring invited me to lunch at Old Town Plantation, site of the original English settlement on the west bank of the Ashley River. The settlers of 1670 had left the site after several years for another location, known then as Oyster Point and now as Charleston. The land had for many years been in the family of his wife, Ferdinanda Legaré Waring. The Warings had recently transferred this tract of immense historical value to the state, with the stipulation that they would remain there the balance of their lives. The exhibition center known as Charles Towne Landing occupies a portion of the tract.

The Warings' old white frame house stood in a setting of spectacular beauty. In front of the house was a tranquil pond, presided over by a majestic American egret perched in a moss-draped live oak tree. Behind the house stood an avenue of widely-spaced live oaks. One sensed immediately that this was one of those rare special lowcountry places created long ago under a different labor system, never to be duplicated after the collapse of the Confederacy.

It was therefore with great surprise that I learned, as many others had doubtlessly learned before me, that all of the landscaping had been carried out within recent memory, under the supervision of Mrs. Waring. The gardens, the pond, and the live oak avenue were her creations. Dr. Waring laughed: "When we planted those trees, we didn't think we'd live long enough to appreciate them."

The Warings were charming and open. Mrs. Waring expressed her continued concerns about the grounds even though the upkeep was now done by state employees. Dr. Waring talked about fishing and about weekends at Wadmalaw Island, where his circle of friends met regularly each Saturday morning to share the local gossip. He recalled how the fear had been expressed by younger pediatricians after World War II that their entering practice might be resented, and how he had quickly dispelled such fears. The sauce for dessert the Warings served that day bore the eponym of a departed friend. This led to a brief discussion of the desirability of avoiding a lingering illness.

Since Dr. Waring's death, I've listened to the recollections of several of his contemporaries. Dr. William Weston, Jr., remembers his contributions to pediatrics and their shared vacations at Highlands, in western North Carolina. Dr. O. B. Mayer remembers his exceptional dedication to the South Carolina Medical Association. Former patients remember him as a kindly doctor who made shots seem painless. Former colleagues remember him as a conservative physician who preached early that penicillin was not a panacea and that tonsillectomies were being done too frequently. Dr. George C. Rogers, Jr., Professor of History at the University of South Carolina, remembers Dr. Waring for the many kindnesses and encouragements given him early in his career. He expressed the sentiment that Dr. Waring may well have been "the last of a breed—the 'talented amateur' who goes on to become a major authority." History, like medicine, is becoming increasingly specialized.

Any serious future historian of medicine in South Carolina must take as the departure point the contributions of Dr. Waring. These contributions become even more remarkable when one considers that his productivity peaked relatively late in life. He demonstrated the need for a systematic approach to medical history, and we can be grateful for the creation of the Waring Historical library and, more recently, of the Waring Library Society. One hopes that funds might become available for an endowed chair at the Medical University—a Joseph Ioor Waring Professorship of the History of Medicine.

Bill's Lesion

J SC Med Assoc 1984; 80: 313-314

*Life is short, and the Art long; the occasion fleeting; experience
fallacious, and judgment difficult.*
                    –The First Aphorism of Hippocrates

The physical examination confirmed my impression: Bill
remained in good health. I could not, of course, assure
him that he did not have significant arteriosclerosis, but I
found no evidence of it and he appeared physiologically much
younger than his 76 years. The laboratory results supported
this conclusion. I complimented him on his excellent habits and
scheduled a return appointment to monitor therapy for his mild
essential hypertension. Finally, for completeness, I told him to
stop by the x-ray department for a routine chest x-ray.

Bill and Anne had raised eight children. Growing up, I had
been about the same age as their three older boys and thus spent
some time at their house. I do not recall a warmer atmosphere.
The children addressed their parents as "Anne" and "Bill," yet
obeyed them to the letter and got along with one another. (What
have the latter-day theorists *really* taught us about parenting?)
Years passed. One day, as a young practitioner, I had the
opportunity to do Bill a small favor. He repaid me a thousand
fold, and became a close and treasured friend. Bill, with his gentle
sense of humor, had a unique way about him, a way of always
putting others first. He was a special person.

My heart sank when, holding the chest x-ray up to the ceiling
light, I first saw the irregular nodule in the left mid-lung field.

That evening, I broke the news to Bill in his living room. I told
him that the x-ray had shown a spot on his left lung, that the spot
could be benign but could also be a tumor, and that he should
stop by the office the next morning and pick up a requisition for
a special kind of x-ray called a tomogram.

Bill did not grimace; he did not blink; he did not bat an eyelash.

Instead, he smiled and said with his customary optimism: "I'll be there." Without another word, he arose and led me down to his cellar to pick out a bottle of his homemade wine to share with Anne in the kitchen.

As soon as the tomograms were available the next afternoon, the radiologist put them up and groaned. "That looks *bad!*" I had to agree. The lesion was solid, without calcium, and sent sinister-looking tentacles into the surrounding parenchyma. I knew the implications: It was probably malignant; thoracotomy would be necessary to obtain a definitive answer; and there might be a 60 to 80 percent chance for surgical cure. Having previously anticipated the worse case, I took Bill into a vacant office and closed the door.

"Bill, the spot could still be benign, but it has features that suggest it's probably going to be malignant." Again, Bill appeared to be completely calm. Choking, I went on. "Bill, I'll be any kind of doctor you want me to be, but I suspect that you'd like for me to tell you what you ought to do. I think that you should plan to go into the hospital this Sunday, and we'll obtain some baseline studies, have appropriate specialists see you and probably have a bronchoscopy done, and probably plan to take out a portion of your left lung next week. I've already made a room reservation."

The only muscles that moved were the risorius muscles and their allies, producing Bill's familiar winning smile. Again, he said: *"I'll be there."*

"Bill," I offered, placing my left hand on his shoulder and fighting back the tears, "I know that if anyone can come through this, you can..."

Bill laughed. "Charley, you're more nervous than I am! I might learn something!"

The baseline studies, the pulmonary function tests, the bronchoscopy, and the CT scans were all normal or unrevealing. All consultants agreed. On Wednesday, the left upper lobe was removed without difficulty. I carried the tissue down to the pathology laboratory and waited breathlessly as the technologist prepared the frozen sections. Soon, the pathologist and I were elated. *Benign! A localized lipoid pneumonia!* The surgery lasted only 45 minutes, and the endotracheal tube was removed before he went to the recovery room.

On the third postoperative day, a routine chest x-ray showed a right upper lobe infiltrate. This appeared to respond to therapy, but although Bill made some progress each day, the progress was slow and he was not eating well. On the seventeenth day, he abruptly developed pulmonary edema. The electrocardiograms and enzymes confirmed a subendocardial infarction. Although the wedge pressures normalized, diuresis was slow and interstitial pulmonary edema persisted. Examination the next evening revealed a left hemiparesis. Two days later, it was evident that he had developed the full-blown adult respiratory distress syndrome.

Bill had requested that his life not be supported artificially should it come to that, but I saw no choice other than placing him on the respirator. Bill fought valiantly, surviving several episodes of shock, but the pulmonary capillaries continued to leak. The edema progressed relentlessly despite the use of every known measure. I was grateful to the nurses, who allowed us to break the rules so that Anne and her children could remain at his side. And in those last hours, I learned what every good nurse already knew, that it is the little things that matter — not the wedge pressures and the blood gases, but the tightness of the tape holding the endotracheal tube, the uncomfortable position of the paralyzed limb. Bill never complained. He would wink at us.

During my occasional moments at home that weekend, I would wander aimlessly, despondent over my judgment and over my chosen profession. Bill had trusted us, and we had failed him. I learned what many families already know, that our most careful risk/benefit deliberations seem irrelevant, that each patient is, after all, a series of *one*, a person whose unique humanity transcends our codified rules for decision-making. I understood how some persons become disenchanted with scientific medicine and seek alternative sources of health care. Bill's enthusiastic assistance with the hospital's purchase of its first CT scanner, as a member of its board of trustees, became an ironic memory. He himself would have been better off had the conventional x-ray machine never been invented.

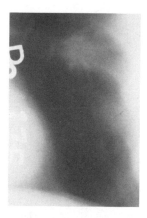

The tomogram

Toward the end, however, I found optimism for the future. Perhaps the anticipated surplus of physicians will enable more and more of us to spend substantial portions of our time with patients and their families during times of crisis, as had been afforded me that weekend. The rewards are mutual. As we attempt to provide comfort, we obtain comfort in turn from those we serve, comfort in their examples, comfort that may someday serve us well when it becomes our turn to join that innumerable caravan.

For whatever small comforts we might have brought Bill during those last hours, he had once again repaid us a thousand fold. The front page obituary described him as a business and civic leader; he was, but I doubt that anyone who knew Bill remembers him primarily that way. Instead, we remember his gentleness, his patience, his way of putting others' interests above his own. And the way he had lived no doubt enabled him, when his summons came quite suddenly and unexpectedly, to confront the prospect of death without batting an eyelash — something I had never seen before, and may not see again. He had shown us the possibility of unfaltering courage. He had attained a final victory over that ultimate challenge posed by our common human predicament.

Fond Memories of Emmett

J SC Med Assoc 1985; 81: 145-146

Orthopedists are among the most likeable of physicians. They tend to be friendly, energetic, positive, and pragmatic. They seem to argue among themselves more than most of us — sometimes coming close to exchanging blows — but they are quick to forgive and forget. Perhaps they appreciate, better than the rest of us, both the toughness and the frailty of human tissue.

Emmett was among the most likeable not just of orthopedists but of men. Driving up in his old car or bouncing down the corridor in his scrub suit, waving "Hello, Sir!" to everyone he met, he made the day a little bit brighter. Emmett had a unique way of treating all people alike yet making each feel special. A recently-arrived resident told his wife how during a weekly morning conference a slightly balding man of medium height would quietly enter the room, sit in a corner, and proceed to make eye contact with every person in the room, affirming each in turn with a wink or hand wave. The resident told his wife: "I don't know who that guy is yet!" Later he learned that the stranger was in fact the most famous person in the room: Emmett Lunceford.

One could easily have worked alongside Emmett for years and yet be unaware of his national and international reputation. He didn't advertise. The casual visitor to his operating room might have mistaken him for an orderly, for he often helped mop the floor between cases. However, orthopedists came from all over the country to learn his methods. His correspondence was worldwide. With characteristic modesty he called his porous-metal hip implant simply "the AML system." Only later did many of us learn that "AML" stood for Austin Moore-Lunceford.

One can envision that Emmett, having neared the pinnacle of success, might easily have moved his practice to Manhattan, living out his life in expensive three-piece suits, operating on the failed hips of the rich and powerful, allowing the world to come to him rather than vice versa. But that, of course, would not

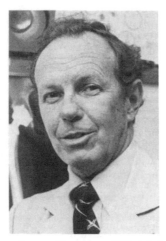

Emmett M. Lunceford, Jr.
(1930-1985)

have been Emmett. With his cowboy hats, his plain metal desk, his directness, Emmett was the quintessential democratic man, sharing his gifts freely with everyone. He continued to spend one morning each week at a Veterans Administration hospital, operating for a pittance. I shall not forget that my last consultation with him, on the day of his death, concerned a Medicaid patient referred to him for infected non-union of the tibia.

The most remarkable aspect of Emmett's career is that as a private practitioner he achieved excellence in all three areas of medicine — service, teaching, and research. The "triple threat" is now a rare commodity even among fulltime academicians; tenure committees now insist on excellence in only two of the three areas. Emmett became not only a consummate surgeon and skilled office physician but also a splendid teacher and gifted experimentalist. Residents praised both his ability to coach them through the most difficult operations without losing time or taking over and also his ability to correct mistakes without damaging self-esteem. Always seeking a better way, taking on new projects, he held appointments and tapped the expertise at all three of our state's research universities — Clemson, USC, and MUSC. Recognizing his excellence, national societies elected him to offices usually reserved for full-time academic department chairmen.

The key to Emmett's huge success was his incredible energy. He was indefatigable. He worked from well before dawn to well after dusk and still found time for his family and his community. There is a story that after undergoing surgery himself he climbed down from the table and made rounds. He was quite possibly the closest thing to the legendary John Hunter to ever cross the piedmont of South Carolina. Even Hunter would have envied Emmett's amazing ability to combine perpetual motion with calm detachment. On one occasion, Emmett spent two hours preparing a delicate bone graft only to have a scrub nurse drop the graft onto the operating room floor. Before setting out to prepare a new one, Emmett's only response was "Oh, jeepers!"

His energy, in turn, must have been due in large measure to his positive attitude. He was never known to say anything negative about anyone, much less criticize a colleague. He was always moving forward, seeking to better the situation. In eastern Tennessee they are still talking about how he managed to steer his crippled Cessna through the sleet and snow, how he steered it through a heavily populated area toward a parking lot only to recognize that his best shot at making it risked slamming into a dormitory. His last decision spared the young women in that dormitory from the consequences of that awful crash.

The theologian Kirsopp Lake once remarked that "faith is not belief in spite of evidence, but life in scorn of consequence." Most of us fail to realize our full potentials because of various doubts—fears of real or imagined consequences. Emmett, putting aside whatever doubts he may have had, doing so much for so many during his allotted time, remains an inspiration. His wife, Caffie, recalled two aphorisms by which he lived: "I only worry about things that are important;" and "If I can't do anything about it, I don't worry about it." Like scores of others, I think I am a better person for having known Emmett.

Real Medicine

J SC Med Assoc 1987; 83: 28-30

From time to time, persons from other states who consider state medical journals to be a dying species ask me why I edit one. My answers range from the laconic to the maudlin, depending on the functional integrity of higher cortical inhibitory pathways. I have always considered one's motives for doing just about anything to be too complex to warrant a single response. However, I usually manage to conceal one motive for editing *The Journal*: an urge to treat authors of unsolicited manuscripts with the respect they deserve.

Some years ago and well before he won fame as "Captain Who?" of the Baltimore Colts, Alex Hawkins traveled from Columbia to the Green Bay Packers' tryout camp. One hot afternoon he became the object of a tongue lashing by the legendary Vince Lombardi. "Mr. Lombardi," Hawkins reminded him with his characteristic insouciance: "I want you to know that I did not deliberately come here all the way from South Carolina to try to ruin your football team." Anyone who regularly submits manuscripts to peer-reviewed medical journals must occasionally feel a desire to express similar sentiments.

Over the years, I have continued to send work to national journals, no doubt compelled by a deep-seated insecurity. Typically, one reviewer likes your manuscript while the other objects to your every use of the semi-colon. Even one's greatest victories are of the Pyrrhic variety, the reviewers having duly extracted their pound of flesh during your successive revisions. Every author's pre-game preparation should include a recitation of Harry Truman's advice to the effect that persons with heat intolerance should stay out of kitchens. As editor of *The Journal*, I've secretly striven to set new standards whereby authors are provided prompt and courteous reviews, always acknowledging that the paper has been read and duly appreciated. But I still play the game. Having a manuscript out at the editor's office piques one's interest in the daily mail.

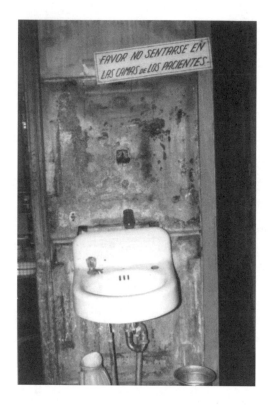

This was the only sink in an open ward for about 30 patients in the Hospital Rosales, San Salvador.

Let us now begin the story. Recently, I was awaiting judgment on a case report submitted to a periodical which we shall call simply *Prestigious Journal A*. *Prestigious Journal A* is bombarded with unsolicited case reports and rejects at least 90 percent of them. I nevertheless considered this one a "can't miss." It was the first well-documented case of a certain presentation of a certain uncommon fungal infection and the presence of a rare congenital immune deficiency presenting in adulthood gave the paper extra pizzazz. I let the manuscript marinate for an entire year, then added the final seasonings. I sought immortalization in *Prestigious Journal A* especially for the resident who had seen the patient with me and had done such a nice job, and felt that surely any reasonable reviewer would share my enthusiasm for such a fine admixture of science and art.

The manuscript had been out for review for about six weeks when one morning Dr. Foster Young poked his head in my office and asked: "Wanna go to El Salvador?" "What?" I exclaimed. "Isn't El Salvador full of guerillas and soldiers shooting at each other?!" Foster got to the point: "The Salvation Army needs people to help with the refugees from the earthquake. I've already spoken to your wife, and *she* wants to go." "Just great, Foster," I told him as I suppressed the matter from higher consciousness. "I'll give it some thought."

Shortly thereafter, the mail arrived. I said to my secretary: "I don't really care what's in it, as long as it's not a rejection letter from *Prestigious Journal A*." There lay the envelope, its large size auguring an unfavorable prognosis. Ripping it open, I learned that one reviewer liked the manuscript and said so in a single sentence. The other devoted an entire page to criticisms of the most minute sort, thereby denying the paper a sufficient priority rating for publication. I felt crushed. Then came the inner voice.

Wait a minute!" it began. "Here you're upset about a case report dealing with some rare entity nobody else in the world has even heard of — while people are dying of *common* problems in El Salvador! What's happened to your priorities?" Are you the same person who once told a medical school admissions committee that he wanted to *help* people?" It didn't take long to tell Foster that my mind was made up. I was going.

The State Department fact sheet advised Americans travelling to El Salvador to "exercise extreme caution." Professor Moss Blachman found time to give us a briefing in between sessions of autographing his new book about the stormy politics of Central America. The history of this small country, containing five million people in an area about the size of Delaware, appeared to be a sad saga of successive wars, atrocities and intrigues. Since 1979, the people have known hardships inflicted by extremists of opposite persuasions. Moss reassured us that the Salvadorans are a friendly, industrious people and that we would probably enjoy the trip as long as we avoided empty side streets.

The first day, I struck out on my own for the large urban medical center, Hospital Rosales. Gaining entrance with my Salvation Army identification card, I strode past the throngs of patients and the ubiquitous soldiers with their M16s and into the director's office. I wished to identify their problems, and see what I might do to help.

We had brought with us a small supply of the latest antibiotics, so my first business was to find out what they were using. "Whatever we happen to have," they said. I then learned that the situation with antibiotics was actually favorable — they did not have any diuretics or antihypertensives. My Salvadoran counterpart, from whom I was to learn a great deal over the next two weeks, escorted me onto the wards. The typical 30-bed unit contained two rows of rusty metal beds, at the end of which stood a single sink. There was no soap. I looked up; a patient with Romañas sign of Chagas' disease smiled pleasantly. My colleague told me that due to shortages, the IVs stayed in "as long as they last" and that much of their equipment was makeshift. There was no blood gas machine. Intensive care facilities were limited, at best. He led me to an isolation room containing a man with suspected rabies, explaining that many of the cases of that disease resulted from shortages of either the vaccine or of the antiserum. I returned to see the man each day, conversing with him privately, and was pleased when his nurse finally announced, "No tiene rabia."

Things were even worse on the surgery service. The Hospital Rosales is the major surgery referral and teaching center for the entire country. Ten of the 13 operating rooms had been destroyed in an earthquake two years ago and lack of funds to rebuild them necessitated that all cases be done in the emergency department. The backlog of patients awaiting surgery was incredible. Sometimes they could not begin cases for lack of an antiseptic scrub solution. Other times they had to terminate cases and close the patient for lack of a new pair of sterile gloves. In the recovery room I was told that the monitoring equipment did not work. The head of surgery pointed to a Spanish version of The Lord's Prayer on the wall and explained that this was sometimes the patients' best hope. The ward for postoperative patients appeared to be about 90 percent occupied. "This is unusual," I was told. "Often we have two patients in each bed and sometimes they sleep on the floor."

Our group received a great deal of media attention back

18

home, about which we felt vaguely uncomfortable for two reasons. First, many South Carolina physicians have done much more with little or no fanfare (I think of Dr. Hal Crosswell's missions to Haiti, for example). Second, although each member of our group did what he or she could, the real heroes were the Salvadorans. They did not complain or cry or curse the world for their phenomenal streak of bad luck. Instead, they were smiling and cheerful—clearly trying to get on with their lives. The physicians were highly motivated and often extremely innovative. They were accepting uncertainties calmly, making decisions that by our standards were incredibly cost-effective. They were practicing *real medicine.*

My Salvadoran counterpart explained that the university's library had not been receiving literature since 1980, causing isolation from developments elsewhere. Seeking verification, I headed for the medical school. Although the earthquake had not destroyed the single building, its safety was questionable. The students were holding classes outside in tents built with their own money and which they proudly called *auditoria.* They had few books and little or no laboratory equipment. And yet they seemed happy and eager to learn. They sat around in small groups, reading or talking quietly, just as one would expect to see on a warm spring day in Charleston or Columbia. They invited me to give them a few lectures and, with the help of an interpreter, I was delighted to oblige.

I learned that the several Salvadoran medical journals had folded, and that this medical library—once the finest in all of Central America—had indeed not received a single issue of a foreign medical journal since 1980. I quickly gave them one, and they seemed very grateful. It was the March 1986 issue of *The Journal of the South Carolina Medical Association*—the issue devoted to antibiotic usage.

Stumbling out of the library, I felt a bit like Commodore Perry opening a small corner of our planet to the outside world. In that moment, I thought that I finally knew why I enjoy editing a state medical journal. I realized that it was a desire to play a part, however small, in the continuous drama of medical information-making—a process that we take for granted, like so many of the other aspects of our lives. But no—the next time someone asks why I edit a state medical journal, I won't use that one, either. It sounds too sentimental.

Eulogy Written in a Country Churchyard

J SC Med Assoc 1988; 84: 94-95

Stories related to the HIV/AIDS epidemic dominated the media coverage of last year's annual SCMA convention, and this year's meeting promises to be a repeat. Already, it appears that two ethical issues will receive top billing. First, do physicians have the right to refuse care of HIV-positive patients? Second, do HIV-positive physicians have the right to practice without restraints? Those who deal with the formulation of "AIDS policies" often find themselves walking on hostile, unfamiliar terrain without a map. The thorny problems force us to choose between worthy but conflicting principles. Finding myself in this position to an increasing extent last summer, I sought refuge in a library.

The library for those lunch hours was the South Caroliniana, located on a corner of the University's historic horseshoe. My project was the history of the Columbia Medical Society. The minutes begin in May 1865 at what must have been the absolute nadir of organized medicine on the North American continent. Seven physicians, defeated, demoralized, and in several instances even homeless as a result of Sherman and the fire met with a single purpose: to be paid for their services. They joylessly resolved to

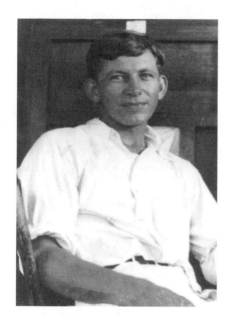

Theodore Brevard Hayne
(1898-1930)

reestablish the antebellum Fee Bill. Then they adjourned. From this lowly beginning, the dusty volumes slowly but surely told the story of a county medical society. But that story is not the purpose of this editorial.

It happened on or about my fifteenth visit to the library. Turning another page, with care not to tear the browning paper, I confronted what seemed to be a routine obituary. It began: "Theodore Brevard Hayne was born August 3, 1893 at Blackstock, S.C. ..." I yawned and began to scan the page as I had scanned my way through countless others in search of patterns. Suddenly, my hairs bristled. I got up from the desk, closed the book, left Columbia, and headed east out the Sumter highway. I had to see it.

I had been down the winding country road a few times, but had never taken the sharp turn to the right. It promised nothing but a few more nondescript houses, a few more fields, and woods. Suddenly, there it was, incongruous with its surroundings: a neat, newly-white wooden church with immaculate grounds. It didn't take long to find the marker. One side of the obelisk carried the message: "THEODORE BREVARD HAYNE, M.D. DIED OF YELLOW FEVER IN LAGOS, NIGERIA, WEST AFRICA.

21

INTERMENT AUG. 24, 1930. GREATER LOVE HATH NO MAN THAN THIS, THAT HE LAY DOWN HIS LIFE FOR HIS FRIENDS." I stood there for a long time, giving no thought to the hot July sun.

Theodore, the son of South Carolina's state health officer, had not set out to be a doctor. But he was keenly interested in science and at the tender age of 16 had carried out a survey of the Little Salkehatchie Swamp in Colleton County. When he graduated from The Citadel in 1920 he took a job with the U. S. Public Health Service in vector-borne diseases. There he was stimulated by the senior investigators whom he impressed in turn, and who gave him credit for assisting with the discovery that mosquito larvae can be killed by Paris Green, a weak arsenical compound. Perhaps more importantly, he single-handedly disproved a prevailing notion that mosquitoes cannot cross large streams. This he accomplished in Chester County by staining anophelene mosquitoes with an aniline dye and afterwards recapturing a stained mosquito a mile and a half away on the other side of the Catawba River.

Inspired, Theodore Hayne went back to Charleston for medical school, graduating from the Medical College of the State of South Carolina in 1927. He did the usual internship, but his first love was still scientific investigation in general and mosquito-borne diseases in particular. It was for that reason that he accepted a position with the Rockefeller Foundation at its center for studying yellow fever in Lagos, Nigeria. The work was by definition dangerous. One bite, resulting from one small break in technique or a tiny flaw in the mosquito netting, could cause the disease with its 25 to 50 percent case-fatality rate. Two previous investigators had lost their lives.

Hayne stayed there for 19 months and then returned to South Carolina, where he married his sweetheart in January of 1930. On March 29, he left for another 18 month tour of duty in Lagos. He discovered that many of the broods of mosquitoes with which he was working contained dwarf variants. He took care to use finely-meshed wire containers. Nevertheless, it is theorized that such a dwarf mosquito escaped and bit him, causing the fatal yellow fever attack from which he died on July 11, 1930. Standing there in the churchyard, I realized an added dimension to the tragedy not evident in the moving obituary. The child from his brief marriage was stillborn, the umbilical cord wrapped around its neck. With only an occasional blackbird looking on, I made no attempt to hold back the tears.

The minutes of the medical society noted that it "was the love of science and not the strains of martial music nor the cheering of his comrades that made Theodore so nobly sacrifice his life, a martyr in the service of mankind fighting an invisible foe." I reflected on the notion that Theodore Hayne had *volunteered* for such dangerous duty. The possibility that one could contract such an untreatable and rapidly fatal illness from routine patient care had disappeared from medicine during this century. Now it has returned in the form of HIV/AIDS.

I suggest no obvious parallels. On the one hand, yellow fever was much more contagious than HIV/AIDS and Theodore Hayne's work was therefore more dangerous than even the bloodiest surgical procedure on an AIDS victim. On the other hand, HIV/AIDS is a different kind of disease. Death does not come swiftly — perhaps almost mercifully swiftly — as it did from yellow fever or bubonic plague. Rather, HIV places a sword of Damocles over the infected person indefinitely, a sword dripping with social stigmata. A different peril for a different age.

Churchill called courage "the first of human qualities because it is the quality which guarantees all the others." HIV/AIDS demands of us, as physicians, a new dimension of courage heretofore was not required by today's world. This is the courage to face with each and every patient contact potential exposure to a chronic but apparently uniformly fatal disease for which there is no cure, that can be transmitted to others for at least 10 years, and that is not considered by most people to be socially acceptable. As I stood there in the country churchyard I wondered what Theodore Hayne would have said. I suspect that he would have taken an interest in our many problems, but without further ado would have gotten about the business of finding solutions. I suspect that he would not have talked and talked and talked about it, as so many persons today seem so inclined to do.

23

"I've Been There"

J SC Med Assoc 1985; 84: 511-512

D r. Joseph Waring told me: "The problem with editing *The Journal* is meeting that deadline." This issue's deadline found me without an editorial. After some hasty consulting, I decided to write about the definition of "hazardous waste." Knowing that the debate would probably be resolved before this issue reaches print, I assembled the materials anyway, sat down at my desk, and waited for inspiration. It never came. My thoughts were elsewhere in a far-away courtroom.

It had been my misfortune the previous week to see a physician subjected to the terrible capriciousness of the tort liability system. I had seen an aggressive plaintiff lawyer make unconscionable *ad hominem* attacks. It brought back all of the arguments that randomly-selected juries are ill-equipped to settle intricate matters about medical decision-making. It brought back all of the concerns that who gets sued and when usually make little or no sense. More importantly, it brought back an issue that receives little or no public attention: the damage done to the physician merely by the fact of being sued.

In recent months, I have had occasion to talk to five physicians who were being sued for the first time. They included a distinguished surgeon, two widely-respected family practitioners, a pillar-of-the-community internist, and a famous medical school professor. In all but one instance, the theory of negligence seemed to revolve around failure to predict the unpredictable. I opened as follows:

"I'm sorry. Let me tell you what I suspect is happening to you. You're not sleeping well. What time you used to call your own is now at the beck and call of lawyers. You've memorized every date, every square inch of that medical record until it seems larger than life. Every patient you see now seems like a potential adversary. You're starting to question your decision to go into medicine in the first place. It's probably spilling over into your personal life. In fact, this matter is disturbing you down to the most basic, deepest core fibers of your being."

Each time, the response was similar. "Gee, how did you know all that?"

I responded: "I've been there."

Ten years have passed. Concerned by these exchanges I hereby break my own self-imposed statute of limitations on the grounds that what I learned might be useful to other physicians. Today my main regret lies exactly where it did when the misfortune occurred: with the patient and the patient's family. Looking back I suppose that I was lucky to have been tested at a relatively young age and in a case in which I could defend my judgment decisions with all of the textbooks and relevant literature. I was in fine company (before it was over, five of us were alleged joint tortfeasors), and I had good lawyers. The matter came to trial but was dismissed as a non-suit. But the proceedings, extending as they did over two years, took their toll. I have concluded that the outcome of malpractice cases is of much less significance than being subjected to the ordeal in the first place.

I have yet to meet a physician who does not feel that his or her first lawsuit was less than a nightmare. The mere accusation of malpractice makes people whisper and demands an enormous redirection of time and energy. But the worst aspect is its challenge to one's identity. The surgeon put it best: "Other people don't realize how *seriously* we take our work." Charging negligence in the practice of medicine is a far cry from charging failure to see a stoplight or to pick up a banana peel. Through the long hours of organic chemistry and anatomy, of internship and residency, there emerges a self-concept strongly wedded to one's commitment and competence. That a trial lawyer with far less training and with little or no certification to do what he or she specifically does can deal such a severe blow to one's sense of self seems grotesquely unfair. But the purpose of this editorial is not to whine "ain't it awful."

I take my text from Churchill: "In life's steeplechase, one must take the hurdles as they come." My purpose is to offer ten suggestions for future hurdlers. Here they are, in no particular order of importance.

1. Be kind to thyself. Remember who you are, what you've

accomplished, and how much you mean to so many people. Get out your old photographs and clippings and consider starting a scrapbook. Remember a corollary of the Golden Rule: you cannot love your neighbor if you do not first love yourself.

2. Take an active role in your defense, but be philosophical. Recognize that to a large extent it's just a game, a game mainly concerned with money and having little or nothing to do with you. Dissociate the theory of negligence from your self-concept as a physician and your self-worth as a person.

3. Prepare *in writing* a list of your long-term goals in the major spheres of life: personal, professional, financial, recreational. File it in a secret place and get it out from time to time to check your bearings. Then, eliminate from your life for the time being whatever will not help you reach these goals and/or does not have a five-year history of importance to you. Say no.

4. Pay close attention to your primary relationships, your immediate family. Go out of your way to meet their needs even when you don't feel like it. Appreciate that it is in giving that we receive.

5. Risk sharing your feelings and frustrations with a friend or two. This is difficult for most of us. When we were young we saw too many John Wayne movies ("Never apologize, never explain; it's a sign of weakness" — *She Wore a Yellow Ribbon*). When we were medical students, interns, and residents, we heard too many tales of the "days of the iron men." But try. Invite someone to lunch. You'll be surprised.

6. Seek solace in whatever body of literature gives you the best access to the eternal truths. For me, it's usually the wisdom literature of ancient Israel (e.g., Psalms, Proverbs, and, Ecclesiastes) or the Stoic philosophers. I still keep in my wallet the first paragraph of the *Enchiridion* by Epictetus. It begins: "Of things some are in our power, and others are not."

7. Get in touch with your position in the life cycle, since your new challenge is but of several. Consult either Gail Sheehy (*Passages*) or Daniel Levinson (*The Seasons of a Man's Life*). Know what's ahead, whether it be the phrase of "becoming one's own man" (age 35-40), the "age 50 transition," or the "late adult transition" (age 60-65).

8. Despite your need for a measure of introspection, don't become a recluse. As Sir William Osler put it, "Seek the cheerful haunts of men and mingle with the bustling crowd."

9. Be a good animal. Compensate for your insomnia by allotting more than your usual amount of time for sleep. Exercise. Elevate those endorphin levels. Avoid habituating tendencies. Get a physical examination, and seek professional help for your emotional problems if necessary. Follow the same advice you would give a patient.

10. Forgive. Work hard at forgiving the plaintiff and the plaintiff's lawyer, however outrageous the allegations may seem. Turning the other cheek may never have seemed like harder advice, but failure to do so hurts only yourself. Recognize that a legal system that allows people to parlay a physician's office visit, procedure, or consultation into small fortunes for themselves is merely symptomatic of deeper problems in our society. And forgive yourself. Even if your medical care may not have met some ideal (and whose always does?), remind yourself that physicians are merely fallible human beings trying to help other fallible human beings. When this ceases to be the case, there'll be no more need for doctors.

Elsewhere in this issue, Dr. Frederick Jones points out our obligation not only to practice good medicine ourselves but also to assure quality care throughout our communities. Unfortunately, it has been difficult to achieve meaningful peer review in medicine as in most occupations. But as medicine becomes increasingly technical and as clinical judgment continues to be subjected to algorithmic analysis, it should become much easier to set criteria regarding the "standard of care." When this happens, we should be in a better position to plead the case for qualified arbitration panels as a viable alternative to the jury system. In the meantime, we must stand as one profession committed to the three C's: competence, consistency, and compassion. We cannot be compassionate to our patients without first being compassionate to each other and to ourselves.

Games Played with Balls

J SC Med Assoc 1991; 83: 30-31

What Thomas Jefferson had to say has generally stood the test of time, but I protest the following: "Games played with the ball ... stamp no character on the mind." Games not only stamp character, they test it. Games give us useful metaphors for the rest of life.

The running back — head down, legs churning, arms cradling the pigskin — shows us how to make it through the day one yard at a time. The infielder — knees flexed, glove low, body square to the line of flight — shows how to handle life's unexpected bounces. The jump shooter — eyes locked on the rim while defenders' arms flail all about him — shows how to block out the distractions. Pick any sport and you'll find the metaphor you need.

We need them not only as individuals but also collectively. As this issue goes to press (early December 1990), drums of war echo from the Persian Gulf while rumors of recession circulate at home. As a profession we brace for sweeping change as we look ahead toward the next century. Looking back over this one, what metaphors might serve us in the near future? Pick any sport.

Yankee Stadium, July 4, 1939. The speeches were over, and all eyes and ears focused on the lone figure near home plate. The whole nation knew the painful truth: the muscle fibers were not made of iron, after all — in fact, they would soon be gone. So what does one say when they hand you the microphone and everybody knows your grim prognosis? Standing tall in his pinstriped uniform, he proudly proclaimed himself the luckiest man on earth. Henry Louis Gehrig, 1903-1941. Lou Gehrig — courage.

The Superdome, New Orleans, March 29, 1982. The big coach watched as the final seconds ticked from the clock, the national championship seemingly his. Then one of his players succumbed to a fake and threw the ball straight into an opponent's hands. So what does one do when the buzzer sounds and one faces the player who threw it all away? Draping a bear hug around the hapless young man, he reminded us all that it was just a game after all, that what matters is not trophies but people. John Thompson of the Georgetown University Hoyas—compassion.

But for a metaphor especially relevant to medicine today, I choose Centre Court, Wimbledon, 1980. It was Bjorn Borg's finest hour in retrospect, but at the time this was far from obvious. In the young John McEnroe, Borg had met his match and he knew it. Point after point he slugged away, his steely concentration a testimony to that most primeval of needs: survival. Then, late in the fifth set, he stopped and searched the crowd for familiar faces. It was the television commentator who conveyed the moment's significance: "He's regrouping."

Regroup. My dictionary tells me that this verb's main usage is a military one: "to reassemble or reorganize (one's forces), as after a battle." Today's usage suggests expanded meaning: to examine one's priorities, to take measure, to stay in focus. The nineties: a time for medicine to regroup.

But I would be remiss to imply that we learn useful metaphors only from the spectator sports. Even more relevant are those we learn the hard way by competing ourselves at whatever level of athletic proficiency. Of the many I've learned that way none proved more useful than one given at just the right time some years ago on a tennis court.

My tennis game was entirely self-taught and nothing to brag about. True, I could hit serves and backhands with reasonable confidence that the ball would remain in play, if without much spin. But the forehand drive—the staple shot in the good player's repertoire—was another story. Demanding extension and pronation of the forearm in perfect timing with shifting weight at the ball's arrival, the shot seemed inordinately complicated. I just couldn't get it right. And it's difficult to enjoy tennis without a trustworthy forehand.

I resolved to take lessons and found a coach. He made one suggestion after another. We tried different methods for hitting the shot including one he called "the loop." Nothing worked. "The doc's forehand" became a standing joke between us.

On a near-freezing and heavily-overcast March day I braced for yet another humiliation on the practice court. Unbeknownst to the coach, I also had a much greater problem than my forehand. The cruel world had dealt me an overhand smash, and I wasn't at all sure that I could battle back. As we began to hit balls, it became obvious that my forehand was worse than ever. Shot after shot sailed into the net or over the baseline—sometimes even over the fence and into the parking lot.

Twenty minutes into the lesson, it began to snow. The coach and I laughed simultaneously. He asked: "Doc, how about another time?" "No," I vowed firmly. "I'm going to stay right here until I get it right this time."

Moments later, the coach came to the net. "Doc, I think I've noticed something. You're coming *in* with your racket, across your body." He drew his racket across his chest to make the point. "Reach out for the ball. *Reach out ... reach out!*"

I did as he said. I began to reach out for the ball. It worked. Soon I was hitting the ball with authority, consistency, and topspin. One hard shot after another cleared the net and nose-dived onto the opposite court. By the end of the lesson, the snow was beginning to stick—and so was my newfound tennis self-confidence.

To be truthful, I never became a good tennis player. A few months later, I tried too hard for a drop shot and came to rest entangled in the net on a dislocated left shoulder. I left tennis but kept the metaphor. My off-court cloud soon lifted. The sun came out of hiding.

Reach out. In medicine, to an extent not found in any other profession, we constantly strive to eliminate our own necessity. Yet it is by reaching out, taking on new problems, incessantly striving to improve the lot of humanity, that we keep right on demonstrating our usefulness. We cannot afford to rest on our laurels. *Reach out ... reach out!*

We know that by the year 2000 there will be many changes, some of them technology-driven, some consumer-driven, some legislation-driven. We know that our own interest and the public interest should coincide to the greatest possible extent. We know that the best way to ensure this desideratum is through participation in organized medicine. It is through organized medicine that we best restore values—not as specialists or subspecialists but as physicians.

Regroup. Reach out. Those are my metaphors for today. But the marvelous thing about games played with balls, Mr. Jefferson, is that the metaphors are nearly endless. I'm learning new ones with a different game; someday, gentle reader, I hope to write one on "The Secret of the Secret." Meanwhile, it's no secret that we can be effective only by acting together. We must share not only common problems but also common inspirations.

Flight 463

J SC Med Assoc 1992; 88: 583

Whether it happened over Texas, New Mexico, or Arizona, I'll never know. I was happily debating what to read next when the announcement came: "Is there a doctor on the plane?" Turning around, I saw the dyspneic elderly woman in the seat behind me. I got up, sat beside her, and accepted the stethoscope and emergency kit from the stewardess. The pulse was strong and regular. There were crackles at the lung bases. I offered her a nitroglycerin tablet. "No thank you. I've just taken my own."

The history was forthcoming: "76-year-old WF with IDDM, s/p CABG X 4 (1982), with stable angina (last attack: four months ago), now with dyspnea, chest tightness, diaphoresis, and 'feeling weak all over' after getting up to go to the restroom." I continued to talk slowly. She gradually improved. The lungs cleared. We were 50 minutes away from the first stop in California. The issue became whether she should be met by an ambulance.

She didn't want one. Her husband of 51 years would be at the airport. He could drive her to the hospital, which was only 20 minutes away. If an ambulance were necessary, he wouldn't let her take trips alone to visit her grandchildren any more. Worse, the ambulance bill wouldn't be covered by her health maintenance organization (HMO), based in the next county. "The last time, they charged me $420 to go two and a half blocks." Although I surmised that her left ventricular ejection fraction was close to its baseline, I also knew that myocardial infarction needed to be excluded especially in the context of diabetes. Should I advise against an ambulance, knowing that if I "guessed wrong" I could be sued for negligence?

My decision: no ambulance. I communicated with the HMO, met the husband, explained the risks and that it was possible I could have "guessed wrong," and reminded him to drive carefully. My reward for this small act was a first-class seat for the 20-minute hop to Orange County. Settling into the comfortable upholstery, I mused that just about every family in the United States has probably had at least one brush with the high cost of medical care (not necessarily involving physicians' fees). I took a small measure of pride that I had not allowed myself to be reduced to a quivering mass of jelly because of the possibility that some California lawyer might sue the heck out of me for having guessed wrong. I remembered my father's words: "Son, just do the right thing and then don't worry about it."

Doctor Weston

J SC Med Assoc 1993; 89: 349-350

He once asked me to call him "Bully" but I never could for reasons I'm just now beginning to understand.

It was not because of the achievements that warranted a front page obituary, impressive though they were. He did it all. He practiced medicine for more than half a century. He held the highest offices in both county and state societies. He ranked nationally in his specialty. He responded to the needs of his city, school, and people when called. He was proudest, of course of his family — three children, 11 grandchildren, and five great grandchildren, all handsome and good as gold. Both sons became not only third-generation pediatricians but also leaders in the profession. Bill the professor, Nelson the chairman of our own Board of Trustees. But all of these things were done or set in motion long before I really knew him.

It was not because of his personality, his energy and effervescence, his charm and charisma, laced with obvious love of humanity. He was always moving forward, even in adversity. And was he ever fun! There was, for example, the time Helen Hayes came to town and we stood around waiting to see what would happen when the two twinkle-eyed octogenarians met. He began with bird call imitations, then crescendoed into his trademark yodel routine. Completely upstaged, the great actress gasped: "My, you're quite a man!" "Yep, I still am ... from the waist up!" There was the time, just before the end, his mind slipping, when I asked him the secret to his longevity for want of a better opener. "I've lived like a cricket — they stay awake and don't try to fool anybody." How wise, how original!

Put simply, it was his ability to touch lives. Scores, perhaps thousands, must have benefited from this gift, and I consider it my infinite good fortune to have been among them. Reader, mark this well: had it not been for the South Carolina Medical Association, the events described below would not have come to pass.

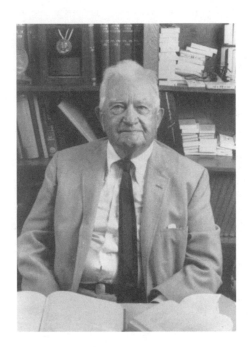

William Weston, Jr.
(1898-1993)

In brief, expressing interest in *The Journal* to Ed Kimbrough one morning in 1975 caused a concatenation of events that led to my being named to the Executive Committee of the newly-formed Waring Library Society at the Medical University of South Carolina. The appointment was, I thought, largely honorary: "We really don't expect you to come all the way to Charleston just for the meetings, just come whenever you can." But another delegate from the backcountry, the late Dr. Waring's longtime friend, was retired and had other ideas. "Charley, why don't we go down to the meeting next month?" What could I say?

To be sure, I had known him or at least of him ever since the Great BB Gun Fight when the excavation for his new house on Adger Road served as my bunker (luckily, we were lousy shots). His office was in the same building as my father's, and I treasured his kind words when Dad died. Entering practice, I heard that he was a kindly but exacting man. One of my partners confided a hard-earned lesson in professional etiquette: "Son, when you call another physician you dial that telephone yourself, don't you have your secretary keep him waiting!" He worked and played by all the rules and, unlike most of us, wasn't afraid to speak his mind. I found him delightful but never really began to know him until the morning of our expedition.

I looked forward to the trip but experienced last-minute pangs of ambivalence, precipitated no doubt by my unfortunate selfishness about time and the usual list of things-to-do. Bob McCardle said just the right thing: "Five years from now, you'll remember going to Charleston with Bully Weston better than you'd remember anything else you might do today." It became the understatement of a lifetime.

The minutes of the Waring Libary Society recorded that "they came all the way to Charleston just for the meeting!" But for us the trip had just begun. On the way back his reminiscences began to soar and he invited me to dinner at his club. The place was empty except for a table of lingering dowagers and we were told in no uncertain terms that the kitchen had closed. He held the line and prevailed. They brought out some leftovers. We had a grand time. Thereafter, he included me in various activities and I always looked forward to being with him. He was incredibly thoughtful.

Time passed. One fall day, he invited me to accompany him and his wife to the Colonial Cup. I accepted, but not because I really wanted to spend an entire Saturday among the jovial steeplechase set. My private life back then was filled with excruciating pain. Reeling from divorce, concerned even about survival, I had turned to woodworking for sublimation and would have preferred to spend the day with the beginnings of a four-poster bed, alone. But I resolved to make the best of it. We were heading out Two Notch Road toward Camden, the three of us, when suddenly and without warning he turned left into a subdivision and said casually, "We've got to pick up Donna." Donna? A year later, he was best man.

There were more good years, then the decline. Visiting the nursing wing, more often than not I would find him asleep. Sometimes I would just stand there or sit, watching him breathe, realizing that nothing that I could do would even begin to repay him. Nothing, that is, except to carry on.

It was not the hearty greetings, the shared friends and family, the wonderful outings, the companionable rounds of golf, the innumerable small favors, the festive occasions, the stories told and retold, nor even the unannounced blind date. It was something visceral, essential, and difficult to convey in words. Perhaps it is best captured by a tale that wells up from the primordial mist, told for thousands of years in many versions in many tongues in many lands. Basically, it goes like this. The young man enters the forest to face the wild boar. If the old men, the grandfathers, are watching, he survives. If not ...

William Weston, Jr., M.D., 1898-1993. Doctor Weston. Thank you.

Nothing Could be Finer

J SC Med Assoc 1997; 93: 459-461

Let's keep it a secret: Nothing could be finer than practicing medicine in South Carolina. Catching up on some reading last summer, I came across two unflattering descriptions of our fair state that help our cause.

First came John Updike's four *Rabbit* novels, the convoluted tale of one Harry (Rabbit) Angstrom's apparently aimless journey through life. Toward the end of the fourth novel Rabbit makes his final flight from responsibility. His one-night affair with his daughter-in-law has just been disclosed to his wife and his son. Rabbit immediately packs his suitcase and heads down I-95 for Florida. He enters South Carolina at Dillon County:

> From here on down to the Florida line Route 95 is like a long green tunnel between tall pines.... South Carolina is a wild state. The first to secede. The pines get taller,

with a tragic feeling. FIREWORKS are offered everywhere for sale. The land gets hillier. Trucks loaded with great tree trunks rumble unstoppably on the down slope and labor to nearly a standstill on the up. Rabbit is nervously aware now of his Pennsylvania plates being Northern. Swerve out of line a bit and they'll throw him in the Pee Dee River. The Lynches River. The Pocataligo River. Animals on this highway are hit so hard they don't squash, they explode, impossible to know what they were. Possums. Porcupines. Some dear old Southern lady's darling pet pussycat. Reduced to fur stains amid the crescent fragments of exploded truck tires. Just think, he lay down for lunch and that was it.[1]

Next came Pat Conroy's *Beach Music*, about high school classmates who try to reconcile relationships shattered by their reactions to Vietnam.[2] The narrator, Jack McCall, is living in Rome with his young daughter, Leah, seeking peace and escape after his wife's fatal leap from the Silas Pearlman Bridge in Charleston. Jack tries to explain to Leah why they mustn't go back:

> "What's South Carolina like?" Leah asked, changing the subject.
> "Horrible. Very ugly and depressing to look at. It smells bad all the time and the ground's covered with rattlesnakes. It has laws making all children slaves from the time they're born until they're eighteen. The state doesn't allow ice cream or candy to be sold inside the state line and requires all kids to eat five pounds of Brussels sprouts a day."
> "I hate Brussels sprouts."
> "That's only the start. All kittens and puppy dogs are drowned as soon as they're born. Stuff like that. You never want to go there. Trust me."

During a flashback to high school days, Jack recalls the arrival of a talented young man from California:

"South Carolina history," Jordan said, shaking his head. "What a contradiction in terms. I've lived all over the world and I've never heard one person ever mention this state's name. It's nowhere, man. A loser state if there ever was one. Nothing's ever happened here."

We, of course, know better. A great deal has happened here. It was here that Europeans first established a settlement in what is now the United States (Winyah Bay, 1526). It was here that Francis Marion and many others chased Cornwallis toward Virginia and surrender at Yorktown. It was here that the first medical school in the Southeast (now MUSC) was founded. We could go on and on about our history, but—reflecting on the tongue-in-cheek accounts of these two great novelists, Updike and Conroy—let's dwell on the present. I've sampled a small portion of what the rest of the world has to offer, and have always come back. Gratefully.

The following reflections, then, derive from various peregrinations over the past half century.

My education at Hand Middle School and Dreher High School in Columbia may have lacked the polish and prestige of St. Paul's School and Groton, but I found I could compete just fine against the preppies.

The beaches at Surfside, Pawley's, and Fripp may lack the reputation and glamour of those at St. Lucia, Waikiki, and Tahiti, but you can't beat our breezes and our brown pelicans flying in formation.

The granite faces at the upstate's Table Rock and Caesar's Head may lack the towering immensity of Yosemite's El Capitan and Half Dome, but you can't beat the catfish dinner at the Table Rock State Park restaurant.

The flowers at Orangeburg's Edisto Gardens and Charleston's Magnolia Gardens and Middleton Place may lack the endless multicolored splendor of Delaware's Longwood and Vienna's Belvedere and Schönbrunn, but you can't beat our camellias and azaleas in springtime.

The scenery along the Little Pee Dee, the Saluda, and the

Edisto may lack the meandering majesty of the Mississippi, the Rhine, and the Danube, but you can't beat our black water rivers for a relaxing canoe trip.

The tabby ruins that dot our lowcountry may lack the marbled mystery of Cos, Rhodes, and Delphi, but you can't beat the peace and quiet to be had beneath the Spanish moss.

The football when Carolina and Clemson go at it in Death Valley or Williams-Brice may lack the pageantry and publicity of the Broncos and Giants going at it in the Super Bowl in Pasadena, but I found the crowd enthusiasm at the latter event dull by comparison.

The Carolina wren, great blue heron, belted kingfisher, and confusing fall warblers that frequent my backyard may lack the novelty of the roseate spoonbills, whooping cranes, black-necked stilts, and scissor-tailed flycatchers I saw in Texas, but you can't beat our wildlife, at least in a state of our size.

The cuisine served up at Columbia's No Name Delicatessen and Kingstree's Brown's Barbecue may lack the elegant sauces and sumptuous deserts at New York's Four Seasons and Philadelphia's Le Bec Fin, but I always come away with less indigestion and a healthier wallet.

The live oaks and loblolly pines that typify our landscape may lack the dizzying heights of California's redwoods and giant sequoias, but the former have always given me as much shade as I can use.

The concert halls that are Charleston's Gaillard Auditorium and Columbia's Koger Center may lack the storied spaciousness of New York's Carnegie Hall or Washington's Kennedy Center, but the white wine they serve at intermission tastes just as good.

The waterfronts at Georgetown, Mt. Pleasant, and Beaufort may lack the architectural gems of Heidelberg, Prague, and Budapest, but the latter don't have shrimpboats — and then there's always the Battery at Charleston.

The Belmont Inn in Abbeville, Claussen's Inn in Columbia, Indigo Inn in Charleston, and Wilcox Inn in Aiken may lack the views and ambience of L'Auberge in Sedona, the Ritz-Carlton in Laguna Niguel, the El Tovar in Grand Canyon, and the Schloss

Hotel in Durnstein, but I slept just as well, thank you.

The greens and fairways at the Links Course at Wild Dunes and the Cotton Dike Course at Dataw may lack the lore and legend of Royal Troon, Carnoustie, and the Old Course at St. Andrews, but the ball bounces and rolls just as well and — for me, at least — is a lot easier to find.

The collections at MUSC's Waring Historical Library and USC's South Caroliniana Library may lack the depth and variety of London's Wellcome Institute and British Museum but I've always found exactly what I wanted.

And this last observation can be generalized. You'll find exactly what you want right here in South Carolina.

Where else can one be within such a short distance from both the mountains and the seashore, and with a change of seasons? Where else can one find comparable cultural and recreational opportunities and diversity within such a confined geographic area? And where else can one find such a generally agreeable place to practice medicine? And where else can one find a more collegial state medical association?

But *shhh*!

Let's keep it a secret!

References

1. Updike J. *Rabbit at Rest.* In Updike J. *Rabbit Angstrom: A Tetralogy.* New York: Alfred A. Knopf; 1995: 1458.
2. Conroy P. *Beach Music.* New York: Doubleday; 1995: 422, 592.

Live as Though Seen

J SC Med Assoc 1999; 95: 77-78

Baltasar Gracián, a worldly Jesuit priest who lived in Spain during the seventeenth century, left us 300 pithy epigrams known collectively as the *Oracle* or *Art of Worldly Wisdom*. The *Oracle* contains common-sense advice for just about any situation. Each time I see a new edition of Gracián, I buy it. If I had the time and money I'd try to acquire a copy of every edition ever published, as William Osler did of Sir Thomas Browne's *Religio Medici*. However, this editorial is not about book collecting. It's about a murder trial.

Gracián's epigram number 297 reads: "Live as though seen." Or, as one of my editions has it: "Always behave as though others were watching." We seem programmed to learn, unlearn, and relearn this simple admonition. Indeed, our national issue-of-the-day reminds us how even the high and mighty should keep it close to their hearts! An updated version of number 297 might read: "Live as though being constantly videotaped," like the character played by Jim Carrey in *The Truman Show*. Alas, the cameras in the video poker parlor weren't working the night the security guard was slain during a bungled robbery.

Few of us welcome the summons to jury duty. The loss of our most precious commodity — time — is only partially offset by the vague sense that we're contributing to our system of justice. I had been summoned to the Circuit Court's last session of the calendar year. Knowing that they seldom call physicians, and almost never call men wearing bow ties, I came prepared. Reporting to the jurors' room, I staked out a table, opened my attaché case, and settled in for a fine week of catching up with paperwork.

First came the preliminaries. We were herded into a large courtroom where our names were called as the lawyers made notes. Several people said they had medical conditions. The judge asked whether they had physicians' statements. They said no and were told to stay. One woman said her husband was a prisoner-for-life in another state and that she could never convict anyone because our legal system is so corrupt. The judge said he understood but would require her presence in the court the entire week. She was escorted out of the room kicking and screaming. The psychiatrist sitting next to me confided the likely diagnosis and the probable circumstances of her marriage to the inmate.

Next came jury selection. I was among about 50 people asked to report to the criminal court. We were told that the case involved an early-morning-hours slaying of a security guard during a robbery. My name was drawn from the rotating drum. I stood up before the lawyers and announced my occupation, confident that I would soon be back at the desk in the jurors' room. Amazingly, neither side struck. Sitting dumfounded in the jury box, I stared at the rotating drum. I admired its miter joints. It was made of solid walnut.

A while later we were told the alleged circumstances of the case. One of two robbers had held a gun to the security guard. The guard resisted and was shot. The second robber ripped the guard's gun from his holster and shot him several more times. He died instantly. Since the video cameras weren't working, the evidence would be mainly from various witnesses. The defense attorney, who did a fine job with the facts at his disposal, told us that all of the evidence presented would be flawed.

Struck with the seriousness of deciding on another human's liberty, I put aside all other concerns. I learned or relearned things I'd rather not know. I learned the meaning of the phrase "do a lick." I learned about the national crime network and about computer-generated lineups. I learned subtle differences between such terms as direct and indirect testimony, larceny and robbery, pistols and revolvers, bullets and cartridges, exit wounds and entrance wounds, latent and known fingerprints. Concentrating as hard as I could, I noted my pulse rate to be about 20 beats per minute faster than usual. Indeed, for the next four days my nervous system behaved as though I were hovering indefinitely over a four-foot downhill, sidehill putt. I was largely oblivious to the bombing of Iraq and the impeaching of the President.

Elected foreman by my fellow jurors, I resolved to do the job as I'd always envisioned doing it. The night before the closing arguments, I prepared for each juror a table with the evidence as I'd seen it, allowing plenty of room for them to make their own notes. I prepared identical sets of 20 ballots, each marked "yes," "no," "abstain," and "I would like to have the following evidence discussed." I bought two boxes of Pentel® roller ball pens. I prepared 12 index cards listing the jurors. I would obtain everyone's participation and allow nobody to dominate. All views would be brought out and respected.

We began our deliberations the next morning with a long moment of silence. Then I explained that—assuming they by and large agreed with the procedure—we would vote and list our concerns in private to the fullest extent possible. We would rotate the role of moderator, whose task would be to call on each juror for his or her opinion on the issue in question. I appointed someone to shuffle the ballots, someone to serve as secretary, and someone to write on the blackboard. Then we began our four and one-half hours of uninterrupted focus.

Did it work? Yes. Was it tense? Yes. Did anyone lose composure? No. Did I eat a single bite of the chicken salad sent in from Lizard's Thicket? No. Did my signature on the guilty verdict look like my usual signature? No. It was compatible with advanced Parkinsonism or hepatic encephalopathy.

Did I learn anything? Absolutely. A renewed sense of confidence in our judicial system—imperfect, like all human institutions, but probably as good as any and better than most. A renewed respect for lawyers and judges and for those who work in courthouses. A renewed ability to listen and to respect divergent viewpoints. And a renewed gratitude to be in a profession where the basic orientation is not "I win, you lose" but rather to help one sick person get well.

Let us return to Baltasar Gracián and epigram number 297.

The defendant nearly went unrecognized. But when the guns were going off and nearly everyone in the video poker parlor was ducking and hiding, one employee came out of his room and moved toward the assailants. His mother, it turned out, was working in the room next to where the shooting was taking place. He got a good look at the defendant. He recognized him as a fellow inmate from a former incarceration. He remembered mixing with him, lifting weights with him, showering with him. He remembered that the defendant bore a tattoo of a smoking gun on the left side of the chest. Ironically the anatomic location of the tattoo corresponded to the victim's fatal wound. Two bullets had destroyed the atria of his heart.

Live as though seen.

I can think of at least three ways to apply this simple admonition.

First, there is the theistic basis for deontological ethics, the transcendent Ought. God is watching. Nothing we do goes unseen.

Second, there is the pragmatic basis for everyday behavior, the likelihood that what we do can and will be seen someday, somewhere, by someone. There is always the possibility of being seen.

Finally, there is the high moral ground for the way we should practice medicine, accountable not only to our patients but also to our profession. I especially like the image used by Dr. Hunter Stokes of Florence during his career as an ophthalmic surgeon. Hunter resolved early on to imagine that a medical student was always stationed right behind him, looking over his left shoulder. The image served him well. Imagine that everything you do is seen, and by discerning eyes.

Live as though seen.

Pew Thoughts While Listening to Pachelbel's Canon in D

J SC Med Assoc 1999; 95: 241-242

My friend Don Bessinger of Greenville suggests we consider Bach as the fifth gospel. A fine thought, and in the same spirit I vote for Johann Pachelbel (1653-1706). True, we know relatively little about this composer. But number me among the millions who find in Pachelbel's canon in D a large measure of solace, comfort, and inspiration not unlike that found in the scriptures. Pachelbel brought a balm to humankind.

Like most great compositions the canon is deceptively simple. It begins calmly and methodically with the familiar I-V-VI-iii-IV-I-IV chord progression. The composer next introduces stress through additional voices, dissonance, and increasing volume. Then comes the resolution, a calming after the storm. For me the canon offers a metaphor for life: birth, challenge, closure. With those who call it trite, overplayed, and exploited in too many commercials, I beg to differ. I can't hear it enough.

Through the years I've collected a number of versions. Some feature string quartets, others Baroque chamber orchestras. One features a piano, another a brass ensemble. One has James Galway on the flute. Another carries in the background the fetching, throaty voice of Cleo Laine, singing "How and where will we touch again?" In yet another, the canon rises and falls above a gentle chorus of ocean surf, an acoustic image of eternal time. But the canon has never soothed me more than it did while sitting in the pew at Martine's funeral. Martine, you see, was Bill's daughter.

This story takes up where another left off 15 years ago (see "Bill's Lesion," *J SC Med Assoc* 1984; 80: 313-314). Bill was a special person, an American original, treasured by all who knew him. He gave liberally of time and talents to family, friends, and community. He and Anne gave to each of their eight children the family trademarks: a novel whistle ("You'd recognize it in

Grand Central Station") and an uncommonly winning smile. I first met Bill through the Cub Scout troop of the same church where I now sat listening to Pachelbel. Somewhere there is a picture of me and my father sitting around at Camp Burnt Gin with Bill and his two older sons, Billy and Johnny. Everyone is smiling, especially Bill.

It was through Martine that as an adult I got to know Bill again. I had come back to town to practice medicine. Late one night I was called in consultation by a neurosurgeon to see a patient whose serum sodium was 173 mEq/L following surgery for a ruptured berry aneurysm. She was asymptomatic but had lost her recent memory. I diagnosed infarction of the thirst center and corrected her life-threatening hypernatremia. Bill brought me a quart of shucked oysters. He took me into his circle of family and friends. That irresistible smile became a constant in my life.

The singular blend of art, science, and probability theory that defines our profession dooms each of us to sadness as well as joy, and the greatest sadness of my career came from Bill's asking me to do his physical examination. I found a coin lesion. I consulted a radiologist, a pulmonologist, an oncologist. We all agreed it had to come out. The lesion proved benign—a localized chronic inflammation caused by mineral oil caused in turn by his habitual use of a nasal salve. Postoperatively he developed pneumonia, then a subendocardial infarction, then the acute respiratory distress syndrome. He died.

It mattered not that Bill was 76 years old and fast approaching the usual lifespan of his family of origin. It mattered not that he had known the risks of thoracotomy. It mattered not that he, like most of us, would probably have preferred to avoid what William Osler called "those cold gradations of decay so distressing to his friends." I never quite recovered. Ever since, I've kept a photograph of Bill in my office, a reminder not only of a special friend but also of fallibility, medicine's and my own.

Martine never got back her recent memory or her thirst sensation but coped reasonably well with both deficits. I tried to be her doctor for a while, even arranging a metabolic analysis of her sodium and water balance, but eventually passed her on to other hands, knowing now all too well the pitfalls of caring for "family." When Martine developed urinary calculi, then renal failure, we all assumed it was because she never drank enough water. As it turned out, though, her organs were riddled with amyloidosis. Hospitalized with pneumonia, she was soon committed to hemodialysis and mechanical ventilation. She had one cardiac arrest after another. Through it all, she flashed that famous family smile. The nurses were amazed.

It was after one of my visits to Martine that I ran into Billy (her oldest brother and Bill's and Anne's first son) and his wife, Ginny. We walked out of the hospital together. It was a splendid autumn day. In the parking lot I emptied my sorrows.

"You know, the greatest regret of my professional career was advising Bill to have surgery."

Billy and Ginny simultaneously turned on me. "Come on Charley, let it go!"

"No," I continued, "not a day passes that I don't think of Bill."

Ginny then gave me the blessing I could never give myself, that I could receive only from a member of the family.

"Charley," she said gently but firmly, "God decided it was Bill's time to go. You're not that important!"

Pachelbel played on.

Editorial Note: I was tempted to use this essay's title, a play on Lewis Thomas's Late Night Thoughts on Listening to Mahler's Ninth Symphony, for the entire collection. "A Hound Dog in Anderson" won out because of its lighter tone.

The English Lesson

J SC Med Assoc 1999; 95: 431-432

Oh the times! Oh the manners!
— Cicero

Manners require time, as nothing is more vulgar than haste.
— Emerson

A year of planning, a week of pleasure. Our foursome — Mac, Wickie, the Mullet, and I — lingered in the pub, celebrating a memorable morning at Muirfield. Wickie had just completed his dream of playing every venue where they'd ever held The Open, and he'd done it in style, breaking 80 with ease. Mac had made an eagle. And the Mullet and I — well, let's just say we had lots of fun, lots of shotmaking opportunities. Ahead that afternoon lay North Berwick, my favorite links in the world. I checked the time. "Let's go, guys, we're running late." But whoops, the coupons were back in the room.

Wickie left the motor running as I dashed into the Marine Hotel. The first task was to retrieve the room key. Over there, they avoid runaway room keys by issuing only one per party, usually attached to a bulky object too large for one's pocket. The custom is to leave the key with the desk clerk when you go out. Two Englishmen stood at the desk waiting for the clerk, who was nowhere in sight.

After what seemed like an eternity, she came back to her station. The first Englishman's request evoked a wee frown. She began to make telephone calls while typing on the computer. Our tee time was now just minutes away. I leaned forward and whispered, "Psst — I just need my room key."

The other Englishman was in my face within a nanosecond. He let me have it. He brayed to the entire lobby, "Over heah we have mannuhs, mind you. You wait your turn. You don't just run over people." There was no defense. I looked him squarely in the eye and said gently but firmly, "I agree."

A driving rain kicked up just as we reached the first tee in the nick of time, adding insult to injury.

The sun came out on the back nine, and — my spirits boosted by the ancient stone walls, the blind shots over hills, the quaint greens, and the splendid views of Bass Rock out in the Firth of Forth — savored yet another near-perfect day. Although I didn't say a word about the incident, I knew the Englishman had left me with a choice. I could add the sorry episode to others in my life brought on largely by ignorance of local ways and customs: the street vendor in London, the baker in Aix-en-Provence, the taxi driver on the island of Rhodes. Or I could take it as a challenge to reflect, to review paradigms, to question attitudes and behaviors, to become a better person.

Finishing my book the next afternoon an hour out of Charlotte, I struck up a conversation with the Englishwoman sitting next to me in the bulkhead.

"Tell me," I asked innocently. "What do you think of Americans' manners?"

"Do you really want to know?"

"Yes."

"We think you're rude."

I then recounted the unpleasantness in the lobby of the Marine Hotel at North Berwick. "Oh yes, lines are very important to us." We reviewed how I might have handled the situation differently, perhaps by asking the two gentlemen ahead of me for permission to speak to the clerk.

When it comes to manners, I had fancied myself somewhere in the upper quartile of *Homo sapiens,* at least when time is plentiful. But therein lies the rub. Pressured by competing time demands, I'm capable of assuming the telephone personality of a snapping turtle, the bedside manner of a barracuda. On occasion I've been reduced to a blithering idiot. Excruciating time pressures have always been for me the downside of medicine. I marvel at the way some family physicians can see 80 or more patients a day without getting flustered, at how some intensivists retain their poise and composure under extreme stress. These people must be made of kryptonite! Yet studies show that small acts of discourtesy make up a large fraction of patient dissatisfaction and are a major reason for changing physicians. Many people will tell you, "Doctors are always in a hurry."

Suboptimal manners are not, of course, unique to physicians. A 1996 *U.S. News and World Report* survey showed that 89 percent of Americans consider incivility to be a serious problem, with 78 percent saying that it had gotten worse over the previous decade. A survey of the recent literature reveals book titles such as *A Short History of Rudeness: Manners, Morals, and Misbehavior in Modern America* and *Civility: Manners, Morals and the Etiquette of Democracy*. The latter author argues that our growing incivility threatens democracy itself. Nor are Americans unique. Prime Minister Tony Blair recently said the same about the United Kingdom. My transgression at the Marine Hotel illustrates the most important etiquette problem in daily life: the Interrupter. Yet stat pages, cell phones, voice mail, e-mail, and the anonymous messengers of managed care condition us to accept interruptions as a way of life. Can anything be done?

The more I think about it, the more strongly I conclude that minding our manners represents a major way by which we can help our profession's image. Here are ten thoughts on the matter, in no particular order (and how I wish I could always take my own advice !):

• Strive to be punctual.
• Cultivate self-awareness of your own manners and those of others.
• Practice small acts of courtesy, such as letting others in line ahead of you.
• Ask, "Is this a good time for you?"
• Be quick to apologize.
• Set aside downtime in your schedule to return telephone calls and the like.
• Try to get a good night's sleep.
• Remember the Platinum Rule: "Do unto others as they would like done unto themselves."
• Treat your office staff courteously, and make it clear to them how much you value courtesy to patients and everyone else.
• Go out of your way to be courteous on the road, whether or not your car marks you as a physician.

Studies indicate that physicians, even in teaching settings, are reluctant to point out breaches of etiquette. We neither reward good behavior nor penalize bad behavior, at least directly. We suffer in silence. We perpetuate the cycle by interrupting our colleagues, often out of impatience or laziness rather than true urgency. John D. Rockefeller, Sr., put it well: "A man has no right to occupy another man's time unnecessarily." This simple rule, I think, is the essence of good professional manners. If we could heed it, how much better we would be, both individually and collectively!

A year later, I conclude that the Englishman at North Berwick did me a favor. I wish there were a way to thank him.

Manners matter. Courtesy counts.

A Hound Dog in Anderson

J SC Med Assoc 2002; 98: 30-31

As this issue goes to press, I ponder *The Journal*'s change to every-other-month publication—a probable sign that, within the foreseeable future (say, 10 to 30 years—but who knows?), our fine publication will someday cease to exist, at least in present form.

As this issue goes to press, I also celebrate my sixtieth birthday—a sure sign that, within the forseeable future (say, 10 to 30 years—but who knows?) Charles S. Bryan will someday cease to exist, at least in present form.

Should either of these events be noted with sadness? Rationally speaking, of course not!

Whenever I start to feel sorry for myself, which is perhaps too often considering my many blessings, I remind myself that the odds against being one's born are greater than 400,000 to one from the perspective of one's mother's ovaries alone. Imagine—400,000 primordial germs cells lined up as potential human beings, and yours rolled down the fallopian tube at just the right time! Conception is like winning a lottery in which everyone in, say, Columbia or Charleston or Greenville-Spartanburg was entered! Toss in the father factor—the odds that a particular spermatozoon found the lucky ovum—and the odds against one's unique personhood become infinitesimally small! Life, even a single day of it, is indeed a miracle!

On those rare occasions when this ovarian imagery fails to cheer me up, I think about a long-departed hound dog in Anderson, South Carolina. If it hadn't been for that dog, Mother and Dad wouldn't have gotten together in the first place.

My father graduated from what is now the Medical University of South Carolina in 1933, the depths of the Depression. After a rotating internship at Roper Hospital he established a general practice in Pelzer. By all accounts he was overworked and underpaid. He charged 50 cents for an office visit, a dollar for a house call, and 10 dollars for a labor case. He met and courted a young woman who was beautiful and talented and who played the harpsichord. Things were getting serious. One night, as he was preparing to take her to a major dance, he was called to see a poor woman in the country. When he finally showed up for his date, she read him the riot act whereupon he said," If that's the way you feel, that's it!" and walked away. (When Dad ran into this lady many years later, the pleasantries included her boast, "I'll bet my children are better looking than yours!" This was probably true, although my two brothers might beg to differ.)

In the meantime my mother had graduated from Goucher College in Baltimore and could not find a job in Washington, D.C., or Alexandria, Virginia, her hometown. Her mother sent her down to Anderson for a short vacation with an older sister who was married to the president of a large textile mill. Her sister's social standing gave Mother entree to an active social life. She met Dad at a party. He called for a date but her dance card was full and she declined.

Mother was the youngest of seven children and her mother — that is, my grandmother — had no doubt chosen her, at least subconsciously, as the one who would care for her in old age. Rumors that Mother was having an exceptionally good time in South Carolina drifted northward. Her mother came down from Alexandria with the plan to stay a week and then take the train back to Alexandria with Mother in tow. The day of the return trip was fast approaching. One morning, Mother set out for her routine walk with the family dachshund up West Whitner Street toward the town square. Just before the square on the left was a filling station, and as she walked by it she noted several men sitting on a bench. In the midst of them was a hound dog.

No sooner had Mother made this observation than the hound dog charged the dachshund. The dachshund held its ground. The hound circled. The dachshund's leash rapped around Mother's legs. The hound drew blood.

Said the sheriff to the bench-sitters: "Okay, boys, whose dog was it that bit Mister Nichols's niece?" Nobody confessed. The dog was nowhere to be found. A doctor ordered Mother to stay in Anderson for a 21-day course of rabies shots. Her mother took the train back to Alexandria, alone. Dad, who was if anything persistent, called again and got a date.

And that's how I owe my existence to a hound dog in Anderson, South Carolina.

When I was about seventeen years old we had one day in Sunday School the obligatory discussion about whether animals have souls. One Bambi Bell chirped: "I believe that in heaven if you want an animal, God will *give* you that animal."

I hope Bambi's right. I want to meet that hound dog.

Thoughts on *The Doctor*

J SC Med Assoc 2003; 99: 112-113

In any profession in any town of any size, one gradually comes to appreciate and respect certain colleagues despite not getting to know them very well. Such has been my relationship over the years with Dr. Melton R. Stuckey who does family medicine in Columbia. He quietly epitomizes what a doctor should be, and I find his faithful attendance at our Internal Medicine Grand Rounds to be especially exemplary. However, this editorial is not written as a paean to Mel Stuckey. It's about a remarkable coincidence concerning Sir Luke Fildes's classic painting, *The Doctor.*

The Doctor features a well-dressed but weary practitioner hovered over a sick child in a modest farmhouse. We sense the physician's unhurried concern, his single-minded focus, his attentive body language. We sense that the child's father, consoling his wife in the shadows of the background, cannot possibly pay this doctor sufficiently for staying up all night. We sense that none of us who write about medical professionalism could capture in a dozen books its essence to the extent that Fildes has done with this wonderful image. In the muted light of that farmhouse, service clearly transcends self-interest.

The Doctor was commissioned by Sir Henry Tate, a Liverpool merchant whose invention of the sugar cube made him fabulously wealthy in a country where they loved their tea. Tate sought a signature painting for the collection he planned to donate to the people of England. He gave Fildes the license to choose his subject. On Christmas morning 1877, Fildes had lost an infant son presumably from one of the acute infectious diseases that so often killed children before the introduction of antibiotics. Fildes set out to immortalize the caring and concern demonstrated by the physician who presided over his son's death. The artist, given a generous budget, constructed an entire sickroom in his studio. The resulting masterpiece has been reproduced—some would say "exploited"—again and again

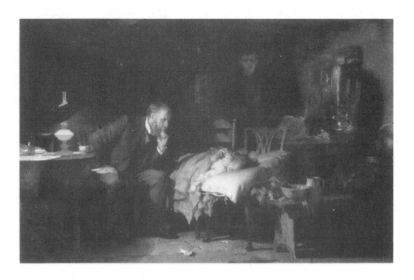

The Doctor *(1891), by Sir Luke Fildes*

through the years as an icon of what medicine should be.

I first saw *The Doctor* in London in 1966, the summer before my senior year of medical school. It's a large canvass, eight feet by ten feet. Standing before it I, like countless others, quietly resolved to live its message as best I could. I bought a handsome print and had it framed. Four years later I gave the print to the neonatologist who took care of my firstborn child. He never acknowledged the gift, and I sometimes wished I'd thanked him another way.

In 2001, thirty-five years after that first viewing, I prevailed on an English friend to swing by the Tate Gallery so that I could see *The Doctor* again. It wasn't there. While I assume that there was a good reason—perhaps it was out on loan—its absence seemed symbolic of the angst now pervasive among physicians, the sense that something is missing. Adding to the irony was the setting of my next encounter with *The Doctor*: the motion picture *Harry Potter and The Sorcerer's Stone,* in which it appears on the wall of the hospital wing at Hogwarts School of Witchcraft and Wizardry. This seemed oddly appropriate, since Fildes and his subjects would find today's medicine magical even by the high standards of Harry Potter's creator, J. K. Rowling.

But therein lies a question. Which doctor would one prefer: Fildes's, who had little to offer except caring and compassion, or any randomly-chosen physician of the early twenty-first century who, however, abrupt, insensitive, and ill-tempered, cures the child with antibiotics? A thoughtful sociologist suggests that the introduction of penicillin into civilian practice during 1945 changed forever the doctor-patient relationship, as patients increasingly sought physicians not for wise counsel but rather for quick technical solutions to whatever ailed them.[1] As scientific advances continue to simplify diagnosis and supply cures, as patients understandably view medicine not as an art contingent upon the physician's largesse but rather as a commodity, and as many people turn to "alternative healers" when we can't solve their functional complaints, one wonders whether Fildes's doctor has indeed become obsolete.

To be sure, Fildes's image is an oversimplification even of late-nineteenth century medicine. In 1891, the year *The Doctor* was unveiled, William Pepper observed: "General medicine and general surgery today are federations of specialties; and the general clinician, even of the broadest gauge, in dealing with obscure and complicated cases, acts but as the leading member in a medical firm."[2] Classically, and as captured by Fildes, medicine consists of a single physician caring for a single patient. Realistically, the doctor has many patients and, conversely, the seriously ill patient has more than one doctor. We are now increasingly concerned about the extent to which third parties — insurance companies, government, and many others — encroach upon the physician-patient relationship. Reflecting on *The Doctor*, Clif Cleaveland speaks of that relationship as a "sacred space" to be ever defended against unwanted intruders.[3] But we digress. Let's return to the remarkable coincidence involving Dr. Melton R. Stuckey.

On January 15, 2003, I made reference to *The Doctor* during a dedication ceremony. My point was the importance of dedicating oneself to certain ideals, even if such dedication runs counter to one's financial self-interest. Fildes was a celebrated artist of his day, best known as a social realist. Why, then, do we seldom hear of him today except for *The Doctor* and a few other canvases? The answer: He concerned himself largely with portraits, which paid well and for which there was great demand. Still, let us be grateful for this singularly fine image of the kind of caring to which we should all aspire.

The next morning—January 16, 2003—Mel Stuckey sought me out after Internal Medicine Grand Rounds. "Did you get that print I left for you?" He had obtained a print of *The Doctor* identical to the one I'd once owned and had no more! And he had given it to *me*! I had it properly framed and was tempted to hang it in my office. Happily, judgment prevailed. I donated it to be hung in a classroom for medical students. Perhaps at least some of them on viewing it will quietly resolve then and there to live its message as best they can in a changing and confusing world.

References

1. Shorter E. *Doctors and their Patients: A Social History*. New Brunswick, New Jersey; 1993: 21-22.
2. Pepper W. Opening address. *Transactions of the Association of American Physicians* 1891; 6: xv-xx.
3. Cleaveland C. *Sacred Space: Stories from a Life in Medicine*. Philadelphia: American College of Physicians: 1998: xvii-xix.

E. Carwile Leroy (1933-2002): *Lacrimae Rerum*

J SC Med Assoc 2003; 99: 114

This year's meeting of the *The Journal's* editorial board won't be the same without Carwile LeRoy, who died in Italy last May after a brief illness. An active participant at our board meetings, Carwile often made suggestions about how we might best meet practicing physicians' educational needs. On a personal note, I shall miss him greatly. Over time, he had become one of my closest friends in South Carolina medicine. My trips to Charleston were incomplete without a round of golf with Carwile at Yeamans Hall, and I was sometimes privileged to stay with Carwile and Dee at their home on Tradd Street. It was Carwile who introduced me to the American Osler Society, which has since become a major interest. After last year's meeting of the editorial board we went to Starbucks on King Street for a cup of coffee. And then, so suddenly, he was gone.

Interacting with Carwile on the editorial board and elsewhere, one would never have suspected his international prominence in the field of rheumatology. When elected a Master of the American College of Physicians, he was praised specifically for contributions to our understanding of scleroderma. Carwile was among the first to show that fibroblasts from patients with scleroderma secrete large quantities of collagen and that the vascular endothelium plays a major role in the disease. Two years before his untimely death, the Medical University of South Carolina made him a Distinguished University Professor. He wrote more than 270 papers and received high honors both from medical organizations and also from his alma maters, which were Wake Forest University and the University of North Carolina School of Medicine. However, I, like countless others, remember Carwile as the quintessential gentleman, always willing to help, always comfortable to be around, gracious and unassuming. His passing leaves a void, but I'm grateful to have known him — which might not have happened had I not become involved in the South Carolina Medical Association.

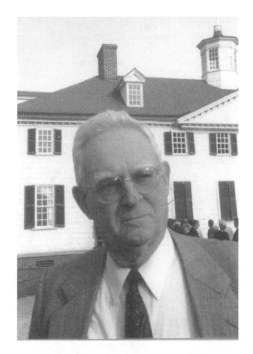

Carwile Leroy at Mount Vernon during the annual meeting of the American Osler Society, April 2001.

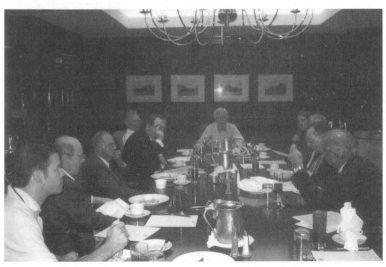

Meeting of the Editorial Board of The Journal of the South Carolina Medical Association, *Charleston, S.C., April 28, 2002. Carwile Leroy is at the far-left corner, to the editor's immediate right.*

His Blood Runneth Orange

J SC Med Assoc 2003; 99: 112-113

Jane Hunter once told me that her husband, Bill, wanted me to write his obituary. How can one even begin to write about a legendary personage with whom one was fortunate to forge a close friendship through the years?

Hold your tears. Bill's isn't dead! Although hobbled and legally blind from the ravages of adult-onset diabetes mellitus, Bill in his ninth decade is very much alive and indeed still sees patients every weekday morning with his son-in-law, Jim Hanahan of Seneca. And he's still very much a living monument in his beloved Clemson, South Carolina, where from his base on the Old Pendleton Highway his energy, enthusiasm, and wisdom have diffused throughout the upstate in both the public and the private communities. Prompting this editorial is my growing conviction since 9/11 and its aftermath that we should celebrate the lives of others while they're still among us! As my medical school classmate Gordon Livingston puts it in his new book *And Never Stop Dancing*, let's not die with the music locked inside us.

William Harvey Hunter was born in Anderson, South Carolina, finished high school in Greenville, and, like most young men of that "greatest generation," had his college career interrupted by World War II. A lieutenant in the Marine Corps, Bill served as a naval aviator. He was one of those brave men who flew combat missions in F4U Corsairs from the decks of aircraft carriers, knowing not only the dangers of enemy fire but also the uncertainties of landing safely on a moving object. He returned to Clemson in 1946 on a football scholarship. Anyone who's spent much time with Bill is sure to have heard at least three great stories.

The first story begins on November 9, 1946. Clemson versus Tulane in New Orleans. The Tigers were without eight of their eleven first-stringers because of illness or injury — and re-

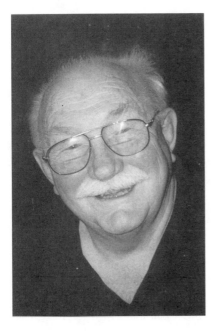

William Harvey Hunter

call that back then the starters played both offense and defense, typically for the entire 60 minutes. During the second quarter, Bill, an interior lineman, suffered an acromioclavicular separation of the right shoulder. He somehow managed to finish the game despite the pain and disability. The final score: Tulane 54, Clemson 13. The team, thoroughly demoralized, took the long ride back to Clemson on the old Southern Railroad sure in the knowledge that they would have to walk from the station back to the dormitories with their heads bowed low. To their great surprise they were met at the station by the entire student body including the marching band! It was then and there that Bill knew that his blood would always run orange.

The second story concerns Bill Hunter's courtship of Jane Gardener. He was working as a lifeguard at Myrtle Beach, across the street from where her family kept an inn. He was taken aback by her long hair and also by her resolve to dive into the ocean from the end of a fishing pier. He told her not to do it, but she did it anyway. She gave him a small consolation present and then challenged him to a swim beyond the breakers. She kept on swimming farther and farther out to sea until an exhausted Bill finally conceded. Although the details of the rest of the courtship have not yet entered the public domain, we do know that Bill, after graduating from the Medical College in Charleston and completing a rotating internship in Greenville, returned to Clemson in 1953 with Jane in tow. This leads us to the third story, how Bill developed his practice.

Establishing a practice was more difficult back then than is now generally the case. There were few groups to join, and commercial advertising was taboo. Bill and Jane waited and waited for patients to arrive. Then one day he was accosted by an anxious man crying out "Daddy's sick." It seems that Daddy lived way back in the hills and that Daddy's regular doctor, on hearing the symptoms of crushing chest pain with nausea, diaphoresis, and shortness of breath, insisted that he be taken to Anderson for hospitalization. Daddy refused. He'd been born in that house and by golly he'd die there as well. Taking Jane with him, Bill arrived at Daddy's homestead with his doctor's bag and an EKG machine whereupon Daddy took one look at the boyish young doctor and muttered, "Well, I guess you'll have to do." Bill confirmed the diagnosis of acute myocardial infarction. He stayed up all night poking medicine into Daddy. The pulmonary edema finally cleared. Stepping out into the breaking dawn, Bill saw what amounted to an entire village keeping solemn vigil beneath the oak trees in Daddy's front yard. It seems that "Daddy" was the patriarch of the entire region! Thereafter Bill never lacked for patients. And the long dinner table at Daddy's birthday invariably featured the preacher on one side of Daddy and Bill on the other.

Bill lasted fifty years in solo practice — no mean feat by any standards. Having visited him in his office, I can testify that he practiced exquisite medicine and had accumulated many pearls of information (for example, he reeled off for my benefit a long list of symptoms attributable to perforation of the tympanic membrane). What is even more remarkable, though, is the way Bill exemplified the vanishing ideal of the small-town family practitioner as the community's leading citizen. He made friends easily among the Clemson faculty, serving them not only as a physician and fundraiser but also as intellectual companion. He teamed with philosophy professor Bill Maker to invite the worldwide community of Hegel scholars to Clemson University, where they were treated to South Carolina barbecue in the Hunters' backyard. More recently he founded Clemson University's Calhoun Lecture Series, which has brought to the campus speakers of national and international renown. He served four years as an advisor for medical education to the National Institutes of Health. And, of course, he was active in the politics of the profession as evinced by his serving as president of the South Carolina Medical Association. For these activities and more, Bill has received just recognition as a Distinguished Alumnus of both Clemson University and the Medical University of South Carolina.

Bill is also an accomplished writer. "Daddy" was published in *The Journal of the American Medical Association*, from which it has been reprinted from time to time as something of a classic. Bill has served on a number of editorial boards including ours. It was he who came up with the idea of offering a reward for the best article in *The Journal of the South Carolina Medical Association* and, as a member of the Roe Foundation's Board of Directors, it was he who saw the idea to fruition. For the past 18 years he's written a regular column for the Anderson *Independent Mail*. Just about everyone in Bill's corner of state, I suspect, is familiar with the story of Patrick Hunter, the autistic grandson whom Bill and Jane have raised and seen through many harrowing episodes. Bill predictably became a leader in the movement to understand and treat autism and, as he modestly suggested in the October 2006 issue of *The Journal*, he was perhaps the first to suggest that autism represents a spectrum of disorders. Bill can no longer see to read, but blindness has not stilled his pen. He's recently brought out a collection of his stories and wisdom under the title *Tales of 17-Mile Hill*.

Well, Jane and Bill, that's a start.

Keep going, Buddy! Or, as they say in your beloved Scotland, "lang may yer lum reek!"

"I'm Not a Missionary"

J SC Med Assoc 2007; 103:

On January 15, 1999, George L. Lundberg was summarily dismissed as editor of *The Journal of the American Association*, allegedly for publishing an article about how college students define sex just as President Clinton was being impeached. Members of the South Carolina delegation to the AMA nominated me as Lundberg's successor. Waiting for the call, I pondered what I'd say to the search committee. To the most obvious question — "If you became editor of *JAMA* what would you do differently?" — here's my tentative script:

(Pause for dramatic effect)

I'd place less emphasis on *JAMA* as the journal *for* the AMA and more emphasis on *JAMA* as the journal *of* the AMA. I'd put less emphasis on competing with *The New England Journal of Medicine* for the week's top medical story by a team of academicians funded by government or industry. I'd put more emphasis on celebrating the rank and file of the American medical profession. To that end, I'd remove the paintings from the cover. I'd do this reluctantly, of course, since the paintings are wonderful and Therese Southgate's cover stories provide a veritable course in art appreciation. But I think it's more important to help practicing physicians feel good about themselves and to reinforce their idealism. I'd grace each week's cover with the photograph of a physician who's contributed to medicine and society above and beyond the call of duty, a physician who exemplifies what I've called "higher professionalism" — service that clearly transcends self-interest. In summary, I'd make it clear that *JAMA* is indeed the journal *of* the American Medical Association and to that end the covers would feature AMA members who exemplify our highest ideals.

(Eye contact with the person who asked the question)

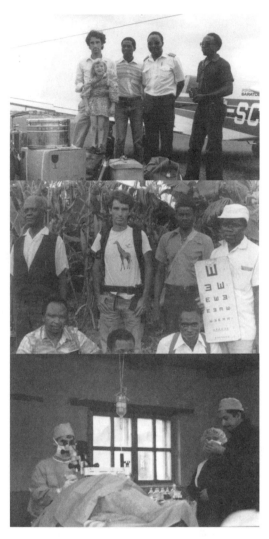

(Top to bottom): Baxter McLendon preparing, with daughter Cordes, to fly in a single-engine airplane to a mission hospital in Tanzania; conducting field surveillance for onchocerciasis in Malawi; and performing surgery in a school classroom in rural Guatemala.

The call never came, which is probably just as well for *JAMA* and for my health.

So why not implement this idea with *The Journal* (that's THE journal — *The Journal of the South Carolina Medical Association*!)? It was to this end that we chose Dr. Todd L. Crump of Lexington, the 2007 recipient of the Community Service Award, for the August issue's cover illustration, and I suggest that we make this a yearly habit. And why not celebrate other physicians and groups of physicians who've performed notable services outside of their practices? In this spirit, the present issue's cover features Dr. Baxter Franklin McLendon of Beaufort, South Carolina.

I first met Baxter at the 1993 annual meeting when he received the Thomas L. and Shirley W. Roe Foundation Award for the best article by a practicing physician during the previous 24-month cycle. Distressed about a patient who'd never seen an ophthalmologist prior to a retinal hemorrhage, Baxter wrote about blindness in South Carolina including services available to people with eye problems. I next met Baxter in his capacity as chair of the Continuing Medical Education Committee, and I ran into him again at this year's annual meeting. He mentioned casually that he planned to sell his practice as soon as possible so that he could go back to working in developing countries. Now that really got my attention! Here's the story as I've pieced it together.

Baxter McLendon, a 1970 graduate of the Medical University of South Carolina, interned in surgery and then, bracing for the "doctor draft" that prevailed through the Vietnam era, sought a job in the United States Public Health Service. "We're sorry," he was told, "there are no jobs left in the Marine Hospital Service. And there are no jobs in the Indian Health Service. Wait a minute—we do have one job at the national leprosy hospital in Carville, Louisiana. Any interest?" He consulted his wife, Susan, who like Baxter is a native of Charleston. They couldn't locate Carville on a map, but concluded, "fine—it's just for two years." Little did they know how their lives would change!

The national leprosarium on the banks of the Mississippi was at that time home to Paul Brand (1914-2003), the legendary hand surgeon and best-selling author (*Fearfully and Wonderfully Made*; *In His Image*; *Pain – The Gift Nobody Wants*), and his wife Margaret, an ophthalmologist. The Brands had come to Carville from India after that country's government with its new independence began to discourage Britons from staying on there. With their cottage just two doors down from the famous couple's, Baxter and Susan got to know the Brands intimately. The Brands stimulated their interest in working with the less fortunate in developing countries. Margaret Brand sparked Baxter's interest in ophthalmology, leading to a residency at the Medical College of Georgia and a cornea fellowship at Oxford University. In 1978, he returned to Charleston for four years of private practice while exploring possibilities overseas.

In 1982, and despite (or perhaps because of) their young family, Baxter and Susan pulled tent and moved to Moshie in Tanzania, East Africa, under the sponsorship of Christoffel Blindenmission in West Germany. There Baxter worked in a hospital, taught in several medical schools, and regularly went to towns and villages, taking with him one or another of the couple's three daughters. These trips, made in single-propeller airplanes flown by bush pilots, could be harrowing to say the least. On one occasion the pilot, whose navigation system consisted of a road map of Tanzania, got lost and they realized they were over Rwanda and with fuel running low. They would probably have crash-landed had it not been for a Dutch pilot who, fortuitously, had turned on his ham radio and heard the plea for directions. Baxter performed hundreds of operations, especially for cataracts and trachoma, diagnosed the first case of AIDS in Tanzania, and tackled reversible causes of blindness such as vitamin A deficiency. Simultaneously ill with typhoid fever and malaria, he had a near-death experience complete with an astral projection. The two years in Tanzania were followed by three years of similar work in Malawi under the sponsorship of the International Eye Foundation. Then came two years in Guatemala, where Baxter helped spearhead efforts to treat onchocerciasis (river blindness) with ivermectin.

In 1991, Baxter and Susan returned to the United States so that their daughters could complete high school and college. For the past 16 years, Baxter has practiced in Beaufort and Hampton and has also taught in the eye residency program at MUSC. However, he and Susan have continued to spend as much time as possible in developing countries such as Haiti (in Leogane and Jeremie, where Columbia ophthalmologist Dr. Hal Croswell has worked regularly for many years), in Namibia (South West Africa), and in Guatemala. With financial assistance from his Rotary Club, Baxter has regularly sponsored visits from physicians in Kenya, Ecuador, Eritrea, and India so that they can observe how ophthalmic medicine and surgery are practiced in the United States. Baxter's honors for these services include the Service Above Self Award from the Rotary Club, the Promotion of Peace and Vision Award from the International Eye Foundation, and the Honor (Achievement) Award from the American Academy of Ophthalmology. If such honors have gone to his head, it doesn't show.

And so now Baxter has sold his practice. The daughters are grown and thriving. Baxter and Susan are looking forward to their next experience. Already he's located an opportunity where he'll be the second ophthalmologist for a population of more than two million.

But when I brought up the word "missionary", Baxter looked up at me incredulously.

"Missionary?!" he exclaimed. "I'm not a missionary!" Indeed, Susan, who is a painter, was once quoted by the press as saying: "Don't picture us as suffering missionaries making big sacrifices. We do it because we want to."

Baxter, in summary, substantiates in spades what most of us told the medical school admissions committee: "I like science and I want to help people." And he likewise illustrates what we secretly felt inside: "… and I can't think of anything that would be more fun!"

The Profession of Medicine

Professional Responsibility

J SC Med Assoc 1977; 73: 232-234

Required courses fill the curriculum of the junior and senior years of medical school: medicine, surgery, obstetrics, pediatrics, and psychiatry, to name but a few. Only one course, we have learned, is required of junior and senior law students. Its title: "Professional Responsibility."

The special articles in this issue of *The Journal* focus on the viability of our professionalism. The purpose of this editorial is to reflect on the need to re-define some of the traditional concepts of professional responsibility in medicine and in law, if our current systems of practice are to survive largely intact.

There are, of course, obvious differences between the professional responsibilities of doctors and lawyers. To borrow from the passage by Roscoe Pound quoted in this issue's essay by Dr. Leon Banov, Jr., doctors deal with "problems of disease," while lawyers deal with "problems of human relations in society."[1] It follows that doctors work in a system of unity of purpose: Everyone tries to help the sick person get well. It also follows that lawyers work in a system of conflicting purposes: an adversary system. I have always considered doctors to be the more fortunate, for our system affords a greater idealism of purpose. In law, there are winners and losers; in medicine, we all win or lose depending on the patient's outcome.

But here we emphasize the similarities. The doctor's only responsibility is to his patient; the lawyer's only responsibility is to his client. At least, these are the usual definitions.

Is there need for change?

The classic statement of the lawyer's responsibility to his client was expressed by Lord Brougham in Queen Caroline's case.[2] Threatening, literally, to destroy the kingdom, Lord Brougham asserted.

> An advocate, in the discharge of his duty, knows but one person in all the world and that person is his client. To save that client by all means and expedients, and at all

71

> hazards and costs to other persons, and, amongst them,
> to himself, is his first and only duty; and in performing
> his duty he must not regard the alarm, the torments, the
> destruction which he may bring to others. Separating the
> duty of a patriot from that of an advocate, he must go
> on reckless of the consequences, though it should be his
> unhappy fate to involve his country in confusion.

The lawyer defends this position, in part, by the presence of a zealous advocate on the other side.

Let us reflect upon Lord Brougham's statement and imagine its application to contemporary medicine. A battle is in progress. Standing over the bed of a seemingly hopelessly ill patient in a busy intensive care unit, the physician confronts the head nurse, the chief of service, the chief of staff, the hospital administrator, the chairman of the utilization review committee, and the representative of the insurance carrier. He shouts:

> This is my patient! I don't care if we use the last drug
> in the pharmacy! I don't care if we use the last unit of
> blood in the blood bank! I don't care if we have to close
> down the rest of the intensive care unit! I don't care if we
> bankrupt the hospital, and exhaust the funds of the entire
> Medicare system! This is my patient, and I am going to
> do everything possible to save him!

The scene is, of course, improbable; it is drawn to illustrate that, carried to its logical extreme, the physician's role as zealous advocate can likewise "involve his country in confusion."

Dr. Claude Emerson Welch in this issue analyzes some of the factors that threaten the framework of medicine as we know it.[3] The factors are many and complex, but surely rising health care costs head the list. Many question whether our economy can continue to support the escalating cost of medical care. This reality may force cataclysmic changes in the system of health care delivery and we may not like them.

I see two major causes of the escalating cost of medical care. Both might be resolved in part, or at least "contained" at an acceptable level, by rethinking what we mean by "professional responsibility."

The first cause is the much-publicized crisis in malpractice

72

liability insurance. Rising premium rates have already palpably affected medical practice. The problem is not unique to medicine. Just as some physicians have been forced out of business by the high premium rates, industries and small businesses are being threatened by the growing problem of "products liability" litigation. Is there need for re-defining "professional responsibility" in the law?

Lawyers argue that their clients' rights are too precious to change the system for one segment of society, however great the cost. They see the lawyer-client relationship just as we see the doctor-patient relationship: something sacred, to be preserved without change. Other thoughtful men in the field of law, however, see the need for change. They see the need for major reforms in the tort-liability system. They see the need to refine traditional concepts of judicial fairness, due process, and equal protection. The problem is how to effect workable changes without sacrificing "fundamental fairness" for each client.

The second cause of escalating medical costs is in our hands to control. This is the problem of the rapidly rising costs of the technologies we use.

Every doctor's desire to do "all that is possible for the patient" must, increasingly, be tempered by financial considerations. Our present system simply cannot support the use of all available technologies for every patient. It has been pointed out, for example, that widespread application of but a few procedures, such as total hip replacement surgery or the coronary artery-saphenous vein bypass operation, would threaten the entire structure of the health-care delivery system.[4] What crisis would ensue should all headache sufferers insist, tomorrow, that their insurance carriers pay the bill for computerized axial tomographic scans of their cranial cavities? Has the enormous rise in national expenditure for laboratory tests (from 5.6 billion dollars in 1971 to 12 billion dollars in 1975) been of real overall benefit to individuals? Thoughtful physicians argue that the problem of cost containment in our profession transcends, in a way, the traditional concept of the doctor-patient relationship.

In 1927, Dr. Francis Peabody delivered a lecture on caring for the patient that has become a classic position statement on the ideal doctor-patient relationship. A medical student recently contrasted the beautiful simplicity of Dr. Peabody's remarks with the situation 50 years later:

> One can no longer consider the caring role of the physician without pondering issues such as how medical care is delivered to the poor, or the wide use of increasingly expensive technology. Caring includes the noble feelings expressed by Peabody, but it also encompasses the hard realities of equity and cost. A real danger in failing to provide education for caring is that too few physicians are trained to grapple with these latter issues.[5]

To deal with these problems in our present society, there is no dearth of articulate spokesmen. A veritable onslaught of new journals and periodicals grapple with the issues of medical ethics, philosophy as applied to medicine and science, and the relationships between medicine and law. But dialogue does not ensure solutions. Dr. Welch relates what happened in China. In reflecting on present problems, I am reminded of America before the Civil War: historians marvel at how many people on both sides were so articulate, but the war came anyway.

At the root of these issues may be the problem of defining the professional's responsibility. How does he see it? How does society see it? How does his patient (or client) see it?

To answer the question posed by the title of Dr. Welch's essay, our answers should all be a resounding yes. We must be optimistic. We should have no problem surviving if our recommendations remain in society's best interests.

References

1. Freeman MH. Are their public interest limits on lawyers' advocacy? *Social Responsibility: Journalism, Law, and Medicine.* Lexington, Virginia: Washington and Lee University; 1976: volume II: 31-39.
2. Fox M. Why people are mad at doctors. *Newsweek,* 10 January 1977: 4.
3. Rippe J. Caring and medical education. *Lancet* 1977; 1: 36-37.

On the Verge of a New Golden Age?

J SC Med Assoc 1988; 84: 38-39

One senses in some quarters pessimism about the future of medical practice. It has been suggested that the Golden Age of American Medicine has come and gone. Characterized by scientific progress and economic prosperity in the post-World War II era, the Golden Age became jeopardized even as it peaked. One historian claims that the high ideals of physicians combined with campaigns against socialized medicine prompted public attempts "to modify the elevated position of physicians in American society."[1] As physicians, we tend to identify other factors. Symbolizing the shaking of confidence was the crisis in malpractice liability insurance, and contributing to the pathogenesis of this crisis were society's growing litigious attitude and distrust of authority figures of any kind. The rise of self-help movements of all descriptions, and the continued presence of groups such as chiropractic, eroded the confidence in scientific medicine. Finally, failure to contain costs due in no small measure to the inability of our society to address squarely the issue of what constitutes entitled health care led to reactions first by government and then by private insurance carriers to curb physicians' incomes. When it was pointed out that physicians' incomes make up but a small fraction of total health care costs, persons in high places in government and business were sometimes unsympathetic.

Against this background, the first glimpse of a recent editorial in *The Journal of the American Medical Association* came as something of a surprise.[2] The title reads: "In Developed Countries, the Golden Age of Medicine is at Hand ..." Then one noted the afterthought: "... for the Patients." Dr. George D. Lundberg outlines ten specific reasons why we should anticipate an unprecedented ability to deliver quality care to our patients, as follows:

• Scientific advances enable us to diagnose and manage even the most serious illnesses.

• New technology abounds. A few examples suffice: prosthetic organs, transplantation services, newer and better imaging techniques, DNA probes and monoclonal antibodies, endoscopy, lasers, home diagnostic tests, and home IV therapy.

• Excellent hospital facilities compete with one another for patients.

• For the first time in this century, the supply of physicians seems adequate.

• Funding for health care is, in general, adequate. The amount spent on health care in the United States whether measured as the percentage of the gross national product (now 11 percent) or total amount exceeds that of any other country.

• The public enjoys multiple options for medical care: private practice, group practice, HMOs, PPOs, IPAs— you name it.

• We now enjoy rapid communication and information systems.

•We are witnessing a new, constructive brand of entrepreneurialism in medicine.

• There is a new wave of science-based preventive medicine.

• We are able to manage our resources more rationally.

Dr. Lundberg makes but brief mention of the problems facing the medical profession, considering these to be too well known to *JAMA* readers to require recitation.

Is it inevitable that the lines of two Golden Ages must crisscross, that is, rising prospects for the patients yet declining prospects for the medical profession? I think not. Further, it is certainly in the public interest that our profession should retain its hard-won high morale. But we must unite behind a high sense of purpose.

Few of today's economic issues are new. In the late 1800s, for example, controversy surrounded the concept of contract practice (yesterday's HMO). Physicians sought contracts by underbidding each other, and the practice continued to grow although opposed by organized medicine. Many physicians crossed lines. Another practice almost inconceivable today but necessary to keep in mind was fee-splitting whereby surgeons sometimes shared the take with referring general practitioners. Commenting on these practices several years ago, Dr. Lester S.

King made some projections about our future:

> The increasing complexity of medical care, the multiplication of specialties, the willingness of the public to pay high fees for surgery but not for medical care, the increasing importance of medical insurance in the payment of fees, the moral fervor of many physicians, the multiplication of professional societies to enhance the "interests" of their members, the legislative intervention to prohibit abuses that refused to remain sharply defined — all these are a few of the strands that have, today, complicated the abuses already widely prevalent in the early 1900s.[3]

Dr. King's analysis clearly indicates the value of history for predicting what we can expect from the future.

Scenario analysis is a new planning technique that takes into account a range of eventualities. The scenario analysis recently formulated by the AMA's Council on Long Range Planning and Development seems especially relevant.[4] In one scenario, the remaining years of the twentieth century are characterized by rapid growth of corporate medicine, with the overall economic growth rate being similar to that of the 1970s. Health care supply will exceed demand and the government will promote managed care systems to reduce spending. The second scenario is that of hard times with a recession economy. The supply of health services will greatly exceed the demand, and there will be a reduction of public and private programs in an attempt to control health care costs and utilization. In the final scenario, there will be a robust economic growth of five percent per year. There would be a stable public policy and health benefits would be generous. Supply and demand would be in balance, and public health issues would be the dominant concerns of Congress. In each scenario, the council concluded that organized medicine would continue to be necessary.

A key conclusion of the Council on Long Range Planning and Development was that the profession must "maintain a strong sense of medical ethics and professionalism in physicians and medical students." One challenge of organized medicine is to provide an adequate forum for dialogue, to allow disagreement, and to work out differences among us. It is easy to project that the self-interests of physicians will become increasingly divergent and divisive: individual physicians versus corporate groups; fee-for-service versus pre-payment plans; specialists versus generalists; hospital- based physicians versus office-based physicians; you-name-it. Organized medicine represents the only valid umbrella for the entire profession. Only by convincing the public of our good intent — our professionalism — can we insure that *their* Golden Age will be, at least to some extent, also ours.

References

1. Burnham JC. American medicine's golden age: What happened to it? *Science* 1982; 215: 1474-1479.
2. Lundberg GD. In developed countries, the golden age of medicine is at hand — for the patients (editorial). *JAMA* 1987; 258: 2415-2416.
3. King LS. Medical practice: Making a living. *JAMA* 1984: 251: 1887-1892.
4. Council on Long Council on Long Range Planning and Development: The future of medicine. A scenario analysis. *JAMA* 1987; 255: 80-85.

William Osler and Medical Societies

J SC Med Assoc 1992; 8: 447-449

Yes, join both the city and county society, and never miss a meeting. Keep your mouth shut too, for a few years, particularly in discussions.

— William Osler

We celebrate this year the centenary of William Osler's *The Principles and Practices of Medicine.*[1] The best-known physician of his generation, Osler continues to inspire: indeed, one author recently suggested: "To the extent that we live up to the Osler hero-myth, our profession will prosper."[2] What was so special about William Osler? What was the fuss about? Of what we now call "the Oslerian tradition," what is truth and what is myth?

Although these questions deserve intricate answers, I'm not sure that they really matter — at least for our daily lives. What matters is not the real William Osler — a complicated human being who, like the rest of us, had his foibles and his problems — but rather the ideal. The medical profession — then and now — needed an idealized William Osler for the same reason that it earlier needed an idealized Hippocrates.[3] Both men stood — and stand — as symbols that medicine is more than a way to make a living. Both men came to symbolize the union of scientific competence and humanistic compassion. Both men cared deeply about medicine as a profession.

Since time immemorial, there have been laypersons who've questioned whether most doctors put the public interest above their own. In truth, an accurate definition of "professionalism" in medicine or for that matter in any other occupation can be as elusive as the snark. However, at least one definition of "profession" seems beyond dispute: "the body of persons in a particular calling or occupation." It follows that standing for professionalism is a corporate responsibility. Each generation — in Hippocrates' time, in Osler's time, in our time — must take its stand for professionalism. Professional organizations constitute the logical starting place.

William Osler was a skilled clinician, a popular teacher, a charming personality, a prolific writer. He excelled in nearly everything he undertook. Yet he said that he had no really exceptional talents and there were those who took him at his word, who attributed his enormous success not to unusual ability but rather to hard work, organization, and a clear sense of priority. In view of Osler's extreme goal-directedness, it may come as something of a surprise that Osler was quite active in medical societies. Why would anyone who placed such a high premium on tangible accomplishment bother to attend the countless meetings, meetings, and meetings that are the stuff of organized medicine? There is a story that once Osler was about to leave for a medical meeting when he turned to a younger colleague and said: "I'm going to the medical society—aren't you coming?" The colleague replied that he was not going because he considered the medical society meetings a waste of his time. Osler replied: "Do you think I don't?" He slammed the door and left for the meeting. In 1889, Osler, recently arrived in Baltimore, was invited to give the annual address to the Medical and Chirurgical Faculty of Maryland. He could easily have given a straightforward scientific paper, but chose instead to enter the fray of medical politics. His topic was a hot potato: whether to regulate medicine through licensure.[4] Osler urged:

> We cannot ... escape from the important fact that in the eyes of the law we all stand equal, and if we wish legislation for the protection of the public, we have got to ask for it together, not singly. I know that this is gall and wormwood to man—at the bitterness of it the gorge rises, but it is a question which has to be met fairly and squarely.

The public interest came first, and the medical society was the appropriate forum to take a stand. In 1903, Osler lectured "On the Educational Value of the Medical Society." He argued that a first function of medical societies is promotion of unity and friendship:

> The first, and in some respects the most important

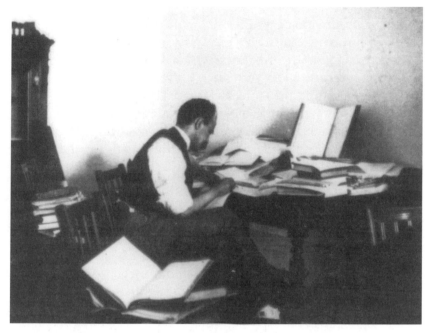

William Osler writing The Principles and Practice of Medicine

function is ... to lay a foundation for that unity and friendship which is essential to the dignity and usefulness of the profession. Unity and friendship! How we all long for them, but how difficult to attain! Strife seems rather to be the very life of the practitioner, whose warfare is incessant against disease and against ignorance and prejudice, and, sad to have to admit, he too often lets his angry passions rise against his professional brother.

A second function was to provide what we would now call continuing medical education:

The well-conducted medical society should represent a clearing house, in which every physician of the district would receive his intellectual rating.... We doctors do not "take stock" often enough, and are very apt to carry on our shelves stale, out-of-date goods. The society helps to keep a man "up to the times," and enables him to refurnish his mental shop with the latest wares.

Finally, Osler urged physicians to participate in all three layers of organized medicine:

> It is not in the local society only that a man can get encouragement in his day's work and a betterment of mind and methods. Every practitioner should feel a pride in belonging to his state society, and should attend the meetings whenever possible, and gradually learn to know his colleagues, and here let me direct your attention to an important movement on the part of the American Medical Association, which has for its object the organization of the profession throughout the entire country.

He recognized that medical societies are the best way to keep up with both the scientific content and also the socioeconomic fabric of medicine.

In 1905, Osler left the United States to become Regius Professor of Medicine at Oxford. His farewell address to the medical profession of the United States, entitled "Unity, Peace and Concord,"[6] provided another strong endorsement of organized medicine. Osler was quite optimistic about medicine's future:

> Linked together by the strong bonds of community of interests, the profession of medicine forms a remarkable world-wide unit in the progressive evolution of which there is a fuller hope for humanity than in any other direction.

However, he again acknowledged that physicians were prone to petty, destructive quarrels. For these, he again saw organized medicine as the best remedy:

> The national and specialty societies, and particularly the American Medical Association, have brought men together and have taught them to know each other and to appreciate the good points which at home may have been overlooked. (Yet) it is in the smaller towns and country districts that the conditions are most favourable for mutual misunderstandings. Only those of us who have been brought up in such surroundings can appreciate how hard it is for physicians to keep on good terms with each other.

In his parting words, Osler spoke of his deep "conviction of the blessings that come from unity, peace, and concord." He emphasized the *community* of medicine.

The fierce public disputes among physicians which characterized medicine at the turn of the twentieth century have, fortunately, become uncommon. However, we can anticipate that if times get tighter and corporate structures become more evident, such acrid rivalries will re-surface. To the old truism that nothing remains constant except change, we might add the truism that adherence to principle is always the best anchor. Osler saw principle in organized medicine. His enthusiasm for medical societies would seem to be an essential part of the legacy we still salute as "the Oslerian tradition."

References

1. Golden RL. Osler's legacy: The centennial of *The Principles and Practice of Medicine. Ann Intern Med* 1992; 116: 255-260.
2. Wheeler HB. Shattuck lecture—healing and heroism. *N Engl J Med* 1990; 322: 1540-1548, 1990.
3. Lloyd GER. The transformations of ancient medicine. *Bull Hist Med 1992; 66: 114-132.*
4. Osler W. License to Practice. *Maryland Med J* 1989; 21: 61-67.
Osler W: On the educational value of the medical society. *Boston Med & Surg J* 1903; 148: 275-279.
5. Osler W. Unity, peace, and concord. *JAMA* 1905; 45: 705-710.

Editorial Note: The above editorial was written as I was embarking on a serious study of William Osler that culminated with *Osler: Inspirations from a Great Physician* (Oxford University Press, 1997), which I still consider my best book. In 1993 Dr. Carwile Leroy introduced me to the American Osler Society, which has led to wonderful friendships and experiences I could scarcely have imagined.

Of Ideals and Heroes

J SC Med Assoc 1994; 90: 193-194

> *The chief ideal of the American people is idealism.*
> — Calvin Coolidge
> *The chief business of the American people is business.*
> — Calvin Coolidge

Capitation. Economic credentialing. Managed competition. Vertical integration. HMOs, HPOs, PPOs. These are but some of the buzzwords that comprise today's lexicon of medicine. Whoops — it's not "medicine" anymore... it's "healthcare" (one word, mind you). Physicians? Well, we're somewhere in the ranks of "healthcare providers." The medical profession? Our annual meeting reminds us to take its definition seriously.

That the structure of American medical practice, the business arrangements through which we earn our livings, will change rapidly is beyond dispute. But the structure of American medical practice has changed before and physicians have emerged all the better for the changes.[1] What seems less clear is the continued survival of the medical profession as we have known it. Yet paradoxically, we have more control over the latter than the former. We cannot stipulate exactly how physicians will function within the fabric of society. But we can indeed stipulate who we are, what we stand for, and how we relate to one another.

In recent months, I've had the chance to discuss this issue — the identity of the medical profession — with colleagues in various forums. One refrain is that we need to promote the idea of a "brotherhood of physicians" or, to be gender-sensitive, a "kinship of physicians." It's a worthy aim and one best achieved within organized medicine. However, any meaningful kinship among physicians is likely to be strained by rising tensions between generalists and specialists.

In 1817 the South Carolina State Legislature accepted as qualified to practice medicine any graduate of a chartered medical school. This established a precedent that became the norm in the United States. Both the medical profession and organized medicine developed in and around the context of general practice. This was in sharp contrast to what happened in Northern Europe, where the medical profession was historically divided and given to pecking orders. However, this century's accelerated development of specialism, subspecialism, and even sub-subspecialism has strained such unity as once existed in American medicine. Thus by 1971, a critical historian could say that "the physician has rapidly become not a core of medical care but only a cog in a complex system" and that the "fractional role for physicians is emphasized in the physicians' own proclivity to uncoordinated specialization."[2] Today, there is a mandate to reverse this trend. And yet ...

And yet it is unclear how changing the generalist: specialist ratio will affect the identity of the medical profession and our relationships to one another. A worst case scenario holds that the role of generalist physicians will be largely subsumed by nurse practitioners while that of specialist physicians will be largely subsumed by technicians. Medicine as we have known it would dissolve and the notion of a "kinship of physicians" would be untenable. The best case scenario, on the other hand, is that the medical profession will remain intact and that we will find new ways to support each other from positions of mutual respect.

The purpose of this editorial is to support the ideal of a kinship of physicians and to encourage the coming generation to find the heroes necessary to defend it. Admittedly, the very notions of idealism and heroism are suspect. H. L. Mencken called idealism the "chief curse of the world," arguing that people "get into trouble by taking their visions and hallucinations too seriously." Mencken similarly declared that the "setting up of heroes is mainly bogus." However, I do not hear such cynicism from medical students and younger physicians. They are as idealistic as their predecessors—perhaps even more so. Our task is to spur them on toward a bright future for medicine in the twenty-first century.

In the history of medicine it is possible to identify epochs with heroes who symbolized the best of what we are about. One thinks of Hippocrates and Galen, of Paracelsus and Paré,

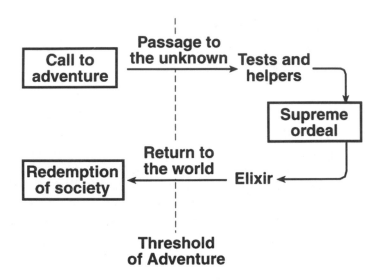

The prototypical hero, called to adventure, must face a supreme ordeal in order to bring back to society a restorative elixir (after Campbell[3]).

of Harvey and Sydenham, of Hunter and Jenner, and, more recently, of William Osler. A century ago, Osler reassured the public that the new scientific medicine retained its humanitarian roots. Simultaneously, he worked hard to promote unity and harmony throughout the profession of Medicine. It is reassuring to note that Osler, like us, experienced pangs of ambivalence on the issue of generalism versus specialism. It is also reassuring to note that his life exemplifies the stereotypical "hero adventure" open to all of us.

The late Joseph Campbell described the great hero adventures of song and story as variations upon a common theme which he called the "monomyth" (Figure).[3] An ordinary person living in his hut (e.g., Bilbo Baggins in *The Hobbit*) or castle (e.g., the prince or princess in most fairy tales) is called to adventure by a mysterious figure who stays with him as a shadow presence. Crossing the threshold of adventure into the dark realm of the unknown, the hero finds one or more helpers and faces a series of tests prior to a supreme ordeal (e.g., the dragon). If he survives the ordeal he obtains a restorative elixir and takes it back to his former world, making it right again. Campbell argued that this pathway is open to everyone. To succeed, we must take risks, find helpers, face our dragons, and bring back our elixirs.

Is the same not also true of professions? We are indeed called to adventure, to leave what seemed until recently to be our safe castle. Our shadow presence is our heritage, our pride and conviction that the medical profession stands for much more than a way to make a living. Yet we must heed the voices of those in other disciplines for they are our potential helpers. At some future date, perhaps in some post-Clinton administration, we may yet face something kin to a supreme ordeal – a test of survival. The elixir that we should bring back to society is the notion of a united medical profession dedicated to the delivery of compassionate yet thoroughly scientific medicine. But, as we are reminded each year at the annual meeting, we must embark on our journey united by a sense of common purpose. None of us can afford to stand apart. We must all participate.

References

1. Rosen G. *The Structure of American Medical Practice,* 1875-1941, edited by CE Rosenberg. Philadelphia: University of Pennsylvania Press, 1983.
2. Stevens R. *American Medicine and the Public Interest.* New Haven, Connecticut: Yale University Press; 1971: 421.
3. Campbell J. *The Hero with a Thousand Faces.* Second edition, Princeton, New Jersey: Princeton University Press; 1968.

What is Professionalism and Can it be Measured?

J SC Med Assoc 1995; 91: 243-244

Medical practice in the twenty-first century will differ dramatically from what we've known. The role of technology will be extremely high but the technology will focus increasingly on prevention of disease and maintenance of organ function rather than crisis intervention. The focus of technology will shift from hospitals to diffuse networks. Most physicians will practice in large organizations and will be reimbursed by capitation, salary, or some combination thereof. Success will be measured, at least in part, by cost-effectiveness. And through all of this the physician-patient relationship will change. One thoughtful reviewer suggests that in 1935 the physician-patient relationship was one-to-one; that in recent years it has been ambiguous; and that in 2005 it will be one-to-n (a concept that suggests that our responsibility is not just to the individual patient, but to all of society).[1] What do these dramatic changes portend for physicians as *professionals*? What do they mean for the medical *profession*?

"Profession" comes from *profiteri*, which in turn comes from *pro* plus *fassfateri*, which means to confess or own to. The original usage of "to profess" in English was to take the vows of a religious order. Thus, the meaning was "to declare openly." To claim to be a professional, then, is "to declare openly" certain attitudes, beliefs, or competencies. But what is a profession and what is not a profession? By one listing, no fewer than 170 occupations purport to be "professions." One authority describes "the professional project" as "the effort of an occupational group to organize itself to maintain a monopoly over a service and control of the market so as to develop a demand for the service in the form it provides," the aim of which is "collective conquest of status."[2] There is general agreement, however, that to be truly "professional" there must be a dedication to the public interest that far transcends socioeconomic gain. A "profession" must meet three criteria: (1) specialized training gained through formal education and apprenticeship, (2) public recognition of the ability to set and regulate practice standards; and (3) commitment to the public good beyond "the economic welfare of the practitioners."[3]

Is it possible to be more specific? What prompted this editorial was the publication by the American Board of Internal Medicine of *Project Professionalism*, an attempt to define and promote professionalism in the training of young physicians.[4] The elements of professionalism were put forth as follows:

• *Altruism*, whereby the ruling principle is the patient's interest, not self-interest;

• *Accountability* not only to patients but also to society and to the profession;

• *Excellence* that includes commitments to exceeding expectations and to life-long learning;

• *Duty* whereby one acknowledges one's availability and responsiveness when "on call";

• *Honor and integrity* whereby one refuses to violate personal and professional codes; and

• *Respect* for others.

What impressed me most about the document was the clear description of certain signs and symptoms that professionalism has been betrayed. These include:

• *Abuse of power*, which can be manifested by betrayal of the trust of patients and colleagues; by bias; by sexual harassment; and by breach of confidentiality;

• *Arrogance*, denoting a haughty self-importance;

• *Greed*, defined as the inappropriate aspiration for money, power, or fame, leaving little room "for understanding, compassion or other qualities necessary for the healing profession";

• *Misrepresentation*, the conscious act of lying or fraud;

• *Impairment* without recognition or acknowledgement;

• *Lack of conscientiousness*, often consisting of doing just enough to get by," such as waiting for the radiology report rather than going to see the x-rays personally; and

• *Conflicts of interest*, whether by self-referral, acceptance of gifts, inappropriate utilization of services, inappropriate collaboration with industry; or compromising the principles of clinical investigation.

This document concludes with specific recommendations for recognizing professionalism and lack thereof, supported by twenty vignettes of real-life examples.

As a third-year medical student, I was told that there were really only three questions of clinical relevance: (1) What is wrong with the patient? (2) What can I do for the patient? (3) What will be the outcome? Thirty years later, I conclude that this list must be expanded to include: (4) What will it cost? and (5) What, specifically, must I do to behave in the best traditions of our profession? The overriding imperative of professionalism is to serve our fellow humans ably and altruistically. In recognizing that we often fall short, we are hardly alone. As one authority puts it: "The professions bitterly disappoint us for failing imperfections of human nature and human institutions. The professional spirit is a ray of hope in the lowering gloom."[2, p. 372] What is professionalism? How can we measure it? How can we foster it? That our medical organizations, at all levels, are paying increasing attention to these vital issues should be a source of comfort, a reason to rejoice, and an impetus for collective self-renewal. What is best for society is, after all, also best for us.

References

1. Greenlick MR. Educating physicians for the for the twenty-first century. *Acad Med* 1995; 70: 179-185.
2. Kultgen J. *Ethics and Professionalism.* Philadelphia: University of Pennsylvania Press; 1988: 100.
3. Sullivan WM. *Work and Integrity: The Crisis and Promise of Professionalism in American.* New York: HarperBusiness; 1995: 2.
4. Stobo JD, Cohen JC, Kimball, HR, et al.. *Project Professionalism.* Philadelphia: American Board of Internal Medicine; 1995.

Sacred Trust

J SC Med Assoc 1998; 94: 190-191

Officers and guests of the South Carolina Medical Association celebrated its sesquicentennial at a banquet on February 14, 1998, which happened to be Valentine's Day. It was fitting that the presiding officer was Dr. S. Nelson Weston, our only third-generation president. Nelson confided:

> I would not have been fulfilled had I not become involved in organized medicine.... I only wish that every doctor in the state could have had my experience, and then they would know what a great organization the SCMA is and will always be.

The path of least resistance leads to indifference and cynicism. To get involved requires energy but reinforces our ideals.

And what are our ideals? They are embraced by that elusive term, "professionalism." When the SCMA was founded 150 years ago, the state of professionalism in medicine was as shaky as that of mid-nineteenth-century medical science. Medical science now prospers as never before, but our future as professionals is uncertain. We worry that we're losing control. We worry whether the medical profession as we've known it will be around a hundred years from now.

Definitions of "profession" generally stipulate a common body of knowledge and a degree of altruism, putting others' interests above one's own. A stricter definition stipulates the so-called "learned" professions: law, medicine, and the ministry. This triumvirate is considered "learned" by dint of having been the subject matter taught in medieval universities. It's always seemed to me that law, medicine, and the ministry command public respect and even awe because their practitioners make difficult judgment decisions in areas of uncertainty. Therein lies the rub.

We will always need lawyers because the outcome of our conflicts with fellow humans will always be uncertain. We will always need ministers because the outcomes of our individual existential dilemmas will always be uncertain. But year by year the relentless advance of medical science makes the outcomes of matters related to health a less dicey proposition. Today's patient wants good technology. Cost aside, that's not all bad. Our task is to make sure that "technician" does not become our only identity.

I recently perused a book entitled *Do We Still Need Doctors?* by Dr. John Lantos, a pediatrician and bioethicist. His points include the following:

• Bioethicists debate whether medicine is mainly a moral enterprise or a technical/scientific enterprise. Many bioethicists conclude that medicine is a technical enterprise rather than a moral one. This view would lead to a "hostile moral takeover."

• Technology is highly seductive. Physicians preoccupied with technical interventions risk losing the historic role of the physician as an interpreter of illness and suffering. Lantos concludes that when disease cannot be cured nor suffering relieved, "doctors are no longer sure what to do or whether they will still have a role to play."

• Society reinforces our love affair with technology. Various social, political, and even moral forces "have institutionalized the doctor's role as one that embodies the values of empiricism, quantification, and objectivity."

• Policy-makers, economists, health-services researchers, and even basic scientists drive us toward the conclusion that medicine is most efficient "if patients are treated as virtually interchangeable and physicians' behavior is confined within strict algorithms."

• In this scenario, physicians who behave as individualists and who cling to the traditional role of wise counselor/teacher in matters of uncertainty risk being marginalized. Successful physicians (at least, "successful" in the usual sense) will increasingly specialize and subspecialize.

Lantos concludes that there will still be a role for the "older type of doctor" especially for patients whose problems don't fit neatly into clinical algorithms. But such physicians may not be rewarded commensurate with their efforts.

What can be done? At least two things.

First, we ran rededicate ourselves as individuals to our main concern: our patients. We can begin each morning by recalling what we told the Admissions Committee, which was basically that "I like science and I want to help people." We can resolve to focus more intensely on our patient, his narratives, his stories of joy and sorrow. We can cultivate self-awareness of our natural tendency to allow compassion to be crowded out by the pursuit of technical competence, even though competence at what we profess to be good at should be our top priority.

Second, we can rededicate ourselves collectively to the ideal of medicine as a profession in the best sense. We can resist the forces that insist that patients' problems should be stuffed into pigeonholes and processed algorithmically through "product lines." We can remind ourselves of what our founding members knew only too well 150 years ago: The boundaries of medical practice must be staked out and defended. And we can remember what Dr. Nelson Weston had to say at our sesquicentennial banquet: The SCMA is a great organization, and getting involved can be an enormously fulfilling experience.

A highlight of each Annual Meeting is the non-denominational worship service on Sunday morning. These services remind us that medicine is indeed a high calling, a sacred trust. Along that line, I strongly recommend a just-published book by Dr. Clif Cleaveland (a colleague with South Carolina roots) entitled *Sacred Space*. Cleaveland makes it clear that despite technology medicine is a deeply personal matter. He concludes that the "sacred space" is the point at which two journeys—ours and the patient's—coincide. The extent to which we defend that space against the forces that encroach upon it will determine, at least in part, the survival of the medical profession as we have been privileged to know it.

References

1. Lantos JD. *Do we Still Need doctors?* New York & London: Routledge; 1997.
2. Cleaveland C. *Sacred Space: Stories from a Life in Medicine.* Philadelphia: American College of Physicians; 1998.

A Very Short History of the Medical Profession, as Told to Patch Adams

J SC Med Assoc 1999; 95: 118-170

Patch Adams is a must-see. As Patch, a maverick medical student on a mission to humanize a teaching hospital over the objections of a stuffy dean, Robin Williams shows why he is arguably the most endearing American actor since the late Jimmy Stewart. But the movie raises some serious questions. What has gone wrong with medicine and the medical profession? Why do audiences usually applaud at the ending?

Convinced of the healing power of humor by a stay in a psychiatric hospital, Patch enters medical school. No sooner is he there than he sneaks onto the wards, puts an enema bulb on his nose, and develops a first-class clown act for the patients and staff. Things take a serious turn when a group of laypersons air their gripes about medicine at a lunch counter. Why do we have to fill out paperwork during an emergency? Why a $250 bill for a sprained ankle, a $1000 bill for antibiotics? Why can't the government provide health insurance for everybody? Patch dreams up a system where doctors and patients will be co-equal partners in a free clinic based on laughter and love. He builds it and they come.

Things go well until Larry enters. Larry is a troubled young man with a history of multiple emergency room visits for self-mutilation. Patch's girlfriend, Corinne Fisher, finds Larry's far-away took disturbing. Patch seems unconcerned: "If we can't show him compassion who can?" One evening while Patch is away pilfering supplies from the teaching hospital, Larry calls for help, for "someone to talk to." Corinne walks into a murder-suicide. Persuaded by his friends not to drop out of medical school in his despondency, Patch graduates to pursue his dream.

Corinne's death, I submit, shows how compassion untempered by competence does everyone a disservice. But the larger point of *Patch Adams* is his confrontation with the medical profession, of "the way things have always been done" as represented by the supercilious Dean Walcott. This prompted me to ask how Patch Adams (by whom I mean Williams's character, not the real-life physician on whom the script was based and to whom no offense is intended) might have responded to different epochs in our collective history.

Let us briefly review the history of medicine from the perspective of what historians and sociologists call "the professional project" — the efforts of those who practice an occupation to define their cognitive, ethical, and institutional frameworks in such a way as to establish a large measure of authority and exclusivity (Table, pages 97-98).

Patch would probably have thrived in classical Greece. Our fuzzy notion that a proud, monolithic medical profession arose there from the mists of antiquity turns out to be an illusion. To be sure the Hippocratic writers would have agreed with Dean Walcott that Patch showed "excessive happiness;" they asserted "the man of uncontrolled laughter and excessive cheerfulness is considered vulgar."[1] But medicine in Greece was hardly synonymous with Hippocrates and his followers. There was in fact no established medical profession. A wide variety of healers of different sects, often peripatetic, competed for those who could afford their services. Patch would have been right at home.

Patch would likewise have enjoyed the Middle Ages, though he would have encountered some of the same problems that bedeviled him at the fictional "Virginia Medical School." Physicians trained in the medieval universities began to organize themselves into guilds. The guilds, subordinate to the universities in principle if not always in practice, developed statutes dealing with apprenticeships, examinations, and licensing designed to enforce the profession's claims to exclusive control over the scope of practice. Patch could have chosen to join either a guild or the swelling ranks of those (including women except for midwives) who practiced extralegally.

During the Enlightenment, Patch might have preferred to live in Scotland. It was there that a young physician named John Gregory, influenced by the philosopher David Hume, reintroduced compassion to medical practice and in so doing may have invented the medical profession as we know it today.[2] Patch might also have sought out the Scottish political philospher Adam Smith (famous for *The Wealth of Nations*), who responded to a growing market in M.D. degrees by questioning the very principle of privilege based on this or that higher degree. We can picture Patch marching down Princess Street in Edinburgh, a merry activist.

Patch would have rejoiced during the early years of the French Revolution during which the guilds, universities, and scientific academies of the Old Regime were abolished. *Laissez-faire*, an extreme form of deregulation, flourished for a decade. Just about anybody could buy a permit to practice medicine. Then came the 1794 National Convention that gave the organized medical profession an effective monopoly over medicine in the cities. Patch might have slipped out of Paris for the countryside to practice among the less-sophisticated.

During the early decades of the nineteenth century, Patch would probably have joined the ranks of irregular practitioners who resisted "heroic therapy" based on bleeding, blistering, and purging. These included the homeopaths with their low doses and the Thomsonians with their herbs. Patch's later difficulties might have begun in 1888 when the Supreme Court of the United States defended the rights of states to require a license to practice medicine. Following the Flexner Report Patch would have found it necessary to embrace rigorous scientific medicine to remain within the law as allopathic practice gained power and prestige. He would have lamented the increasing domination of medicine by specialists. He would have been concerned about rising costs, and would sense the inevitability of regulation of medical practice by government and business.[3]

But I believe that, if given the chance to live during any era and in any place, Patch would choose the here and now: 1999 in the United States.

The movie's redeeming moment comes when Patch and Dean Walcott square off before the Board of Medical Examiners with Patch's career at stake. Friends and patients line the balconies and foyer. The Board concludes that while Patch's

Some Landmarks in the History of the Medical Profession

Classical Greece	1. Schools of medicine are organized, generally around a founding persona. 2. There is considerable professional fragmentation around various sects.
The Middle Ages (sixth through fifteenth centuries)	1. Medicine, law, and theology become institutionalized within universities. 2. Practitioners organize themselves into guilds; statutes deal with apprenticeships, examinations, and licensing.
Renaissance and early modern periods (sixteenth and seventeenth centuries)	1. Boards of physicians (protomedicato) are named by the crown and given power to examine, license, and police (Sicily, Italy, Spain). 2. Colleges of physicians separate from medical school faculties are founded; guilds are vested with licensing authority (England).
The Enlightenment (eighteenth century)	1. State patronage gives status and autonomy to various guilds and healers; divisions of labor increase. 2. Later, the power and autonomy of guilds are undermined from opposite directions by central government and free enterprise.
The French Revolution (1789-1799)	1. Guilds, universities, and academies are abolished, allowing *laissez-faire* medicine to flourish for about ten years. 2. A central "School of Health" is formed in Paris and a strict, uniform licensing system is put in place.
The nineteenth century in Britain	1. The Apothecaries Act (1815) sets standards for professional education. 2. By the 1880s, higher standards are established through a system of examinations by the royal colleges, along with certification for general practitioners.

International trends during the nineteenth century	1. National medical societies are founded in most Western nations with the notable exception of Germany; these include Britain (1832), the United States (1847), and Canada (1867). 2. Most Western nations evolve toward a two-tiered medical profession with an elite and a broad spectrum of lesser practitioners.
Rise of medicine in the United States during the nineteenth century	1. States create licensing boards; the rights of states to require a license to practice medicine is defended by the Supreme Court (1888). 2. Scientific advances and aseptic surgery confer new legitimacy to medical practice.
Course of the medical profession in the United States during the twentieth century	1. The location of medical practice shifts to physicians' offices and hospitals. 2. Specialists begin to dominate practice based on experimental science. 3. Third party payers come between the physician-patient relationship. 4. Medicare and Medicaid legislation (1960s) reduces the charitable component of medicine but places medicine increasingly under government scrutiny and control. 5. Medicine becomes increasingly expensive and therefore burdensome to society and to business. 6. Physician autonomy decreases; patient autonomy increases; the bioethics movement with its emphasis on patient autonomy echoes other "rights movements" within society.

refusal to conform may not be entirely admirable, his passion for healing, his "pure flame," should not be extinguished. As for the dean — well, he should loosen up and learn to laugh. Thus, the medical profession embraces Patch despite its reservations. Patch's future patients will be much better off for his decision to stay in school, to become an orthodox physician (at least in his own way) as opposed to veering off toward one or another brand of alternative medicine.

Dr. Jordan J. Cohen, president of the Association of American

Medical Colleges, recently wrote, "The key to valuing the profession is to profess its values."[4] Each generation has the chance to reinterpret these values within the context of its own times. Each generation of physicians should enter dialogue with its public. Organized medicine, like all human institutions, may have its flaws yet remains the optimum forum for such dialogue. The board's verdict on Patch is a wonderful affirmation of organized medicine's willingness to listen, to learn, to love, and to risk change. But please—no enema bulbs.

References

1. Longrigg J. *Greek Medicine: From the Heroic to the Hellenistic Age.* New York: Routledge; 1998: 103.
2. McCullough LB. *John Gregory and the Invention of Professional Medical Ethics and the Profession of Medicine.* Dordrecht, The Netherlands: Kluwer, 1998.
3. Starr P. *The Social Transformation of American Medicine.* New York Basic Books, 1982.
4. Cohen JJ. Leadership for medicine's promising future. *Acad Med* 1998; 73: 132-137.

What is a Doctor? Reflections on the Physician Charter on Professionalism

J SC Med Assoc 2002; 98: 327-329

The future of medicine as a service to humankind is bright indeed. The future of the medical profession is unclear. To what extent will physicians retain their autonomy, self-regulation, status, privileges, and prestige? Others with less training and little or no knowledge of molecular biology can do most if not all of the things doctors do, usually at lower cost. Will health care delivery soon consist mainly of mid-level practitioners referring to technicians? The perceived threats to the medical profession are, of course, part and parcel of pervasive challenges to authority and status throughout Western culture. Yet the case of the medical profession in the United States may be an extreme case. Seldom, if ever, has a profession risen so fast and fallen so precipitously in the public eye as has American medicine during the twentieth century.[1,2]

These overarching concerns no doubt explain, in part, the surging interest in medical professionalism that began sometime during the early- to mid-1990s. Tangible evidence of this interest includes numerous journal articles, conference proceedings, task forces, and curricular revisions. Government and business forces increasingly favor what amounts to a hostile takeover of traditional professional values by capitalistic values. Government favors increasing regulation of medical practice, submitting physicians to extensive paperwork and strict penalties for perceived non-compliance. Business favors standardization of medical practice and treatment of physicians as salaried workers.[3] Although many patients still value their special relationships with primary care physicians, others seek out the latest sub-subspecialists with the newest technologies and, when still unsatisfied, alternative care providers whose methods contain little if any scientific rationale. In short, the surging interest in medical professionalism echoes a wider concern about the future of medicine as a profession — a calling, not a business.

Against this background, three prestigious medical organizations recently issued a Physician Charter on Professionalism, published in the *Annals of Internal Medicine* and elsewhere.[4] The charter puts forth three fundamental principles:
• Primacy of patient welfare
• Patient autonomy
• Social justice
These principles are followed by 10 specific commitments:
• Professional competence
• Honesty with patients
• Patient confidentiality
• Maintaining appropriate relationships
• Improving the quality of care
• Improving access to care
• Just distribution of finite resources
• Scientific knowledge
• Managing conflicts of interest
• Professional responsibilities
So far, so good. Is anything missing?

The Charter, as I understand it, was intended to be an important first step. Physicians throughout the world were invited to react to it and are now doing so. My concerns are basically three, as follows.

First, and as emphasized by Stephen H. Miles, the Charter pays relatively little attention to physicians' broader social roles and responsibilities. Miles asks, "Whose profession is it anyway?"[5] Like everyone else, we as physicians agree that the essence of medical professionalism consists of subordination of the physician's self-interest to the interests of patients and society.[6] But do our actions usually reflect this desideratum? Libertarian philosophers question the usefulness of altruism in human behavior.[7] Sociologists question the ulterior motives of would-be "professionals," describing "the professional project" as the collective efforts of any occupational group to gain power and status.[8,9] Miles and also the historian Rosemary A. Stevens[10] stress that physicians can retain and enhance their professionalism by assuming larger roles in the health of disadvantaged persons, especially in the developing world. To do so, we must act collectively.

Second, the Charter pays relatively little attention to caring and compassion as generally understood. Reflecting the current penchant for rights- or duty-based ethics as opposed to virtue- or character-based ethics, the charter places great emphasis on patient autonomy. The emphasis on patient autonomy reflects the fallout from the bioethics movement that began during the 1970s. The generally accepted principles of the new biomedical ethics include "beneficence" and "autonomy" but do not specifically include caring and compassion.[11] Caring is perhaps best understood by a hierarchy of terms, in ascending order of difficulty as follows:

• *Beneficence* (from the Latin, "well-doing"), defined as doing good or active kindness.
• *Empathy* (from the Greek, "in-feeling"), defined as the ability to comprehend another's feelings and emotions.
• *Sympathy* (from the Greek, "fellow-feeling"), defined as being affected by the misfortunes of another.
• *Compassion* (from the Latin, "suffer with"), defined as participation in another's feelings of misfortunes to the extent that one becomes a fellow sufferer.[12]

Effective technologies reduce the need for compassion in the strict sense of "suffering with" in daily medical practice. We are called to compassion mainly when relevant technology is unavailable, unaffordable, or unsuccessful. The term "compassion" is often used cheaply, but I suggest that we can define it in specific operational terms: for example, giving care without reimbursement, giving care when one would rather be doing something else, and giving care that involves emotional or physical risks to ourselves.[13] Demonstrating compassion in these ways makes the strongest case for professionalism — service above self.

Finally, the Charter pays little if any attention to the relationships of physicians with one another. Competition among professionals — in medicine as in athletics — should be based on excellence and good sportsmanship with adherence to clearly articulated rules and guidelines. Competition among professionals should not thrive on the motive of self-aggrandizement, or driving others out of the local market. Early codes of medical ethics such as those articulated by Thomas

Percival in 1803 and by the American Medical Association in 1847 are sometimes criticized on the grounds that they deal mainly with "etiquette" — yet are not etiquette and civility not indispensable to any claims of professionalism? Recalling that the AMA's Code of Ethics broke new ground,[14] we must continue to underscore mutual support and collegiality despite others' efforts to drive wedges between us and our colleagues.

The Physician Charter on Professionalism is an excellent first start and its authors are to be congratulated. Yet much remains to be done. Elsewhere,[13] I have argued that medical professionalism defies a "one size fits all" definition. Rather, medical professionalism involves a spectrum of behaviors defined by the incredibly wide range of tasks and behaviors that comprise medical practice. But the take-home point is that however we define, practice, and promote it, professionalism matters. The future of medicine as a profession, as opposed to a mere commodity, hinges to a large extent on our collective response.

References

1. Lantos JD. *Do We Still Need Doctors?* New York: Routledge; 1997.
2. Krause EA. *Death of the Guilds: Professions, States, and the Advance of Capitalism, 1930 to the Present.* New Haven: Yale University Press; 1996: 29-78.
3. Hoff T. The physician as worker: What it means and why now? *Health Care Management Review* 2001; 24(4): 52-87.
4. Project of the ABIM Foundation, ACP-ASIM Foundation, and European Federation of Internal Medicine. Medical Professionalism in the new millennium: A physician charter. *Ann Intern Med* 2002; 136: 243-246.
5. Miles SH. On a new charter to defend medical professionalism: Whose profession is it anyway? *Hastings Center Report* 2002; 32(3): 46-48.
6. Reynolds RP. Reaffirming professionalism through the education community. *Ann Intern Med* 1994; 120: 609-614.
7. Rand A. The objectivist ethics. In Rand A. *The Virtue of Selfishness.* New York: Signet; 1964: 13-39.
8. Larson MS. *The Rise of Professionalism.* Berkeley: University of California Press; 1977: 8, 66, 105.
9. Kultgen J. *Ethics and Professionalism.* Philadelphia: University of Pennsylvania Press; 1988: 100.
10. Stevens RA. Public roles for the medical profession in the United

States: Beyond theories of decline and fall. *Milbank Quarterly* 2001; 79: 327-353.

11. Beauchamp TL, Childress JF. *Principles of Biomedical Ethics.* Fifth edition, New York: Oxford University Press; 2001.

12. Bryan CS. Care carefully. In Bryan CS. *Osler: Inspirations from a Great Physician.* New York: Oxford University Press; 1997: 133-160.

13. Bryan CS. HIV/AIDS, ethics, and professionalism: Where went the debate? *Trans Am Clin Climatol Assoc* 2003; 114: 353-367.

14. Baker RB, Caplan AL, Emanuel LL, Latham SR, eds. *The American Medical Ethics Revolution: How the AMA's Code of Ethics Has Transformed Physicians' Relationships to Patients, Professionals, and Society.* Baltimore: The Johns Hopkins University Press; 1999.

Editorial Note: In January 2002, after serving eight years as chair of the Department of Medicine at the University of South Carolina School of Medicine, I succeeded Dr. Donald E. Saunders, Jr., as director of the University's Center for Bioethics and Medical Humanities. Dean Larry R. Faulkner charged me with the task of developing a vertical curriculum in professionalism (that is, a curriculum that cut across all four years of medical school). "Professionalism" was then *au courant* in medical education circles and a special interest of the American Association of Medical Colleges. Medical professionalism — how to define it, how to teach it to students, how to promote it among faculty and practicing physicians — therefore became an area of focus, as reflected in the preceding editorial and in those that follow. I consider my major possible contributions to this field of interest to be (1) a distinction I've called "basic" or "generic" professionalism (in brief, doing the right thing well) and "higher" professionalism (in brief, service that clearly transcends self-interest); and (2) a renewed emphasis on the seven classic virtues of antiquity (as opposed to inventing virtues *du jour* as one goes along).

Advancing Medical Professionalism.
I. Our Public Image

J SC Med Assoc 2004; 100: 60-62

There are men and classes of men that stand above the common herd: the soldier, the sailor, and the shepherd not infrequently, the artist rarely, rarelier still, the clergyman; the physician almost as a rule. He is the flower (such as it is) of our civilization.... Generosity he has, such as is possible to those who practice an art (and) never to those who drive a trade; discretion, tested by a thousand embarrassments; and what are more important, Heraculean cheerfulness and courage.
— Robert Louis Stevenson

The medical profession is not different form any other: its members are, for the most part, ordinary empty-headed dolts, ready to see what is not there and to deny the obvious.
— Thomas Mann

Professionalism has become a major issue for physicians, medical educators, and medical organizations. Since the early 1990s, task forces have been created, conferences convened, medical school curricula revised, residency program accreditation requirements re-written, and articles published in most leading medical journals. Several organizations have sponsored a Physician Charter on Professionalism, which has been widely disseminated and well received.[1,2] Yet some external critics suggest that "medical professionalism" is now an oxymoron. Physicians' services, these critics imply, no longer require uncommon levels of formal education, technical know-how, judgment, compassion, and insights into the human condition. Medicine is merely another commodity, or "something useful that can be turned to commercial or other advantage."[3] What's going on, and what can be done about it?

The eminent social historian Rosemary Stevens maintains that it is time for the American medical profession to move beyond "theories of decline and fall."[4,5] It is time to cease lamenting that we have plummeted from positions of power, prestige, and

Some Forces Impacting Negatively on the Medical Profession, with Suggested Strategies*	
Force	**Suggested Strategies**
Intrusions by government and business interests on physician autonomy	Work with government and business to define health care policies that promote quality and access and contain costs
Ongoing efforts of alternative health care providers to expand their scopes of practice	Insist on evidence-based practice not only for alternative health care providers but also for physicians
Perceptions that some, pehaps many, physicians are unduly concerned with personal gain*	Re-commit, both individually and collectively, to the ideal of caring and competent service that transcends self-interest
Perceptions that physicians, as a group, are not especially concerned with the public welfare*	Publicize medicine's track record of constructive activities toward the public welfare, with renewed commitment to public service at all levels
Balkanization of organized medicine into dozens, perhaps hundreds, of special interest groups*	Support of local, state, and national umbrella organizations by all physicians, with promotion of dialogue and agendas toward positive change

*It is in these areas that interventions are most likely to succeed in the long run. Strictly speaking, the perceptions of others (that is, our reputations) are not within our power to control; the classic expression of this principle can be found in the first paragraph of the *Enchridion* by the Stoic philosopher Epictetus. The optimistic position taken here is that widespread and genuine efforts of physicians to address these issues will have a favorable impact on the public image of the medical profession.

personal influence. It is time to acknowledge that we are indeed co-dependent on business interests and government. It is time to form new strategic alliances and new visions of what constitutes the common good. We must assert our claims to professionalism by asserting our leadership toward helping re-shape America's health care delivery system. However, to be credible we must enhance our public image ("*image*: the character projected to the public ... especially as interpreted by the mass media"[3]), which is best done not by waging publicity campaigns but rather by enhancing our private reality ("*reality*: the quality or stage of being actual or true"[3]).

Stevens suggests that the theories of decline and fall may be just that: *theories*. A popular mythology holds that the power, prestige, and public image of the American medical profession peaked during the 1950s and 1960s and began to decline shortly after the passage of Medicare legislation. In 1970 the sociologist Eliot Freidson contended that American physicians functioned in a "splendid isolation." In 1975 the philosopher Ivan Illich called medicine a conspiracy against the public. In 1982 the sociologist Paul Starr traced the rise of a "sovereign profession" soon to be unraveled by MBAs and "the coming of the corporation." In 1996 yet another sociologist, Elliott Krause, argued that, while the professions have been under assault in all of the Western democracies, American medicine represents the most extreme case, indeed the "fall of a giant." According to Stevens, "All of the criticisms seem to come together in one powerful myth of rise and fall, where professionalism had been (on top), and where it was going (downhill). The message was resolutely downbeat. Doctors, once heroes, even kings, had fallen from the pedestal of public adulation." She goes on to say that this popular mythology of decline and fall needs serious reappraisal.

Stevens, like other commentators, acknowledges the impact of government and business interests on medicine as an autonomous profession. Medicare and Medicaid legislation heightened the demand for services, eventually leading to government insistence on labyrinthine rules and regulations that squeeze much of the joy from medical practice. Business concerns that the cost of medical care had spun out of control eventually led to the managed care revolution with its incessant questioning of our judgment about what is best for our patients. However, Stevens differs from those prophets of doom who suggest that physicians emerged the clear losers from their three-way tug-of-war with government and business interests. She suggests that although "organized medicine has become conspicuous politically by its marginality among a cacophony of players, demoted from center stage and seen as just another self-interested player," this grim scenario does not need to be the final act:

In theory, at least, a revived, socially confident medical profession, exerting moral leadership at the national level, might help create reform coalitions and build practical consensus among otherwise competing groups. Despite recent negative critiques, the American medical profession actually has a long history of public service, though that history has been submerged in recent years. In short, the profession's public roles are overdue for updating.

"Medical professionalism" is a multifaceted construct. No one person, group, or organization holds all the answers, at least for now. Historically, we as physicians have resisted the intrusions of government, business interests, and alternative health care providers. However, such resistance tarnishes our image to the extent that laypersons see us as primarily interested in our own welfare, not theirs. We must convince them otherwise. We must also re-commit ourselves to the ideal of service that transcends self-interest. And we must advocate at multiple levels, both individually and collectively, for better systems of care and population health.[7] Finally, we must convince all of our colleagues to support the efforts of organized medicine to insist on ethical, competent, cost-effective, and socially responsive health care for all of our citizens. To quote Stevens one more time: "The responsibilities of professionalism today are awesome. Can the profession overcome the burdens of its received history? Are professional organizations sufficiently competent and poised to forge ahead?"[5] The answers are yes only to the extent that all of us become involved.

References

1. Project of the ABIM Foundation, ACP-ASIM Foundation, and European Federation of Internal Medicine. Medical Professionalism in the new millennium. A physician charter. *Ann Intern Med* 2002; 136: 243-246.
2. Bryan CS. What is a doctor? Reflections on the physician charter on professionalism. *J SC Med Assoc* 2002; 98: 327-329.

3. *The American Heritage Dictionary of the English Language.* Third edition, Boston: Houghton Mifflin Company; 1992.
4. Stevens RA. Public roles for the medical profession in the United States: Beyond theories of decline and fall. *Milbank Quarterly* 2001; 79: 327-353.
5. Stevens RA. Themes in the history of medical professionalism. *Mount Sinai J Med* 2002; 69: 357-362.
6. Sullivan WM. What is left of professionalism after managed care? *Hastings Center Report* 1999; 29 (2): 7-13.
7. Gruen RL, Pearson SD, Brennan TA. Physician-citizens — public roles and professional obligations. *JAMA* 2004; 291: 94-98.

Advancing Medical Professoinalism.
II. One Size Does Not Fit All

J SC Med Assoc 2004; 100: 89-92

Several blocks from my office, a carwash and automobile detailing shop beams its name with a single word: "Professional" (Figure). Having thought for many years about the derivation and definitions of "professional" and "professionalism," I stopped by one day to get the proprietor's take on these matters. His answers were as good as any I've heard: "Be the best you can be," and "It's not the job, it's the attitude." His answers also reminded me of a recent book title: *Professionalism is for Everyone.*[1] And why not? Surely, *everyone* should do his/her best at whatever services he/she does for others, especially when reimbursement is expected! Members of the classic "learned professions" — medicine, law, clergy, and the university professorate — have no right to restrict the use of "professional" and "professionalism."

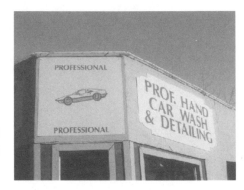

Signage for an automobile carwash and detailing shop (see text).

Still, most of us claim medicine to be a higher calling, not just another way to make a living. We justify our claim by the length of training—11 years of higher education is now the minimum and 15 or more years are not unusual. We justify our claim by the levels of skill and judgment required for much of what we do. We justify our claim by the moral and ethical sophistication demanded by the unequal power relationships between doctor and patient in matters of great consequence for the latter. Yet patients, third party payers, and the general public increasingly regard our services as commodities to be bought and sold like everybody else's. Can we claim to be "professionals" in a larger sense than, say, the claims made by "professional salesmen" or "professional hairdressers"? If so, why and how?

What distinguishes medicine from the other classic learned professions such as law and the clergy is our intimate relationship with ever-evolving technologies. New technologies continually enhance our capacity to serve our fellow humans. New technologies also heighten public expectations and even demands. Lawrence J. Henderson famously said, "Somewhere between 1910 and 1912 in this country, a random patient, with a random disease, consulting a doctor chosen at random had, for the first time in the history of mankind, a better than fifty-fifty chance of profiting from the encounter." Henderson died in 1942, the year penicillin G was introduced into medical practice. It has been said that the introduction of penicillin marked a dramatic change in the doctor-patient relationship; thereafter, patients would generally turn to physicians not for wise counsel but rather for technical solutions to whatever ailed them. New technologies, I suggest, also affect what we mean by "professionalism." This point was driven home to me by the HIV/AIDS epidemic.

The HIV/AIDS epidemic afforded infectious diseases subspecialists like myself the opportunity to experience first hand what can be described as a truncated history of medicine. When the first cases were described in 1981, we were essentially clueless about what was killing our patients. As more and more patients came to us and died, we found ourselves in roles we'd never imagined. My medical school classmate Donna Mildvan, who was the first to recognize AIDS in New York City, likens those early years of the epidemic to medieval times. Our time, concern, and—yes—compassion were about all we had to offer. Most of us had gone into infectious diseases because we liked to solve problems but did not especially want to assume open-ended responsibility for people with long, drawn-out, inevitably fatal illnesses. We did not want to be, for example, oncologists with their terminally ill cancer patients, nephrologists with their hemodialysis clinics, or pulmonologists with their waiting rooms full of "pink puffers" and "blue bloaters." We wanted to be pure consultants, called in by other physicians to make diagnoses and recommend treatments. Or perhaps we wanted to be like surgeons: "Get in, fix it, get out!" The HIV/AIDS epidemic swept us into roles we'd never imagined. We made house calls, delved into difficult personal and social issues, assumed primary care for patients doomed to miserable deaths, and reassured a nervous public as best we could. Most of us found those early years to be enormously fulfilling. Our lives were changed, usually for the better. But the patients kept coming and dying, the initial promise of AZT monotherapy proved illusory, and most of us developed burnout.

Then, in 1986, the introduction of the protease inhibitors launched the present era of highly active antiretroviral therapy (HAART). Thus, within a mere 15 years, AIDS moved from the status of a deadly, untreatable scourge of unknown etiology to a specific infection that could be defined, staged, and treated successfully using the latest tools of molecular biology. Incredible!

Basic (Generic) and Higher Professionalism*

	Basic Professionalism	Higher Professionalism
Brief definition	Service that is competent, timely, and just	Service that clearly transcends self-interest
Nature of work	Occupation	Calling
Purpose of work	Often well defined and circumscribed	Often poorly defined and open-ended
Applicability	All situations in which one is reimbursed for performing services	Situations calling for action "above and beyond the call of duty"
Compensation	Usually well-defined (*quid pro quo*)	Usually absent or insufficient
Power relationships	Power between provider and client is usually equal or nearly equal.	The provider often holds significant power over the client's welfare
Usual ethical framework	Rights- and duty-based	Virtue-based (in addition to being rights- and duty-based)
Level of caring	Beneficence (doing good), combined with empathy and sympathy when appropriate	Compassion in the strict sense of becoming a fellow sufferer
Requisite virtues	Cardinal virtues (prudence, temperance, justice, and fortitude), to assure excellence in function	Transcendent virtues (faith, hope, and love) in addition to the cardinal virtues, for service at a higher level
Personal risks to the provider	Few if any	Often substantial

*Adapted from (2)

Reflecting on the HIV/AIDS epidemic, I have concluded that medical professionalism is not amenable to a one-size-fits-all definition. Rather, it should be viewed as a tiered construct with at least two levels, which for simplicity I call "basic" (or "generic") professionalism and "higher" professionalism (Table).[2] Basic professionalism can be understood as *doing the right thing well*. Higher professionalism can be understood as *service that clearly transcends self-interest*. These levels require different types of caring. Caring, as I understand it, embraces the following concepts in ascending order of difficulty: *beneficence* (doing good), *empathy* (understanding intellectually another's feelings), *sympathy* (experiencing feelings similar to another's), and *compassion* (which literally means "to suffer with," to become a fellow sufferer). The word "compassion" is often used carelessly; as Flannery O'Conner put it, "It is a quality which no one can put his finger on in any exact critical sense, so it is always safe for anybody to use."[3] However, I believe that "compassion" in medicine can be defined in concrete terms, such as (1) care for which one is unpaid or poorly paid; (2) care when one would rather be doing something else, such as staying in bed at 3 o'clock in the morning; (3) care that puts one at emotional risk; and (4) care that puts one at physical risk. In the early years of the HIV/AIDS epidemic, we did all of these, and more.

The key elements of medical professionalism are competence and caring. As the Hippocratic aphorism puts it, "Where there is love of humankind, there also is love of the art." However, the balance between competence and caring — that is, the relative importance of competent service versus "caring" for the task at hand — depends on the availability of relevant technology. Between 1981 and 1986, technologies for dealing with HIV were woefully inadequate. Having little to offer but ourselves, we cared and cared and cared. The protease inhibitors gave us HAART and, in so doing, "medicalized" the disease. Today, for those patients who can understand their disease and adhere to their regimens, HIV/AIDS has become highly treatable. The frequent house calls and lengthy counseling sessions have become unnecessary. During those early years of the epidemic, my colleagues and I worried whether we were giving our patients sufficient emotional support. Now we worry about whether we are using the new drugs and other technologies correctly. Most patients who are doing well with high CD4 lymphocyte counts and undetectable HIV-1 viral loads seldom need nor want the "compassion" of yesteryear.

These, then, are my conclusions:

• "Basic" or "generic" professionalism may be all that is necessary when the following conditions are met: (1) The problem is well defined; (2) technology to deal with the problem is readily available and affordable; and (3) an uncontroversial algorithm outlines the standard approach to diagnosis and treatment. The clinical situation requires *benevolent competence*. "Compassion" in the strict sense of "suffering with" is unnecessary and perhaps even undesirable, except in rare circumstances.

• "Higher" professionalism is desirable when any of the following conditions are present: (1) The problem is poorly defined; (2) relevant technology is lacking or unaffordable; (3) adequate reimbursement is unlikely to be forthcoming; (4) caring for the patient compromises the physician's other activities and interests; (5) caring for the patient puts the physician at emotional risk; or (6) caring for the patient puts the physician at physical risk — even the risk of contracting a fatal disease.

• Our claims to being professionals exhibiting a level of professionalism greater than that required of those engaged in most other walks of life depends largely on the extent to which we engage in higher professionalism, both individually and collectively.

The issue of professionalism matters to the future of the medical profession, and, as this series continues, I welcome the ideas and insights of my fellow SCMA members.

References

1. Ball JR. *Professionalism is for Everyone: Five Keys to Being a True Professional*. Reston, VA: The Goals Institute; 2001.
2. Bryan CS. The Theodore E. Woodward Award. HIV/AIDS, ethics, and medical professionalism: Where went the debate? *Trans Am Clin Climatol Assoc* 2003; 114: 353-367.
3. O'Conner F. The nature and aim of fiction. In: O'Conner F. *Mystery and Manners: Occasional Prose, selected and edited by Sally and Robert Fitzgerald*. New York: Farrar, Straus & Giroux; 1970: 86.

Advancing Medical Professionalism.
III. Bearding the Evils of Specialization

J SC Med Assoc 2004; 100: 205-207

A friend recently gave me a copy of a book by M. Scott Peck, the psychiatrist and popular writer, entitled *People of the Lie: The Hope for Healing Human Evil.* I found it to be a rather dull read until, in one of the late chapters, Peck proposes that a major cause of evil in our society is specialization. He writes:

> I am thoroughly convinced that much of the evil of our times is related to specialization and that we desperately need to develop an attitude of suspicious caution toward it. I think we need to treat specialization with the same degree of disgust that we bring to nuclear reactors.[1]

Peck takes as his main example the massacre at MyLai during the Vietnam Conflict. American troops of Task Force Barker, stressed, confused, and angry, killed several hundred unarmed villagers in the name of pacification. Peck suggests that specialization promotes evil by delegating authority, fragmenting conscience, fostering narcissism, and creating confusion about the overarching moral purpose of an enterprise among those whose lot it is to do the actual work. Writing 21 years before the recent events at Abu Ghraib and elsewhere, Peck predicted that the moral lapses at MyLai would happen and haunt us again. What goes wrong? How do the well-intentioned policies of a democratic and idealistic nation lead to actions that few Americans would condone?

And if Peck is correct, how does his thesis that specialization promotes evil apply to medicine?

"Evil" is a highly nuanced word. The usual definitions are (1) something that is morally bad or wrong; and (2) something that causes or constitutes misfortune, suffering, difficulty, or woe. All of us would, I think, agree that medical specialization is by and large a good thing, responsible for most innovations and for our ability to deliver sophisticated, up-to-date care. Watching various specialists and subspecialists converge upon a patient's problem constitutes one of the joys of practicing medicine in the United States. Flagrant moral lapses are uncommon, and, when they do occur, our profession usually recognizes and reprimands the perpetrators. Yet does specialization sometimes promote evil in the sense of bad results, undesirable outcomes? Yes, of course. Consider, for example, two patients referred to me for refractory mouth ulcers.

Case 1. A young woman was referred for painful mouth ulcers of more than a year's duration, unresponsive to various treatments including multiple courses of acyclovir. I diagnosed unusually severe aphthous stomatitis and prescribed a four-day course of high-dose prednisone. She returned a week later, the mouth ulcers completely gone, and asked, "Why didn't my doctor know to do what you did?"

"Look," I told her, "your doctor is one of the very best family doctors in South Carolina. I could not do what your doctor does — treat dozens of sick people every day. I happen to be a specialist. Other doctors send me patients with very unusual problems like yours. Now, you go back to your doctor, and I'll of course be happy to see you again if he wants me to."

She came back a year later, 40 pounds heavier and overtly cushingoid. She had not taken my advice, had not gone back to her doctor, and someone had kept on giving her prednisone.

Case 2. An elderly woman was referred for painful mouth ulcers of more than a year's duration, unresponsive to various treatments including multiple courses of acyclovir. I pressed for more tissue and diagnosed pemphigus. She and her son, who was her only living first-degree relative, did not want referral to a tertiary care center. After simple measures failed, I decided to admit her to the hospital for intravenous administration of high-dose immune globulin. I admitted her to a teaching service on which I was not the attending physician.

She experienced chest pain during the first infusion. She had been having chest pain off and on for months, and I favored continuing the infusions at a slower rate. However, the housestaff, reciting something about the effect of high-dose immune globulin on the glycoprotein IIb/IIIa receptor, refused to give her the infusions without first performing coronary arteriography. The catheterization somehow resulted in a massive retroperitoneal bleed. She then developed the acute respiratory distress syndrome and died several weeks later of multiorgan failure.

I came away from both of these cases with the uneasy sense that specialization, to which I had been a participant, had been the primary cause of a bad result. In Case 1, specialization prompted the patient to distrust her primary care physician and led to inappropriate treatment from someone else. In Case 2, specialization promoted an algorithmic approach to management which, as often happens, may have been insensitive to the actual scenario and to the meaning of illness and suffering in the patient's life (both the patient and her son felt that continuing the infusions was well worth the risk of a heart attack).

Little has been written about the effect of specialization on medical professionalism. My MEDLINE search of the literature between 1966 and 2004 revealed only 9 articles in which these terms were cross-referenced, and 6 of the 9 articles pertained to other types of health care providers. In 1994, Reynolds concluded that specialization may undermine the medical education community's ability to reaffirm professional values.[2] More recently, Frankford et al. suggested ways to foster commitment to professionalism within the context of multispecialty practice organizations.[3] Defining medical professionalism as "an ethical system supported by an appropriate institutional infrastructure," they recommend that we must learn the skill of "reflective practice" whereby, as individuals and in groups, we examine what we do and why we do it.

Specialization in medicine as in just about everything else will continue to increase. My chief concern, which I suspect is shared by most readers of *The Journal*, is the fragmentation of medical care that sometimes ensues when patients seemingly go from one specialist to another with nobody in charge. What, if anything, can be done? Here's my own short list of suggestions:
• Seek to understand the clinical scenario from the patient's perspective, including the meaning of illness.

• Always ask, "What is really in this patient's best interests?" Be wary of the phenomenon of "groupthink."
• When referring a patient to a specialist, state as precisely as you can what you wish to be done.
• When seeing a patient as a consultant, justify and prioritize your recommendations.
• Communicate, communicate, communicate.
• Respect your colleagues, but be willing to ask questions and to stand up for what you feel is in the patient's best interests.
• Reflect, reflect, reflect.
• Promote systems of medical practice that encourage both thoughtful, unhurried primary care and also judicious and reasonable referrals to specialists.

References

1. Peck FS. *People of the Lie: The Hope for Healing Human Evil*. New York: Touchstone; 1983: 213-253.
2. Reynolds PP. Reaffirming professionalism through the education community. *Ann Intern Med* 1994; 120: 609-614.
3. Frankford DM, Patterson MA, Konrad TR. Transforming practice organizations to foster lifelong learning and commitment to medical professionalism. *Acad Med* 2000; 75: 708-717.

Advancing Medical Professionalism.
IV. Why Higher Professionalism Hurts

J SC Med Assoc 2004; 100: 265-267

Earlier in this series we made a distinction between "basic or generic professionalism" and "higher" professionalism.[1] We gave a brief definition of higher professionalism: service that clearly transcends self-interest. To clarify further the concept of graded professionalism — that is, professionalism that becomes progressively more difficult to achieve — let us consider some ethical dilemmas developed a decade ago by the American Board of Internal Medicine in its impressive document, *Project Professionalism*.[2] The authors of that document chose not to give their opinions regarding the best answers to their multiple choice questions, their purpose being to stimulate discussion (Linda L. Blank, personal communication). However, Daniel Barry and his colleagues at the University of Colorado Health Sciences Center agreed upon the "best response" and an alternative "acceptable" response to six of the scenarios, presented below.

Case 1. A pharmaceutical company approaches you about a clinical research project involving your office patients. Your patients with high blood pressure will be eligible to be treated with a new medication that has just been released by the FDA. The object of the study is to evaluate risk and benefits of this medication in an unselected office population. The pharmaceutical company will pay $250 per patient for the expenses generated by the study and one year's salary for a data manager, and will supply the drug free of charge. Meetings to discuss the initiation of the study and follow-up results will be held in New Orleans and Honolulu. Your spouse will be invited as the company's guest to attend these meetings since they will take you away from home.

Participating in the study would be considered appropriate professional behavior if:

A. Your patients sign an informed consent.

B. Your patients sign an informed consent and your partners approve the study.

C. An oversight committee of the hospital where you have privileges or your regional medical society approves the study.

D. None of the above.

Barry and colleagues deemed "D" the best response, with "C" the best alternative response.

Case 2. You are practicing hematology and oncology in a suburb of a large metropolitan area. Currently, you refer your patients who require radiotherapy to one or two hospitals in the city depending on where the patients live and the type of problem. A radiotherapist whose knowledge and skill you respect informs you that she will be joining a for-profit national radiotherapy company that is thinking of locating in your area. This new company will bring both the latest equipment and upgraded service to your community. She informs you that an excellent opportunity now exists to invest in this company and that the larger the number of investors from the area, the greater the likelihood the company will locate in your community.

Which of the following statements most accurately assesses the possibility of conflict of interest regarding your investment in this company?

A. *An investment will pose a conflict of interest, and you should not take it.*

B. *Your investment will pose no conflict of interest for you because the new radiotherapy unit will offer superior treatment and will be available to your patients.*

C. *There is a possibility of a conflict of interest that requires that you inform your patients of the investment.*

D. *Your investment will pose no conflict of interest if you avoid referring patients to the new radiotherapy unit.*

E. *There will be no problem of conflict of interest for you if your spouse makes the investment.*

Barry and colleagues deemed "A" the best response with "C" the best alternative response.

Case 3. A friend's 16-year-old daughter visits your office requesting birth control pills. Her family is Catholic and against birth control and premarital sex. She requests you do not discuss this with her parents. After concluding the visit, you return to your desk where you find a message to call the patient's mother. In the past you have always discussed the daughter's health and concerns openly. What will you do?

A. *Call the mother back and disclose the reason for her daughter's visit.*

B. *Return the call and tell the patient's mother you can't discuss the matter, knowing this will look suspicious to her.*

C. *Return the call but be evasive when questioned about the nature of the call.*

D. *Don't return the call.*

Barry and colleagues deemed "B" the best response with "C" the best alternative response.

Case 4. You are the chief of service at a hospital and a medical student informs you that she smelled alcohol on the breath of an attending physician during morning rounds on more than one occasion. Another student and a resident confirm this report. How do you proceed?

A. *Approach the physician in question and ask if he/she has a drinking problem.*

B. *Talk to friends and family members of the physician to see if they suspect a drinking problem.*

C. *Review the physician's file and monitor him/her closely.*

D. *Report the physician to the State Board of Medical Examiners.*

Barry and colleagues deemed "D" the best response with "A" the best alternative response.

Case 5. During your rounds with the housestaff team, a male staff member comes up to the group, places his arm around the waist of a female house officer, and thanks her for the terrific job she did taking care of one of his patients. You sense that the house officer is made uncomfortable by the gesture. An appropriate first response would be which of the following?

A. *Do nothing, on the basis that the faculty member was simply showing his appreciation for a job well done.*

B. *Report the incident to the program director as an example of sexual harassment.*

C. *Tell your colleague, the faculty member, that you thought the gesture was inappropriate and that you were made uncomfortable by it.*

D. *Ask the resident if the gesture made her uncomfortable.*

E. *Ask the resident if there are actions she would like you to take on her behalf.*

Barry and colleagues deemed "C" the best response and "E" the best alternative response.

Case 6. An established patient of yours presents with symptoms of depression. This is the second time in three months that the patient has visited you for these complaints. You wish to start treatment with an antidepressant medication. As you are filling out the prescription the patient asks you not to document the diagnosis or medication in the chart. She is concerned that her employer will find out about her diagnosis and she could potentially lose her job like a coworker did. She knows that her insurance company has access to her diagnosis. How do you proceed?

A. *Inform the patient that you must document the diagnosis to provide any treatment.*

B. *Agree to not document the diagnosis but prescribe the medication anyway.*

C. *Agree to not document the diagnosis but refuse to provide the prescription.*

D. *Terminate your relationship with the patient because she is inhibiting your ability to provide adequate care.*

E. *Document an alternative diagnosis, such as fatigue, and provide the prescription.*

Barry and colleagues deemed "A" the best response and "C" the best alternative response.

These are tough questions. Barry and colleagues determined the percentage of best or acceptable responses to be 40% for first-year medical students, 58% for fourth-year medical students, 52% for third-year residents, and 65% for more advanced residents and fellows. I've given these scenarios to 248 graduating medical students over five years, and determined that they gave the best or acceptable responses 72% of the time. I've also discussed several of these scenarios with colleagues well versed in medical ethics. They disagreed among themselves, sometimes violently so!

Note, however, that the best responses as determined by Barry and colleagues invariably demand self-sacrifice:

• Refusing gifts — denying oneself extra income and paid vacations even when the offer does not seem to be inconsistent with good patient care (Case 1).

• Shunning potential conflicts of interest — denying oneself an excellent investment opportunity, even when the firm in question might benefit the community (Case 2).

• Preserving confidentiality involving mature minors — denying oneself the unqualified admiration and friendship of peers in order to protect the privacy of an adolescent (Case 3).

• Addressing possible physician impairment — denying oneself smooth sailing in a relationship and freedom from possible legal entanglements even when there is no evidence that patients have been harmed (Case 4).

• Confronting sexual harassment — denying oneself a peaceful morning or afternoon and risking potential repercussions, such as behind-the-back criticism and lack of referrals (Case 5).

• Maintaining honesty in documentation — denying oneself compliance with a patient's well-meaning and well-reasoned wishes, even when the patient's concerns seem reasonable and the potential response of employers and other third parties may be unreasonable (Case 6).

Fortunately, most of the things most of us do during daily rounds seldom pose ethical dilemmas such as those given in these scenarios. Hence, our "basic" professionalism — competence and caring — usually suffices. Yet I suspect most physicians have grappled with scenarios similar to those presented here.

In summary, higher professionalism usually requires sacrifices of one kind or another — financial, social, emotional, and even the risk of litigation. To say that "professionalism means putting others' interest ahead of one's own" sounds platitudinous, and indeed is often just that. To practice higher professionalism requires courage, patience, a high level of ethical sophistication, and a willingness to choose a clear conscience over comfortable circumstances and success, as the world is wont to measure it.

Higher professionalism hurts.

References

1. Bryan CS. Advancing medical professionalism. II. One size does not fit all. *J SC Med Assoc* 2004; 100: 123-125.

2. American Board of Internal Medicine. *Project Professionalism*. Philadelphia: American Board of Internal Medicine; 1994.
3. Barry D, Cyran E, Anderson RJ. Common issues in medical professionalism: Room to grow. *Am J Med* 2000; 108: 136-142.

Advancing Medical Professionalism. V. The Social Contract, and Why Tort Reform is Essential

J SC Med Assoc 2004; 100: 265-267

On February 28, 2003, Dr. Carlo Urbani, a 46-year-old Italian physician working with the World Health Organization, examined a patient with an unusual flu-like illness in the Vietnam French Hospital in Hanoi. Dr. Urbani diagnosed what is now called the severe acute respiratory syndrome (SARS), a highly contagious illness that begins like the common cold and often leads to acute respiratory failure. The disease spread through the hospital, with more than half the cases and all of the subsequent deaths being among health care workers. Dr. Urbani chose to stay with the doctors and nurses who quarantined themselves to protect their families and the community. He told his wife and childhood sweetheart, Giuliana, to go back to Italy with their three children, saying, "This will be the end for me." On March 11, Dr. Urbani developed symptoms of SARS during a flight to

Bangkok, Thailand, where he was to attend a meeting. He died eighteen days later.[1]

The cause of SARS was found to be a novel coronavirus that jumped from feral animals to humans in the Guangdong province of China. The first isolate was named the Urbani strain in honor of the physician who sounded the alarm.[2] By July 2003, when the chain of human transmission was apparently broken, the disease had affected at least 8437 persons in 26 countries with 813 deaths. Health care workers developed the disease and sometimes died in numbers far disproportionate to the general population. In Hong Kong, where the greatest number of cases occurred, nearly 25% were in health care workers, as were 65% of the cases in Canada. Thus, beginning with Dr. Carlo Urbani, SARS posed a problem that has recurred from time to time throughout the history of medicine: Do I put myself at risk to care for patients affected with a new and apparently dangerous disease?

In June 2004 a team of Hong Kong physicians and surgeons reported six cases of SARS complicated by spontaneous pneumothorax. All four of the patients who accepted chest tubes developed air leaks or recurrences, which might have been indications for procedures such as thoracoscopic repair. These patients were managed medically. The authors candidly reported that among their reasons for not operating was the potential danger to surgeons and other personnel. They concluded, "The benefits of surgical management must be balanced against the potential risks to health-care workers."[3] Indeed, two members of their cardiothoracic surgery team had previously developed SARS and nearly died.[4]

An editorial by Dr. Gregory A. Felice, who is chief of the Infectious Disease Section of the Veterans Affairs Medical Center in Minneapolis, Minnesota, accompanied this report of six cases of pneumothorax. Dr. Felice registered his concern that the Hong Kong doctors had abstained from surgery in part because of the potential risk to operating room staff. After briefly reviewing the mixed responses of physicians to contagious diseases through the course of history, he observes:

As medicine became a rigorous scientific discipline in the

twentieth century, physicians gained increased respect and power, and the medical profession became more cohesive and developed integrated, widely accepted ethical codes. A social contract developed between physicians and society, whereby in return for substantial income, high social prestige, and professional autonomy, physicians are expected to go to great lengths to provide optimal care even in perilous times.

Dr. Felice went on to cite the American Medical Association's Declaration of Professional Responsibility, which tell us to "apply our knowledge and skills when needed, though doing so may put us at risk."[5]

The purpose of this editorial is to assert that (1) Dr. Carlo Urbani exemplifies our finest traditions — what I have previously called "higher" professionalism, as opposed to that expected in everyday circumstances; and (2) Dr. Felice's invoking "a social contract" requires clarification especially as it affects the growing problem of tort liability as applied to medicine.

Mentioning social contract theory brings back memories of college courses in which we learned how Thomas Hobbes (1588-1679) traced the origin of government and laws to a hypothetical State of Nature. People way back yonder, according to Hobbes, accepted limits to their behavior (government) in return for a measure of security from the Law of the Jungle. Others, notably John Locke (1632-1704) and Jean-Jacques Rousseau (1712-1778), modified Hobbes's theory in response to their own political agendas. Scholarly discussion of social contract theory now flourishes after decades of dormancy. In 1971, John Rawls of Harvard University published his influential *A Theory of Justice*, in which he argued for the concept of "justice as fairness."[6] Rawls and others support a concept of justice as "reasonableness" to all affected parties.

Returning to the dilemma faced by the Hong Kong physicians and reviewed by Gregory Felice, what risks can be reasonably expected of physicians? Consider these scenarios:

• *Scenario A*: A procedure carries a 99.9% chance that the patient will benefit and a 0.1% chance that the surgeon will acquire a fatal disease.

• *Scenario B*: A procedure carries a 90% chance that the patient will benefit and a 10% chance that the surgeon will acquire a fatal disease.

• *Scenario C*: A procedure carries a 50% chance that the patient will benefit and a 50% chance that the surgeon will acquire a fatal disease.

• *Scenario D*: A procedure carries a 10% chance that the patient will benefit and a 90% chance that the surgeon will acquire a fatal disease.

• *Scenario E*. A procedure carries a 0.1% chance that the patient will benefit and a 99.9% chance that the surgeon will acquire a fatal disease.

Most people, I think, would draw two conclusions. First, it is naïve to suggest that physicians must assume extremely high risks when the likelihood of benefiting their patients is slim. Second, and on the other hand, to stipulate when and under what circumstances physicians must assume such risks introduces a "slippery slope" of moral reasoning. Thus, there are no clear answers. It is for this reason that we should take the physician's character and courage into account. We thereby enter the domain of virtue ethics—ethics over and above those stipulated by the usual deontological (Kantian) and consequentialist (utilitarian) frameworks.

Dr. Felice refers to a social contract obligating physicians to accept certain risks in exchange for power and privilege acquired during the twentieth century. This assertion fails to account for the mounting threats to medicine (and, indeed, to other professions) in Western culture. Dr. Abigail Zuger, who was among those who during the early years of the HIV/AIDS epidemic argued for such risk-taking, recently wrote: "The profession of medicine has taken its members on a wild ride during the past century: a slow, glorious climb in well-being followed by a steep, stomach-churning fall." Dr. Zuger ranks the "rising tide of medical-malpractice litigation" high among the causes of widespread physician dissatisfaction.[7] If we are to use social contract theory to require risk-taking on behalf of patients, we should review with the rest of society what constitutes an adequate exchange. Data do not support the loose notion

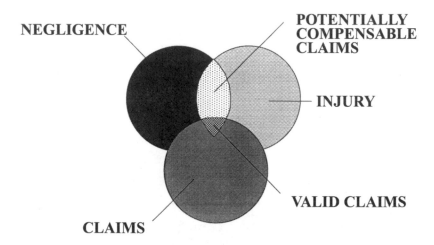

NEGLIGENCE

POTENTIALLY COMPENSABLE CLAIMS

INJURY

VALID CLAIMS

CLAIMS

Hypothetical relationship between negligence, injury, and malpractice claims (not to scale; the relative sizes of the circles and the extent of their overlaps are unknown). Ideally, neither injury that is not due to negligence nor negligence that does not result in injury should be the basis for claims. Ideally, there should be an easier and more cost-effective way to identify and adjudicate cases of negligence that result in injury. Such a system, combined with caps on rewards above and beyond actual damages, would be fairer than the present lottery system not only for physicians but also for patients and society.

that medicine is an easy way to become wealthy. Indeed, data suggest that medical education gives a poorer financial return on educational investment than either business or law.[8] The tort liability system as applied to medicine should be overhauled in such a way as to assure justice as "reasonableness" not only to physicians but also to patients and society. The current lottery system rewards a few at the expense of many (Figure).

The courage and heroism exemplified by Dr. Carlo Urbani and others beckon us to aspire to a virtue-based ethic, a higher professionalism that transcends our own self-interests. However, such professionalism will thrive only to the extent to which society reciprocates by setting reasonable limits for all affected parties.

128

References

1. Reilley B, Van Herp M, Sermand D, et al. SARS and Carlo Urbani. *N Engl J Med* 2003; 348: 1951-1952.

2. Ksiazek TG, Erdman D, Goldsmith CS, et al. A novel coronavirus associated with severe acute respiratory syndrome. *N Engl J Med* 2003; 348: 1953-1966.

3. Sihoe ADL, Wong RHL, Lee ATH, et al. Severe acute respiratory syndrome complicated by spontaneous pneumothorax. *Chest* 2004; 125: 2345-2351.

4. Sihoe ADL, Wong RHL, Yim APC. *Primum non nocere* (letter). *Chest* 2004; 126: 2026.

5. Felice GA. SARS, pneumothorax, and our response to epidemics (editorial). *Chest* 2004; 125: 1982-1985.

6. Rawls J. *A Theory of Justice*. Revised edition, Cambridge, Massachusetts: The Belknap Press or Harvard University Press; 1999.

7. Zuger A. Dissatisfaction with medical practice. *N Engl J Med* 2004; 350: 69-75.

8. Weeks WB, Wallace AE, Wallace MM, et al. A comparison of the educational costs and incomes of physicians and other professionals. *N Engl J Med* 1994; 330: 1280-1286.

Advancing Medical Professionalism.
VI. Summing Up

J SC Med Assoc 2005; 101: 115-116

> *No physician, insofar as he is a physician, considers his own*
> *good in what he prescribes, but the good of his patient; for*
> *the true physician is also a ruler having the human body as a*
> *subject, and is not a mere moneymaker.*
>   — Plato, *The Republic*

My wife, Donna, is a devotee of the television program *ER*, and sometimes I'll watch it with her. The scriptwriters are said to consult with the faculty of a prominent institute for medical ethics, and it shows. On a recent episode, Dr. John Carter, whom we've seen progress from medical student to resident to senior attending physician in the big city emergency room, cares for a teenaged girl whose kidney transplant came from her father. She enters the emergency room with acute renal failure. Dr. Carter quickly surmises the problem to be acute tubular necrosis caused by a drug she's getting to control her seizures. The drug, prescribed by her neurologist, is extremely expensive. Her father had to obtain a second job in order to afford it. The drug's manufacturer had recently sent a letter to all physicians in the United States warning about the possibility of acute renal failure. Dr. Carter asks the hospital pharmacy to investigate. The neurologist enters and insists that the cause of acute renal failure is transplant rejection, not drug toxicity. Dr. Carter oversees a kidney biopsy, which shows classic changes of tubular necrosis. Questioned by Dr. Carter, the neurologist then admits that he's an investigator for the drug company and is being paid to enroll patients in a post-marketing study. The patient's distraught father offers to donate his remaining kidney. The physicians advise him that their code of ethics forbid it. The father then kills himself in front of the two physicians so that his daughter can get the kidney.

In this series of editorials, we have distinguished between "basic medical professionalism" (in brief, doing the right thing well, as is mandated by any quid-pro-quo business relationship) and "higher medical professionalism" (in brief, service that clearly transcends self-interest, and which is at times self-damaging). Dr. John Carter clearly shows the latter. His supervisor becomes furious about his asking the pharmacy to investigate, since drug companies constitute a major funding source for the hospital. The neurologist, who not long ago studied under Dr. Carter, goes away with hurt feelings and we sense that their relationship will never be the same. For John Carter, virtue clearly becomes its own, and perhaps only, reward.

Here are some of the points we've covered in these editorials:

• Medical professionalism is increasingly threatened by such outside forces as government, business, alternative health care providers, and perceptions in some quarters that physicians are not especially concerned about the greater public welfare.

• Medical professionalism is increasingly threatened by the balkanization of organized medicine into dozens, perhaps hundreds, of specialty organizations and special interest groups.

• Medical professionalism poses numerous personal and ethical questions on a daily basis. Conflicts of interest and obligation are part and parcel of much of what we do. Ethical dilemmas often have more than one "acceptable" solution. What constitutes "professionalism" can often be viewed as a tiered construct rather than an all-or-none construct. Higher medical professionalism, as opposed to the *quid pro quo* transaction required of basic professionalism, usually demands self-sacrifice (altruism).

• Our claims that medicine is more than just another way to make a living depend in large measure on the extent that, individually and collectively, we contribute to the welfare of others well beyond the *quid pro quo* of ordinary business relationships.

• Our claims that we represent a great and noble professional tradition depend in large measure on the extent that we treat not only our patients but also each other with mutual respect, resisting the temptation to succumb to the "we versus them" mentality of competing specialties, practice organizations, and institutions.

• Medicine does not belong to us. It belongs to society. Ultimately, society will get the kind of medical profession it supports and deserves. Reform in the tort liability system as it affects medical practice is essential to the long-term viability of medical professionalism as we now know it.

• We should celebrate the lives and examples of colleagues such as the late Dr. Carlo Urbani who remind us that medicine is indeed a higher calling, a benefit to our fellow humans, a responsibility that summons us to strive continually to be the best we can possibly be.

Our ability to offer the world's best medical care is increasingly offset by problems of cost and access. It is now predicted, for example, that by 2014 health care costs will amount to 19% of our gross domestic product if nothing is done. It is now pointed out, for example, that to make an automobile in the United States the manufacturer must pay more for health insurance than for steel. It continues to be pointed out that millions of Americans are uninsured or underinsured, and that debts related to health care now constitute the leading cause of bankruptcy.

This issue of *The Journal* coincides with our annual meeting. The next issue (June 2005) coincides with the centenary of this publication, one of the oldest of its kind in the United States. Reviewing all of our back issues, I'm impressed with the thoroughness and thoughtfulness with which South Carolina physicians through the years have articulated the concepts outlined above. Reviewing current opinion, I'm impressed with the urgent need for physicians to assume leadership roles in the articulation of a reasonable ethic for health care delivery in the United States.

Higher medical professionalism requires individual virtue, as was exemplified by Dr. John Carter on the television program I watched that recent evening. However and as also illustrated in *ER* and throughout our media, medical professionalism should summon us to act collectively to assure fair and just health care for all of our citizens.

"I Like Science and I Want to Help People" — Introductory Remarks on Professionalism for Freshman Medical Students

J SC Med Assoc 2005; 101: e301-e306

(Address given on August 9, 2005, to the Class of 2009
at the University of South Carolina School of Medicine)

Most of you, I suspect, gave the Admissions Committee some variation on the theme, "*I like science and I want to help people.*" Few if any of you replied: "I want to be a doctor because I think it would be cool." I hope to explore what we mean by the phrase, "I like science and I want to help people," and to reinforce your suspicion that few if any human endeavors are cooler — that is, more challenging and more rewarding — than the practice of medicine.

You now take your place on the shoulders of giants who have made possible today's scientific medicine — people like Hippocrates and Galen, Thomas Sydenham and William Harvey, Ambrose Paré and John Hunter, William Withering and Edward Jenner, Louis Pasteur and Robert Koch, and, in more recent times, Sir William Osler and Harvey Cushing. Rather than bore you with an overview of the history of medicine, I'd like to focus on two monuments right here in Columbia, South Carolina.

First, I take you to the grounds of the state capitol building, and more specifically to the corner of Gervais and Assembly Streets. There one finds with his back to the sidewalk the bust of J. Marion Sims, the marble man of South Carolina medicine. Sims, the son of the county sheriff in Lancaster, South Carolina, chose medicine almost by elimination. To use the later words of President Daniel Coit Gilman of the Johns Hopkins University, he considered himself "too weak to farm, too stupid for the law, and too immoral for the pulpit." Sims graduated from South Carolina College, now the University of South Carolina, where (according to his autobiography) his career was remarkable only for good behavior. He graduated in medicine from the University of Pennsylvania, tried and failed at general practice in Lancaster, and moved to Alabama where he gradually became known as a gifted surgeon. One day he was called to see a young slave woman named Anarcha, who had lost control of both her bladder and her rectum as a result of traumatic childbirth. Sims examined her reluctantly; he later wrote: "If there was anything I hated it was examining the organs of the female pelvis." He made the diagnosis of vesicovaginal fistula — that is, an abnormal communication between the vagina and the urinary bladder. His first reaction was that the lesion was "a surgical curiosity, although a rare one."

Vesicovaginal fistula was in 1845 the stumbling block to further progress in operative gynecology. No one had repaired it with consistent success. Indeed, no one had managed to visualize it satisfactorily in a living patient. Afflicted patients, with their urine leaking continually into the vagina, were miserable. Some even committed suicide. Shortly thereafter, Sims was called to see two additional patients with this condition. He took all three of them to his infirmary, examined them, concluded there was nothing to be done, and told them: "Tomorrow I shall send you home."

He decided to give it one last try. He bought the largest pewter spoon he could find, bent the handle, and used it to examine one of his patients a second time. As he later wrote: "Introducing the bent handle of the spoon I saw everything as no man had ever seen before. The fistula was as plain as the nose on a man's face. The edges were clear and well-defined … as if it had been cut out of a piece of paper. The walls of the vagina could be seen closing in every direction; the neck of the uterus was dilated and well-defined, and even the secretions from the neck could be seen as a tear glistening in the eye…. I said at once, "Why cannot these things be cured?" Sims invited all of the doctors in Montgomery, Alabama, to attend his operation, which consisted simply of paring the edges of the fistula and drawing them together with thread. It worked — but the suture line broke down and the symptoms recurred. For the next three years, Sims, at his own expense, kept the three women in his infirmary and operated again and again trying to repair the fistulas. The other physicians lost interest. The three women took turns assisting him with his surgery. His brother-in-law pleaded with him to give it up to support his family. Finally, he hit upon the idea of using silver wire for suture material. The silver sutures held. Sims went on to become the first physician to specialize in gynecology, to found the first hospital devoted exclusively to diseases of women, to be decorated by several courts in Europe, and to become widely known as the father of modern operative gynecology.

Next, I take you to a country churchyard about six miles east of where you now sit (the campus of the University of South Carolina School of Medicine). I take you there to see an obelisk in memory of Dr. Theodore Brevard Hayne, who died in 1930 while studying yellow fever in West Africa. Let us examine briefly the status of yellow fever in 1930. In 1900, a United States Army Commission (headed by Walter Reed but with the real breakthroughs made by Reed's colleagues, Jesse Lazear, James Carroll, and Aristides Agramonte), determined that epidemic yellow fever is transmitted by a common household mosquito. This observation led to the elimination of yellow fever as a threat to the major seaports of the Western Hemisphere. However, the disease remained widespread in parts of South America and Africa. The causative virus was isolated in West Africa in 1927, but a vaccine was still unavailable. It began to be apparent that mosquitoes other than the common household mosquito *Aedes aegypti* could transmit the disease. Four Rockefeller Foundation researchers had already died studying the disease.

Theodore Hayne grew up in Congaree, South Carolina, just down the road from where you now sit. By all accounts he was an extremely likeable young man. He loved the out of doors, and as a teenager he became interested in the mosquitoes that cause malaria, which was then still an important problem in South Carolina. He was not an especially good student. When he entered The Citadel, he made a bet with his best friend, one "Shrimp" Hasell, as to which of them would finish last. It was close. After his graduation Hayne did malaria research and then decided to go to medical school. He graduated, did an internship, and joined the Rockefeller Foundation's West African Yellow Fever Commission near Lagos, Nigeria. After an eighteen month tour of duty he returned to South Carolina and married his sweetheart, Roselle Hundley. He returned to Nigeria with the plan that she would join him. Hayne took on the task of caring for broods of mosquitoes infected with the deadly yellow fever virus. He knew that one mosquito escaping from the netting could cause him to get yellow fever, with its 25 to 50 percent case-fatality rate. He received word from home that Roselle was pregnant, which meant that she could not go to West Africa anytime soon. He agonized over whether to resign from the Rockefeller Foundation. He decided to stay and complete his research. He developed yellow fever and died.

We will return later to J. Marion Sims and Theodore B. Hayne. Let us now examine what we mean by the term, "Professionalism."

Just about everyone in today's society aspires to professional status. Consider, for example, a car wash just down the street from Palmetto Health Richland, where I work, and across the street from the School of Medicine's Family Practice Center. The signage simply says, "Professional." I stopped by one day and asked the owner what "professional" meant to him. He beamed two splendid definitions: "Be the best you can be," and "It's not the job, it's the attitude." His insights and his obvious pride in his work are indeed exemplary, yet beg the question whether medical professionalism differs substantially from professionalism in other walks of life. What IS medical professionalism, and how can we best promote it?

In recent years there has been a tremendous surge of articles in the medical literature dealing with "professionalism," which has become a buzzword among educators. A recent author, who examines how "professionalism" will necessarily differ for your generation compared to those who've gone before you, observes:

> Most of these articles define professionalism as a set of
> virtues, including altruism, honesty, compassion, and
> integrity, then create behavioral definitions under each
> of these virtues that are quantifiable in physicians....
> Although valuable in the debate, these attempts... fall
> short of capturing its essence.

The author goes on to say: "The core of professionalism is the personal transformation of self that takes place in stages during the early years of medical training and practice."[1] The author thus intimates that professionalism is somehow related to what we might call *character*, and a field of inquiry known as *virtue ethics*.

In the second year of medical school you will be introduced to medical ethics, to ways of thinking about various quandaries that arise in clinical practice. Suffice it here to note that there are two major frameworks for looking at ethical dilemmas: deontology (that is, rule-based ethics), and utilitarianism (or consequentialism, that is, outcome-based ethics). Ethical discussion and debate often seems interminable and inconclusive in part because the participants fall back to one or the other of these frameworks. For example, a deontologist might say "Thou shalt not kill," whereas a consequentialist would justify killing in certain circumstances such as self-defense. Virtue ethics is arguably a third option. It is generally seen, however, as an alternative to utilitarianism whereby one is concerned not only with isolated actions but also with the character of the agent.

My interest in virtue ethics was piqued some years ago during a game of Trivial Pursuit ® with my wife. She usually wins because I can't answer questions in the Entertainment category. One night, however, I was close to victory. I need to answer only one more question: "What are the three cardinal virtues?" I knew the answer cold; indeed, I'd just read a book on the subject. However, I suspected the answer on the card might be wrong, since there are four of them, not three. Indeed, it was. The card gave as the answer: "Faith, hope, charity." These are not the cardinal virtues.

Since that evening I've asked many people including entire audiences and learned persons in philosophy and theology whether they can name the cardinal virtues. Few can. The four cardinal virtues, first enumerated by Plato in *The Republic*, are: prudence (wisdom), temperance, justice, and fortitude (courage). These are distinct from (but complementary to) the theological virtues (or, as I prefer to call them, the transcendent virtues) enumerated by St. Paul in 1 Corinthians 13:13: faith, hope, and love (or charity). I would ask you to memorize these seven virtues. I would also ask you to memorize today's four commonly used principles of medical ethics, as enumerated by Tom Beauchamp and James Childress: beneficence (to do good), nonmaleficence (to do no harm), justice, and autonomy. Note that justice is the only one of these principles that is also a cardinal virtue.

"I like science and I want to help people." The essence of medical professionalism, I suggest, consists of *competence, caring, and social responsibility*—a slightly more sophisticated version of what you told the medical school Admissions Committee. For many of us, the most durable image of professionalism is a painting by Sir Luke Fildes entitled *The Doctor*, which you'll find in one of your conference rooms in the medical school library. Yet which is more important: caring (as wonderfully evinced by *The Doctor*) or competence? Some years ago as a rhetorical exercise I ranked "the C's of medicine" in the following order: (1) courage, which as Sir Winston Churchill put it is the virtue that makes the others possible; (2) competence, which is the physician's first responsibility to the physician acting *as a physician* as distinct from a concerned layperson; and (3) compassion. I argued that in a sense, benevolent competence *is* compassion, whereas compassion without competence is fraud. Let us examine these briefly.

Courage has been defined by the Canadian philosopher Douglas Walton as the use of both moral and practical reasoning to achieve a socially-desirable goal. Moral reasoning takes altruism as its principal facilitating virtue. Practical reasoning takes persistence as its principal facilitating virtue. J. Marion Sims exemplifies especially practical reasoning, facilitated by his incredible persistence. Theodore B. Hayne exemplifies especially moral reasoning, facilitated by his altruism—his willingness to risk his life in the service of scientific progress.

Competence as understood in medicine is now being redefined. The Accreditation Council for Graduate Medical Education identifies six areas of competence: patient care (including clinical reasoning), medical knowledge, practice-based learning and improving (including information management), interpersonal and communication skills, professionalism, and systems-based practice (including health economics and teamwork). I especially like the following definition by two physicians at the University of Rochester: "Professional competence is the habitual and judicious use of communication, knowledge, technical skills, clinical reasoning, emotions, *values, and reflection* in daily practice for the benefit of the individual and community served (*emphasis added*)."[2] Note that according to this definition, competence embraces caring and social responsibility.

Compassion is more problematic. The term "compassion" is used freely and cheaply by most people today, including those of us in medicine. The Southern writer Flannery O'Conner wrote: "Compassion is a word that sounds good in anybody's mouth and which no book jacket can do without. It is a quality which no one can put his finger on in any exact sense, so it is always safe for anybody to use."[3] I believe it is more useful to consider *caring* as a hierarchy of behaviors which in ascending order of difficulty are as follows:

• *Beneficence* (which from the Latin means simply "active kindness," and which we previously noted to be one of the four principles of today's medical ethics).

• *Empathy* (which from the Greek means "in feeling," the ability to understand how someone else feels).

• *Sympathy* (which from the Greek means "like-feeling," the ability not only to understand but also to experience feelings similar to someone else's).

• *Compassion* (which from the Greek means "suffering with," to become a fellow sufferer, to take on someone else's burdens).

I suggest, however, that physicians exemplify in at least some respects compassion in this strict sense of becoming a fellow sufferer, as in (1) rendering service for which one is not reimbursed, or is poorly reimbursed; (2) rendering service when one would rather be doing something else; (3) rendering service that involves emotional risks; and (4) rendering service that involves physical risks.[4] To put it differently, compassion consists of deeds (not words) that risk compromising one's own financial, social, emotional, or physical well-being. This resonates, and at a high level, with an understanding common to nearly all definitions of "professionalism": placing the interests of the patient (or client) above one's self-interests.

Competence, caring, and social responsibility. My thinking about this triumvirate received momentum from reflections on the great epidemic of our times, the HIV/AIDS epidemic. Infectious diseases specialists like me were privileged to participate in what amounted to be an overview of all of medical history, truncated between 1981 and 1996. In the span of 15 years, we went from being in a "black box" to being able to understand and treat the disease with the latest tools of molecular biology. In these 15 years, we also experienced an emotional roller-coaster ride. At first we were perplexed but fascinated. As patients kept coming and dying, we became confused and despondent. In the late 1980s, after the causative virus was isolated and AZT (azidothymidine, now known as zidovudine) was introduced, we enjoyed an enormous sense of public usefulness and personal fulfillment. But the promise of AZT proved illusory, the patients kept on coming and dying, and most of us burned out. The introduction in 1996 of a new class of drugs known as the protease inhibitors made the disease somewhat analogous to insulin-dependent diabetes mellitus—a nuisance, yet one that patients can live with very well provided they become knowledgeable and follow prescriptions to the letter. During these 15 years, we infectious disease specialists went from a work ethic based largely on compassion to one based largely on competence. During the early years, we found ourselves in roles we'd never imagined. We made frequent house calls, dealt with some of society's most sensitive issues, and gave emotional support not only to patients and their families but also to society at large. As one of my colleagues put it, we rediscovered why we went into medicine in the first place. My main self-doubts during those early years concerned whether I was giving my patients sufficient emotional support, offering enough compassion. On a Sunday afternoon, should I enjoy myself or should I drive 30 miles out into the country to see one of my patients who is close to death? Today, my main self-doubts concern whether I am making optimal use of the cornucopia of available drugs. The disease has become "medicalized."[4]

I tell this story in order to distinguish between what I call "basic" professionalism and "higher" professionalism. Basic professionalism as I understand it means bringing to bear in full measure the cardinal virtues—wisdom, temperance, justice, and courage — to one's occupational task. Higher professionalism calls into play the transcendent virtues — faith, hope, and especially love (or compassion, in the sense of shouldering another's burden, of becoming a fellow sufferer). Some people argue that "professionalism is for *everyone*" — and why not? Why shouldn't *everyone* exemplify what the owner of the car wash told me: "Be the best you can be," and "It's not the job, it's the attitude." We admire *The Doctor* by Sir Luke Fildes because its subject has obviously become a fellow sufferer. As dawn breaks through the window of a modest farmhouse, Fildes's doctor, who has evidently stayed up all night, continues to contemplate his patient, a sick child probably suffering from a life-threatening infection. Yet who among us would prefer Fildes's doctor to the gruffest, most insensitive physician alive today who, nevertheless, gives the child a curative antibiotic?

Basic professionalism, I suggest, is all that is required of the physician when the problem is clear-cut and when there is adequate technology to deal with it. Higher professionalism becomes desirable when the problem is not clear-cut and/or when adequate technology is lacking. Basic professionalism is rights- and duty-based, whereas higher professionalism is also virtue-based. Basic professionalism takes competence as its primary requisite, whereas higher professionalism summons into play compassion and courage. Basic professionalism is facilitated by the cardinal virtues, whereas higher professionalism summons into play the theological (or transcendent) virtues, and, especially, love.

Does "higher" professionalism remain relevant to what we do? Let us briefly consider the three so-called "learned professions": law, medicine, and ministry. These three occupations are called "learned professions" because they happen to have been the subjects taught in medieval universities. However, the common denominator of these three occupations consists of performing services and rendering judgments on behalf of our fellow humans in matters of importance in which there is considerable uncertainty about the outcome. But therein lies the rub for medicine. We will always need lawyers, for the outcome of a matter brought before a court is never certain. We will always need ministers, for we will never know exactly what happens to us when we die. Medicine alone among these occupations is inseparably wedded to science and technology. Medicine as a "profession" in the sense that I've just defined it is uniquely vulnerable because science and technology steadily reduce the uncertainty. Hence, the question arises: "Will we still need doctors?" Most of the things physicians do can in fact be done by other people, and with less training. Will the future of medicine consist mainly of mid-level practitioners referring to technicians? Each generation of physicians must re-define and defend the concept of "professionalism" in the context of changing times and new technologies. We can already identify some of the broad challenges that face your generation. These include the transition to the so-called post-modern era, the transition from a utilitarian ethic to a virtue ethic, the replacement of the traditional doctor-patient dyad with a society-doctor-patient triad, and the need to address not only the quality of medical care but also the pressing problems of cost and access.

Some of you may recall from your undergraduate psychology course the premise of the humanistic psychologist Abraham Maslow that all of us have certain needs, which constitute a hierarchy. Maslow divided these needs into (1) "deficit needs" — physiological needs, safety needs, belong needs, and esteem needs — and (2) "being needs," which for him were synonymous with self-actualization. I suggest that Maslow's deficit needs correspond to "basic" professionalism — doing the right thing well, in return for which one makes a living. "Higher" professionalism" — on the other hand — calls into play "being all that one can be," rendering service that clearly transcends self-interest.[5]

Let me close with 10 suggestions for you toward achieving self-actualization, that is, toward "higher" professionalism, being all that you can be.

First, maintain high ideals and principles. I recommend that you start (if you have not already, and less than 5 percent of the population has) a written system of time management. Place in writing your basic principles, your long-term goals, and your short-term goals. What we call *character* is, in a sense, having one's principles, goals, and actions in perfect alignment (congruity). Yet it's important to have written goals in all of the major areas of life, not just your work. Most of us (and speaking especially for myself!) are guilty of putting too much emphasis on one or another area, and to our own detriment. Ideally, one should develop written principles, goals, and action steps around a major definite purpose, your response to the opening question you'll soon find yourself asking patients, "Why are you here?" Studies indicate that the students who best resist the cynicism fostered by the so-called "hidden curriculum" of the clinical years of medical school are those who best protect and nurture the principles and values they brought with them.

Second, set limits to your deficit needs. Maslow became increasingly concerned that success in the United States was being defined largely in material terms, which continues to be the case. Studies indicate that happiness plateaus at an annual income (in 2005 dollars) of about $105,000; thereafter, additional income buys relatively little additional happiness. Most of you will graduate from medical school with substantial debt. Some of you will find in your late thirties that you enjoy enormous earning potential. If you're not careful, greed will take over your life. Resist it.

Third, keep a journal. The overarching purpose of our vertical curriculum on Ethics and Professionalism is to encourage as a lifelong habit reflection on what you do and why you do it. Cultivate a sense of ethical awareness and what is now called "reflective practice." Make notes on critical incidents, including episodes that bother you. Make notes on role models, both positive and negative, behaviors to emulate and behaviors to avoid. Many are the murky areas of medical practice. Strive to become ethically sophisticated.

Fourth, pursue beauty and truth. Medicine by definition will expose you to a disproportionate share of suffering and sorrow. Perhaps it was no accident that John Keats, who left us those immortal lines "Truth is beauty, beauty truth/That is all you know on earth and all you need to know," was a onetime medical student. My favorite advice for medical students is this quotation from Sir William Osler: "Spend the last half hour of the day in communion with the saints of humanity." Shun late night television and whodunits for literature that heightens your awareness of the human condition. Also, seek beauty in the edifying aspects of our culture according to your tastes, such as art, music, dance, or theater.

Fifth, seek out and treasure peak experiences, those moments in which we gain insight into the eternal, the transcendent, and the sacred. You'll find a lot of these in clinical medicine. It's been said, "The world is a great show, and physicians have a front row seat."

Sixth, maintain a healthy sense of humor, not the usual type based on circulating jokes with their surprise endings but rather the gentle, self-deprecating kind of humor that celebrates the nuances of everyday life, the foibles and frailties of the human condition including your own shortcomings. You'll find your sense of humor to be a wonderful counterweight to the stresses and strains of medical school and medical practice and also to the growing realization of your own mortality.

Seventh, strive to be self-accepting and accepting of others. Medical schools have an unfortunate tradition of being less than supportive environments. Indeed, many have written about a "culture of abuse" — the tendency of faculty and residents to berate students unnecessarily. All too often, those whose self-esteem has been damaged try to damage the self-esteem of others. Avoid this tendency. Strive toward what the humanistic psychologist Carl Rogers called "unconditional positive regard" for your fellow humans, what others have called "the sacredness of each individual."

Eighth, learn teamwork. Traditionally, medical practice has been the province of the rugged, solitary individual. Solo practice is now the exception, but even if you ultimately choose to practice alone you'll find the need to function efficiently within a complicated network of often-competing groups and individuals. Learn to be a good leader and also a good follower. Relate to nurses and other health care workers from a posture of mutual respect.

Ninth, promote social progress. You will find in our curriculum a number of opportunities to participate in projects such as the Free Medical Clinic. Our claims to a higher professionalism, being worthy of the honor and privileges bestowed upon us by society, demand our demonstrating a high sense of social responsibility. The most pressing issue for physicians today is the need to address problems of access to medical care. We must also redouble our efforts to educate the public about ways to prevent illness. It has been said that medicine is the only occupation that, through its progress, seeks constantly to eliminate the need for its own existence.

Finally, love your work. Abraham Maslow suggested that self-actualized people tend to regard work as "creative play." One of your tasks these next three years is to figure out which among the many medical specialties best meshes with your natural aptitudes and offers you the most joy. Recognize, of course, that your work will not always be play. As Maslow put it, "Discipline, hard work, postponement of pleasure, forcing himself, all become necessary even for the 'born physician'."

"I like science and I want to help people." This is indeed the essence of medical professionalism. This attitude combined with scientific advances of the twenty-first century will lead you in directions that none of us can even imagine. But the fundamental principles will remain unchanged. They are captured in the first aphorism of Hippocrates, carved beneath the bust of J. Marion Sims: "Where there is love of humanity, there also is love of the art." They are captured in scripture, carved on the tombstone of Theodore B. Hayne: "Greater love hath no man than this, that he lay down his life for his friends." Both of these quotations express the idea that love, highest of the three transcendent virtues, should always inform prudence (or practical wisdom), highest of the four cardinal virtues. Thus, we might best see ourselves as constantly striving to become better *loving persons of character*.

"I like science and I want to help people." These ideals have been expressed in Latin as *philanthropia* and *philotechnia*, the twin pillars of caring and competence.

Strive to never forget what you told the Admissions Committee.

Oh, and by the way, have fun.

Medicine is indeed a cool thing to do.

References

1. Smith LG. Medical professionalism and the generation gap. *Am J Med* 2005; 18: 439-442.
2. Epstein RM, Hundert EM. Defining and assessing professional competence. *JAMA* 2002; 287: 226-235.
3. O'Conner F. The nature and aim of fiction. In: *O'Conner F. Mystery and Manners: Occasional Prose, Selected and Edited by Sally and Robert Fitzgerald.* New York: Farrar, Straus & Giroux; 1970: 86.
4. Bryan CS. Theodore E. Woodward Award. HIV/AIDS, ethics, and medical professionalism: Where went the debate? *Trans Am Clin Climatol Assoc* 2003; 114: 353-367.
5. Bryan CS. Medical professionalism and Maslow's needs hierarchy. *Pharos* 2005 (spring): 4-10.

Editorial Note: The patient reader will recognize immediately that this essay constitutes an amalgam of thoughts published elsewhere in this volume. It appeared as an article in an electronic issue of *The Journal* (unlike the other essays herein, which appeared as editorials in hard-copy issues). I wrote it consciously and perhaps self-indulgently as an attempt to emulate the introductory addresses that were much in vogue and often published during the nineteenth century — for example, those by Charleston's Samuel Henry Dickson and Boston's Oliver Wendell Holmes. I resisted the temptation to quote the following from one of Holmes's 1871 commencement address at Bellevue Hospital College:

> I warn you against all ambitious aspirations outside of your profession. Medicine is the most difficult of the sciences and the most laborious of the arts. It will task all your powers of body and mind if you are faithful to it. Do not dabble in the muddy sewer of politics, nor linger by the enchanged streams of literature.... The great practitioners are generally those who concentrate all their powers on their business. If there are here and there brilliant exceptions, it is only in virtue of extraordinary gifts,

The Virtues in Medicine

The Limits of Altruism

J SC Med Assoc 1978; 74: 337

At the annual meeting, the House of Delegates of the South Carolina Medical Association passed a resolution suggesting that Medicaid recipients should pay a portion of their bills. Behind the resolution was the notion that assumption of partial fiscal responsibility might act as a deterrent to excessive use of health care services. The president of the SCMA was quoted in the lay press as acknowledging that this resolution was not entirely altruistic. This acknowledgement has already been used by some to fan the flames of fashionable criticism of organized medicine.

The same week, national news magazines gave prominence to a special article appearing in the *New England Journal of Medicine* — an article that could have been amplified by any practitioner.[1] The article averred that the physician's ideal, like that of Faust, is to "know all, love all, heal all." Among the factors that sometimes thwart the realization of such an ideal stands "the hateful patient." The author identified four types. First comes the *dependent clinger* who exhausts the physician's stamina by his bottomless need for medical services. Next comes the *entitled demander* (a lawyer was cited as the example) who intimidates and threatens the physician to provide more and more services. The third type is the *manipulative help-rejecter* who insists on trying new remedies but also insists that nothing helps; this is the common "crock." Finally, there is the *self-destructive denier* who derives great pleasure in thwarting the physician's efforts to help him.

Such patients inevitably evoke negative feelings in their physicians. The thrust of the essay was that physicians should acknowledge these feelings, that in fact these negative emotions constitute an important part of the patient's data base. Such insights may be helpful, but it seems likely that most physicians will continue to recognize that, as one of my colleagues puts it, "five percent of patients cause 95 percent of my headaches."

We do not suggest that such "hateful patients" are more prevalent among Medicaid recipients. We do suggest, however, that the purest altruistic motives become contaminated when such patients receive a *carte blanche* to medical services and assume no fiscal responsibility themselves.

Are there limits to altruism? The subject would be worthy of lengthy debate in the grand Socratic style. For practical purposes, however, the major conflict is the old issue of "need" versus "right." Health care providers, like others in the "helping professions" (including teachers, counselors, and social workers), view services in terms of needs. Altruism, then, could be defined as the refusal to deny needed services even at personal cost. On the other hand, many others (including some lawyers, politicians, and rights advocates) view services in terms of rights. It is not up to the provider to ascertain whether or not need exists; the patient has a right to services whether they are needed or not.

The issue seems basic, and it's comforting to know that it's receiving serious discussion among sociologists and others.[2] We feel that our profession must remain altruistic when clear need exists. But if altruism must also apply to alleged "rights" irrespective of *bona fide* need it seems doubtful that the resources of either our profession or of society will ultimately suffice. It is the nature of man that a few will perceive bottomless needs, irrespective of what really ails them. Unfortunately, any system for financing health care delivery must take into account the incessant demands of these few.

References

1. Groves JE. Taking care of the hateful patient. *N Engl J Med* 1978; 298: 883-887.
2. Gaylin W, Glasser I, Marcus S, Bothman DJ. *The Limits of Benevolence*. New York: Pantheon Books. 1978.

To Care and Not to Care

J SC Med Assoc 1979; 75: 28-29

My prosperous businessman cousin leaned back from the Thanksgiving dinner table and opined: "The problem with medicine nowadays is that doctors are too scientific and don't seem to care about their patients and take the time to talk to them." I replied meekly that there are only so many hours in the day. Given the choice between the best scientific medicine and caring talk, I'd prefer to pay my doctor for the former. My health matters more than my doctor's sympathy. I went on to elaborate about some of the complexities of the doctor's many dilemmas — knowing all the while that my extroverted cousin would insist on the last word. He did.

In this issue of *The Journal*, Dr. Oliver Kepler discusses some of the problems of teaching human values to medical students. He met many frustrations in teaching an elective course, which had been designed to provide the students "more insight into themselves, their patients and the patient-doctor relationship." "The wonder of it all," Dr. Kepler tells us, "is that so many physicians do become caring and concerned practitioners and eventually lose most of their earlier cynicism."

Each of the points made by my cousin, and most of the issues raised by Dr. Kepler, were raised 51 years ago by Dr. Francis Peabody in his eloquent commencement address at Harvard Medical School. Peabody acknowledged the criticisms that medicine had become "too scientific" at the expense of compassion, that approximately one-half of patients who present themselves to physicians' offices bring with them symptoms for which no organic basis can be diagnosed, that medical training provides little foundation for dealing with many of the problems encountered, and that the treatment of a disease process differs from the management of a patient. Peabody's last sentence earned him literary immortality: "One of the essential qualities of the clinician is interest in humanity, for the secret of the care of the patient is in caring for the patient."[1]

Teachers with Peabody's insight and eloquence are rare. One such teacher, Dr. Philip Tumulty of The Johns Hopkins University School of Medicine, retired this year and, like Peabody, gave a commencement address which may linger on to inspire future generations. Beginning with the simple fact that the patient is, first of all, a person, Dr. Tumulty elaborates that the patient "is a very special kind of a person because he is a sick person." Few teachers have surpassed Tumulty's ability to enumerate the factors that contribute to effective patient management. Pertinent to caring in our era, this reminder by Dr. Tumulty stands out: "Such terms as primary care, secondary care or tertiary care are, in fact, meaningless. There is really a choice between only two kinds of care: good or bad, adequate or inadequate, complete or incomplete."[2]

Can caring be taught? Can a course aimed at conveying the principles of caring compete for the student's interest with rigorously scientific subject matter? Is it better to defer the lessons in caring to some later date in the physician's education — perhaps to the years of residency training, or perhaps to the trial and error of practice?

A great deal has been written about these issues. The acceleration of technology and of medical knowledge has made Dr. Peabody's famous passage seem simplistic. The decisions faced by today's physicians are often extremely multifacted. The thoughtful physician might, for instance, care considerably about whether to have his patient undergo computerized tomography as part of a headache workup. But will the patient actually appreciate the depth of the physician's thinking that went into the decision that the patient's (or more likely his insurance carrier's) money might be invested more wisely, since the headache is much more likely to represent tension than meningioma? Probably not.

Recently, a medical student wrote about the need for more scientific information about caring as part of the medical curriculum.[3] Arguing that "the notion that caring comes naturally to the physician in training is a fantasy," he went on to tell us:

Caring ... (now) carries different connotations and responsibilities from those of 50 years ago when Peabody wrote about it. One can no longer consider the caring role of the physician without pondering issues such as how medical care is delivered to the poor, or the wise use of increasingly expensive technology. Caring certainly includes the noble feelings expressed by Peabody, but it also encompasses the hard realities of equity and cost. A real danger in failing to provide education for caring is that too few physicians are trained to grapple with these latter issues.[3]

This author and others[4] agree that the notion of caring encompasses a number of aspects of human behavior that should be amenable to scientific study.

Surprisingly few who have written about caring in medical practice seem to have defined their word. The usual synonyms for "caring" would be "concerned" and "interested." A practical problem for the physician — given the limitations of his or her time — is that she must be genuinely concerned and convey this concern to the patient. Let us assume that a physician has only ten minutes to spend with a sick person before he must hurry to another commitment. Is it preferable to spend that time obtaining a crucial bit of scientific information — for instance, examining the peripheral blood smear, urine sediment, or sputum gram strain — or should he spend that time reassuring the patient and his relatives that everything possible is being done? If he chooses the former, he has probably done what is best for the patient's health but risks losing the patient's confidence. If she chooses the latter, she gains the patient's confidence for the moment, but knows that she has, in fact, not done her best work. The physician is in a classic double-bind situation. The sad truth is that there's just not enough time in the day to practice medicine without shortcuts.

Caring takes time. As Dr. Tumulty states, "Time personally spent with the patient is the most essential ingredient of excellence in clinical practice. There are simply no short cuts and no substitutions." A sad commentary of our era is that "caring time" is seldom if ever recognized by third party payers as an allowable charge. As a practicing internist puts it, "A system of physician compensation has developed in this country so that the less a doctor talks to you and the more he does to you the more he is paid."[5] One should not assume that the technical doers do not care. They often care a great deal, and their pride in technical excellence is certainly in the patient's best interest. One should not even assume that physicians who seldom if ever talk to patients don't care. I think especially of a famous surgical pathologist (the late Bill Shelley, who like Philip Tumulty was one of my teachers) who rarely saw patients, but could remember the names of the persons associated with his slides and bits of tissue years later. But we should insist that the considerable time needed for caring and conveying our sense of caring deserves some reimbursement (my businessman cousin was quick, after all, to place a monetary value on *his* time).

Finally, the notion of how to care appropriately deserves attention in the medical curriculum. How, for instance, should the student be taught to care for the patient with literally bottomless needs for human sympathy and compassion? Such patients, familiar to all physicians' offices, have the potential to drain their doctors' emotional and physical resources to the point that appropriate care for all of their patients becomes compromised. The professional person's caring demands some degree of detached objectivity.

Yes, Peabody's famous passage is a bit simplistic. Caring must be learned, and hopefully can be taught. At the very least, it should be modeled. Its limits require better definition. As T.S. Eliot put it in "Ash-Wednesday": "Teach us to care and not to care...."

References

1. Peabody FW. The care of the patient. *JAMA* 1927; 88: 877-882.
2. Tumulty PA. The art of healing. *Johns Hopkins Med J* 1978; 143: 140-143.
3. Rippe J. Caring and medical education. *Lancet* 1977; 1: 36-37.
4. Engel GL. The care of the patient: Art or science? *Johns Hopkins Med J* 1977; 140:222-232.
5. Fox M. Why people are mad at doctors. *Newsweek*; 10 January 1977: 4.

"Reverence for Life" — A Unifying Field for Ethical Decision Making?

J SC Med Assoc 1987; 83: 83-84

As for man, his days are as grass; as a flower of the field, so he flourisheth. For the wind passeth over it, and it is gone; and the place thereof shall know it no more.
— Psalms 103: 15, 16

The skilled gardener waters his grass and flowers until death and decay, the common fate of living things, become inevitable. Accepting this outcome, he begins to prepare the soil for next year's crop. The physician, reflecting the values of society, continues to nurture the dying patient long after it's plain to all of the caregivers that the patient no longer profits from his labors. We often hear that our nation's expenditures for health care are entirely unrealistic and that one-half of these expenditures take place in the final year of life, often for limited gain if gain is to be measured in terms of human happiness.

In this issue of *The Journal*, Dr. C. D. Bessinger, Jr., examines the concept of "reverence for life" as a unifying basis or "field" for ethical decision making. Taking his cue from Dr. Albert Schweitzer's *Philosophy of Civilization* (1923), Dr. Bessinger previously proposed that "reverence for life" applies not only to the care of the dying patient but also to the unborn patient, the proper use of scarce resources, corporate decision-making, and medical experimentation. He argued that "reverence for life does not yield to a generalized protocol" but rather "must be viewed as the field itself, in which clinical decisions are always formed in an attitude of 'sincere thought.'"[1]

In the present paper, Dr. Bessinger illustrates this concept with a specific case history. A child born with hydrocephalus underwent successful shunting but required life-long custodial care by his parents until death occurred at age twenty-nine years. The discussion revolves around the decision, two months prior to death, to place this patient on a ventilator and to administer intensive care. Dr. Bessinger argues the "the patient's condition had been acknowledged to be irreversible and progressive." At that point, the concept of "reverence for life" would have dictated that the dignity of the patient's remaining life be preserved but that ineffective and unnecessary interventions (presumably including placement of the patient on the ventilator) might best have been avoided.

In these two thoughtful papers, Dr. Bessinger seeks a unifying basis for resolving many of the difficult problems faced by clinicians and ethicists. He proposes the concept of "reverence for life" as an alternative to various other appeals to higher authority—such as *primum non nocere*, one or another specific oath, "laws of humanity," societal convenants, "boundary of the human," "community of values," "quality of life," utilitarianism, and situational relativism. In an editorial accompanying his first paper, Dr. Nora Bell, a philosopher, suggested that the discipline of medical ethics will assume increasing importance in medical schools and hospitals.[2] This is already becoming the case.

Dr. Bessinger's thesis should appeal to many persons who similarly seek a unifying principle for difficult medical decision making. Steeped in religious heritage and age-old truths, this concept or attitude has long colored the discussions between physicians and their patients or patients' families. Taken broadly, the concept of "reverence for life" might lead us to involve not only formally-trained ethicists but also (and perhaps most significantly) the clergy in these processes.

There remains the problem of how "reverence for life" should actually be utilized in day-to-day practice. However appealing the concept of letting go of life that has been largely used up, with limited potential for creative consciousness and happiness, in order to make room for new life, may seem in theory, there are strong ethical, emotional, and legal impediments to its use. The case described in this issue merely illustrates "what might have been done" rather than what was actually done for this specific patient. We see once more the potential for a family's financial ruination by medical care rendered with the full knowledge that the patient will never again enjoy the warm rays of the noonday sun.

We badly need a comfortable framework for thoughtful clinical application of age-old ethical, philosophical, and religious principles such as those skillfully articulated by Dr. Bessinger.

References

1. Bessinger CD Jr. Medical ethics and "reverence for life." *J SC Med Assoc* 1986; 82: 405-407.
2. Bell, NK: Health care's moral quandary (editorial). *J SC Med Assoc* 1986; 82: 411-413.

Peace and Good Will

J SC Med Assoc 1989; 85: 580-581

Among the blessings of the holiday season is the opportunity to set priorities for the coming year, to reflect on what really matters in our lives. Looking back on 1989 and looking forward to 1990, two observations give special meaning to this year's reflections.

Looking back, there was Hugo. The current volume of *The Journal* opened last January with a reminder by our association's president that South Carolina is a poor, small, and "very provincial" state — usually at or near the bottom in various national rankings.[1] It seems cruel and ironic that our state should have borne the brunt of the most costly natural disaster in the history of the United States. The hurricane's terrible capriciousness gave compelling proof that we are never in full control of our individual or collective destinies.

Looking forward, this year's holiday season marks the beginning of the last decade of the second millennium — A.D. (*Anno Domini*) or C.E. (Common Era), however one chooses to call it. Two thousand years might seem like a rather trivial span from the anthropologist's perspective that our species is some 4.5 million years old. Yet judging from the way things have been going lately, the prospects for another two thousand years do not seem especially bright for *Homo sapiens*. Within our lifetimes we have already seen the appearance of two unique and unprecedented threats to species survival: nuclear weapons and AIDS. We can anticipate that the nineties will be, among other things, a time for reevaluating our collective worldview.

In Hugo's wake, a substantial portion of South Carolina now seems makeshift. We have makeshift homes for some of our people, makeshift dunes for some of our beaches, and even makeshift shelters for endangered species such as the red-cockaded woodpecker. We might recall that *Time* magazine began 1989 by naming Earth "planet of the year" — a fragile planet assaulted on many fronts by twentieth century human activities.[2] We, like the red cockaded woodpecker, live within narrow parameters — parameters paradoxically threatened by scientific progress. Can we, as physicians, offer any special insights into how to make scientific progress somehow compatible with the long-range interests of humanity and of life on earth?

Perhaps. The most optimistic point of view, I suggest, is that put forward two years ago in *The Journal* by Dr. C. D. Bessinger, Jr., of Greenville: the concept of "reverence for life" as applied to our daily clinical practices.[3] Within this concept in mind, we have as physicians a unique opportunity to grapple first-hand with the tension between what might be called the scientific and the religious (in the very broadest sense) approaches to the human predicament. It may be useful to review briefly the history of this tension (Figure).

In Western thought, the tension arose on opposite shores of the Mediterranean in the ancient world. To explain nature's apparent order and purpose (*telos*), the Israelites turned to Yahweh. Meanwhile, Greeks such as Democritus and Aristotle turned to science. The uneasy truce forged by the early Christians, who wrote and thought in Greek, was consummated by

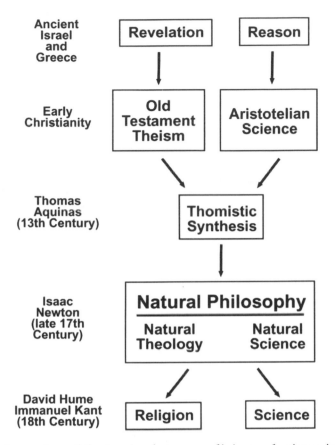

Ancient Israel and Greece	Revelation	Reason
Early Christianity	Old Testament Theism	Aristotelian Science
Thomas Aquinas (13th Century)	Thomistic Synthesis	
Isaac Newton (late 17th Century)	Natural Philosophy — Natural Theology / Natural Science	
David Hume Immanuel Kant (18th Century)	Religion	Science

A brief overview of the tension between religion and science in Western thought (see text).

St. Thomas Aquinas' brilliant synthesis whereby all of nature attests to the glory of God. Thomas Aquinas, it has been said, baptized Aristotle. Regrettably, the church failed to understand that science is a way of thinking, not a body of facts—a verb rather than a noun. Hence, the discrediting of scientific dogma was unacceptable and Galileo had to go. Sir Isaac Newton tried valiantly to bring all of knowledge back together but his argument ultimately failed. Today both physicists and molecular biologists attribute the smallest, most fundamental events to random chance—just as Democritus in ancient Greece had pre-

159

dicted would be the case. To an ever-increasing extent, science and religion have come to be viewed as separate, watertight compartments of human thought.[4]

Whatever our perspectives may be on the Big Question — the question of ultimate *telos* or First Cause — we should rejoice that as physicians we can combine these competing traditions on a daily basis. In no other profession is it so easy to practice what William Osler called *"philanthropia* and *philotechnia* — the joy of working joined in each one to a true love for his brother."[5] Today, we joyfully use such tools as lasers, nuclear magnetic resonance, and monoclonal immunoglobulins in daily medical practice. Simultaneously, the new science brings unprecedented ethical quandaries. Hence, in both areas (*philanthropia* and *philotechnia*), the challenges have never been greater nor more exciting. In perhaps no other profession is it so readily feasible to combine the two traditions by using, as Dr. Bessinger suggests, "reverence for life" as a unifying principle. In no other profession is it so feasible to lose oneself in the service of others and — in so doing — to teach by example, to instill the value of having values.

"Reverence for life" is not a passive quality, but rather an extremely active process. Its facilitating virtues include courage and humility. But to be effective, we must have a clear sense of priorities. For ourselves, for each other, and for our patients, the traditional salutation of the holiday season seems a good place to start. Peace on earth, good will towards men.

References

1. Rowland TC Jr. Lowest is best. *J SC Med Assoc* 1989; 85: 3.
2. Planet of the year: What on earth are we doing? *Time,* 2 January 1989.
3. Bessinger CD Jr. Reverence for life in clinical practice. *J SC Med Assoc* 1987; 83: 69-71.
4. Provine W. Scientists, face it! Science and religion are incompatible. *The Scientist,* 5 September 1988.
5. Osler W. The old humanities and the new science. *Brit Med J* 1919; 2: 8-33.

High Tech, High Touch

J SC Med Assoc 1990; 86: 114-115

We've heard it before and we'll hear it again: despite our technical progress we must not forget the healing role of the physician's personality. We must not allow medicine to become depersonalized. In this issue of *The Journal,* the Reverend Joe Baroody of Florence offers some well-reasoned and practical suggestions in his article,"Fast Medicine and High-Tech Healing." He reminds us that fast medicine reflects a fast society. People seek quicker, more efficient ways to do just about everything and often don't want close personal contact. A few observers suggest that high technology will eventually cause the end of the medical profession as we now know it.

For three reasons, I suggest that the situation is not nearly so bad as sometimes presented and that such pessimism is unwarranted.

First, the good old days weren't all that good. The Reverend Baroody begins his article by alluding to the ideals of William Osler extant around the turn of the century. We sometimes forget that these were only ideals. Osler's eloquence and charisma were matched by few even in his own day. By 1900, when Osler was in his prime, people were already bemoaning the decline of the wise, compassionate family physician. By 1915 affluent citizens in the larger cities usually preferred specialists.[1] Many people were already bemoaning the passing of "the good old timey physician who made house calls."

Even Osler is perhaps not an apt role model for most of us. As happens with many great men, we confuse William Osler the man with the ideals projected in his writings and by his many followers. Few of us enjoy what for Osler was a tremendous advantage: to have been the youngest son in a large and caring family. Now understood in Adlerian terms, this unique birthright enables its possessor to "read the vibes" and relate to others quickly, effectively, and humorously. It might comfort us to know that not everybody was pleased even by Osler's bedside manner.[2] We should also remember that Osler cautioned his students not to make definite diagnoses when they could not prove them and not to use drugs of dubious efficacy. I suspect that he would have gladly traded in his era for ours.

Second, the present isn't all that bad. Today's hospitals and physicians' offices are much friendlier and less imposing places compared to their predecessors of only a few decades ago. The increasing sophistication of our technology finds a parallel in the increasing warmth of the health care setting. We have piped-in soft music, warm colors, and—yes, soft and warm touch.

That the technical and humanistic aspects of medicine should develop in parallel is predictable. John Naisbitt called this parallel "high tech/high touch" in his best seller, *Megatrends*:

Whenever new technology is introduced into society, there must be a counterbalancing human response—that is, high touch—or the technology is rejected. The more high tech, the more high touch.[3]

Perhaps the most spectacular testimony to Naisbitt's premise has been the emergence of family medicine as a formal specialty. Several decades ago, as everyone talked about the potential for organ transplantation and open-heart surgery, it was widely predicted that general practice would soon be obsolete. Today, patients are gently guided through a maze of technology by a thriving new breed of family practitioners. The success of the family medicine movement illustrates how people still need the reassurance of "high touch" — and that we are providing it to an ever-increasing extent.

Third, the future looks bright. Our technology will give us still-better and safer diagnostic and therapeutic modalities. Yet we will be using much of the sophisticated technology in the outpatient setting and even in patients' homes. Patients who require hospitalization will be served by caregivers far better-trained than their predecessors to offer compassion and empathy. The rise of hospital pastoral care as a specialty within the clergy bears witness to this trend. Nurses, social workers, and many others understand the theory and practice of "high-touch" just as they appreciate "high-tech." But what about us?

This past holiday season, I was moved by two notes. One came in a book inscription: "Thank you for allowing me to die gracefully." She died Christmas Eve. The other came from parents whose son died five years ago: "We will never forget you and your kindness." In both instances I had stood by helplessly, with nothing to offer but compassion. Nobody wrote: "Thank you for your deft use of synergistic antibiotic combinations." Perhaps—just perhaps—our predecessors are remembered especially for their compassion because they so often had little else to offer.

Personally, I thank the Reverend Baroody not only for writing down his ABCs but also for forcing me to ask this question: which is more important, competence or compassion? I'm contemplating the issue now—as an editorial for the April issue of *The Journal.* Stay tuned.

References

1. Loudon I. The concept of the family doctor. *Bull Hist Med* 1984; 58: 347-362.
2. Harrell GT. Osler's practice. *Bull Hist Med* 1973; 47: 545-568.
3. Naisbitt J. *Megatrends: Ten Directions Transforming Our Lives.* New York: Warner Books, Inc.; 1982: 39-53.

Editorial Note. Looking back on this editorial 17 years later I recognize the seeds of what became a major research interest, namely the perceived tension between detached objectivity ("high tech") on the one hand and humanistic caring ("high touch"). This issue formed the basis, in part, of my distinction between a basic or generic professionalism ("Doing the right thing well") and a higher professionalism ("Service that clearly transcends self-interest").

The V-Word and the Four Cs

J SC Med Assoc 1990; 86: 259-260

My wife nearly always beats me at Trivial Pursuit® — on the entertainment questions, I'm helpless. Although I usually accept defeat gracefully, a recent game was played under protest. The question in dispute: "Name the cardinal virtues."

I knew the answer cold. There are four cardinal virtues: prudence, justice, temperance, and fortitude (courage).[1] First mentioned as such in Plato's *Republic*, these have been the cardinal virtues ever since. I also knew that Trivial Pursuit would probably give a different answer. It did: faith, hope, and charity (love). For the record, these are not the cardinal virtues, but rather the "theological virtues" mentioned a single time in the New Testament (I Corinthians 13:13). But who was I to argue with Trivial Pursuit? Point, set, match.

I forgive the authors of Trivial Pursuit for their error. One seldom hears "virtue" — the V-word — in polite conversation. Hardly anybody teaches "virtue" in the schools anymore. Even moral philosophers concede that constructing a virtue-based ethics (as opposed to results-based, duty-based, or rights-based ethics) has become a dubious enterprise. Following the lead of Alasdair MacIntyre[2] they tell us that it's now "after-virtue time." We can no longer even name the virtues, much less know what they are all about or how to teach them.

In the February issue of *The Journal*, the Reverend Joe Baroody of Florence offered us an excellent list of ABCs for improving our relationship with our patients. The essence of the Reverend Baroody's message was that in our age of sophisticated technology we must remember to be compassionate. Reflecting on his article in my editorial, I promised to provide some further thoughts on the following question: Which matters more, our competence or our compassion? Here goes.

As a serious issue, this question first struck me late one night during my residency. The patient was a frail, elderly woman with an acute myocardial infarction. She was going into shock, and we called a cardiologist. Entering the intensive care unit, having never seen the patient before, the cardiologist abruptly announced. Mrs. Jones, I'm Dr. Smith, and I'm going to put this catheter in your heart."

Now I suppose that many persons would criticize Dr. Smith (not his real name) on the grounds that his bedside approach epitomizes our profession's present-day shortcomings. Namely, we've made great strides in technical proficiency but along the way we've lost our human touch. Surely, Dr. Smith should have talked quietly with the patient, given a reassuring pat on the shoulder, and sought out her relatives in the waiting room before inserting the catheter.

I felt that way for a while, but I now disagree. I now feel strongly that Dr. Smith's first obligation to Mrs. Jones was to insert the catheter safely and competently. I now feel strongly that he would have done Mrs. Jones a disservice had any attempts to be "compassionate" detracted from his ability to rivet his attention on the technical problems at hand. I now feel, in retrospect, that it is best for me to assume that he was just as tired as I was late that night, and that he was wise to conserve his energies. The rest of us could reassure Mrs. Jones and talk to the family. That was our job.

This may seem harsh. However, I submit that this opinion is not only consistent with good medicine but is also consistent with the concept of "virtue" as applied to medicine. Namely, our first obligation to our patients is to perform competently that which we allow others to pay us to do. This may vary according to the nature of our specialty.

At one extreme, those reimbursed primarily for procedures do their patients a disservice to the extent to which "compassion" detracts from competent performance of those procedures. At the other extreme, those reimbursed primarily for rendering compassion (such as pastoral care-givers) do patients a disservice to the extent to which fascination with technology detracts from their ability to impart the human touch. The truly wonderful thing about medicine is that most of us most of the time can do both. But in striking a balance, we should always strive to do well the things people pay us to do.

The four C's? I would rank them in this order: (1) courage (which makes the others possible); (2) competence (which establishes credibility); (3) consistency (which ensures that competence will become reality); and (4) "compassion." On the one hand, "compassion" without competence at what one claims to be able to do is fraud. Robert M. Veatch notes: "Naked virtue can produce a messianic complex in those who are not really messiahs."[3] On the other hand, I submit that the consistent application of competence *is* compassion.[4]

As we gather for our annual meeting, we continue to hear criticisms of our profession from various quarters. Let's be positive. The secret of caring for the patient is to be able to do something for the patient and to do it well. And never before has it been possible to do so much for so many.

References and Note

1. Pieper J. *The Four Cardinal Virtues*. Notre Dame, Indiana: University of Notre Dame Press; 1966.
2. MacIntyre A. *After Virtue*. Notre Dame, Indiana: University of Notre Dame; 1981.
3. Veatch RM. Against virtue: A deontological critique of virtue theory in medical ethics. In: Shelp EE, ed. *Virtue and Medicine: Explorations in the Character of Medicine*. Dordrecht: D. Reidel Publishing Company; 1985: 329-345.
4. I would also hold that compassion is a facilitating virtue for courage and a motivating virtue for achieving competence. Hence, we have a feedback loop. Or, to quote Groucho Marx: "These are my principles ... and if you don't like'em, I've got others."

First Among the Cs

J SC Med Assoc 1990; 86: 461-463

In the February issue of *The Journal*, the Reverend Joe Baroody of Florence reminded us that high-tech medicine does not replace the need for compassion. Reflecting on this message, I promised to answer the following question: "Which matters more, our competence or our compassion?" In the April issue, I argued that while both are clearly important and necessary, competence at what we are licensed and paid to do should have top priority. In his letter to the editor in the current issue, my good friend Dr. Lawrence Jowers takes me to task. Caring, he argues, comes first.

I am convinced that our difference is more semantic than real. Only a misanthrope would suggest that we not exercise compassion at every turn. Still, I defend my position that for physicians qua physicians, competence comes first. I'll also still hold that applied competence *is* compassion, while compassion without competence is fraud. Nonetheless, I respect Dr. Jowers' point of view and acknowledge that I can defend the above positions only by taking recourse to extreme situations.

Consider a patient presenting to the emergency room after the abrupt onset of fever, headache, and stiff neck. The triage nurse can choose between two physicians. Physician A can be expected to curse and snarl; physician B can be expected to heap upon the patient layer after layer of compassionate concern. Physician A can also be expected to complete the lumbar puncture and have penicillin G dripping into the patient's veins within 20 minutes. Physician B can be expected to postpone the lumbar puncture until the CT scan has been completed and then—hours later—prescribe the wrong drug. If assigned to physician B, the patient will probably die of meningococcal meningitis. Physician C, known for both competence and compassion, is unavailable.

Choose between physicians A and B.

Still, I think that any difference between Dr. Jowers and me

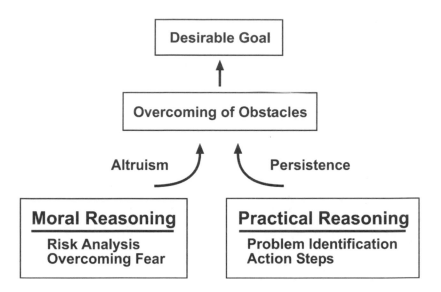

Courage, according to the Canadian philosopher Douglas Walton, involves both moral and practical reasoning to overcome obstacles toward the attainment of a socially desirable goal. Moral reasoning utilizes altruism as a facilitating virtue; practical reasoning utilizes persistence.

can be resolved by appealing to a higher court. In the April issue I ranked the four Cs as follows: (1) courage (which makes everything possible); (2) competence (which establishes credibility); (3) consistency (which ensures that competence will become reality); and (4) compassion. In a footnote, though, I noted that compassion can be an enabling virtue to both courage and competence. Let's consider the foremost of these virtues, the first among the Cs: courage.

What *is* courage? This problem has preoccupied moral philosophers for at least two millenia. Most of them have agreed that courage is not synonymous with bravery, nor does courage imply the absence of fear. Rather, courage requires consummate use of our ability to reason, to be rational in the face of uncertainty and danger. Aristotle held that the courageous act must also be a critically thought-out one. Thomas Aquinas

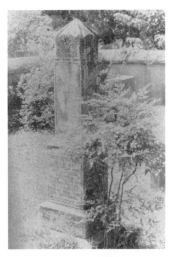
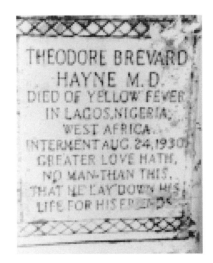

An obelisk in St. John's Episcopal Church, Congaree, South Carolina, marks the grave of Dr. Theodore Brevard Hayne (1898-1930), the last person to die of yellow fever while studying the disease. The same verse of scripture (John 15:13) occurs on other monuments to yellow fever victims (for example in the Martyrs Park in Memphis, Tennessee).

ranked prudence (or wisdom) first among the cardinal virtues since it so heavily influences the others. More recently, the philosopher Douglas N. Walton has argued for a concept of courage "like what the British call 'muddling through' — keeping one's head and doing a creditable job of deliberately acting sensibly and appropriately despite dangerous, painful, or very adverse circumstances."[1] Walton's analysis (Figure, preceding page) merits further consideration.

Taking his illustrations mainly from military anecdotes, Walton argues that courage is present when, through reasoning, obstacles are overcome to achieve a desirable goal. The courageous act requires two kinds of reasoning: moral reasoning to determine that the goal merits the risk and practical reasoning to design a plan of action. Note the presence of two facilitating virtues: altruism and persistence. Now we're getting somewhere!

In or near Columbia stand two monuments in memory of South Carolina physicians. Both were born in small towns;

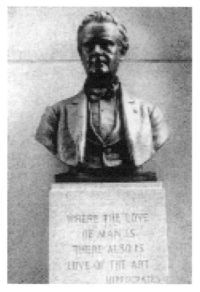

A monument to the memory of Dr. J. Marion Sims (1813-1883), whose discovery of a cure for vesicovaginal fistula paved the way for modern operative gynecology, stands on the South Carolina State House grounds at the corner of Gervais and Assembly Streets. The inscription is attributed to Hippocrates: "Where the love of man is, there also is love of the art [of medicine]."

both became fired with ambition to contribute to medical science. One succeeded and became famous; the other did not. Both displayed enormous courage, in quite different ways.

In the northwest corner of a country churchyard in Congaree, S. C., stands an obelisk in memory of Dr. Theodore Brevard Hayne.[2] Fascinated by mosquito-borne infectious diseases, Hayne took a position with the Rockefeller Foundation in Lagos, Nigeria, to study yellow fever. Four previous Rockefeller investigators had died. Hayne knew the risk. He pressed forward with his research even after discovering dwarf variants among his broods. A French journalist recently wrote: "The ultimate courage is the willingness to sacrifice our own existence. It is that rock on which all other possible kinds of courage can be based."[3] Theodore Brevard Hayne, M.D. *Altruism*.

In the northwest comer of the statehouse grounds stands a monument to Dr. J. Marion Sims, founder of modern operative gynecology. Vesicovaginal fistula had been the great stumbling block to further progress in women's surgery. The stories of how Sims visualized the fistula and devised sutures that held have been told many times. Not so frequently told, though, is the record of how many times he failed—and kept on trying.

For four years, he kept at his own expense a small infirmary in his backyard and operated over and over again on its three occupants. Colleagues lost interest; relatives pleaded with him to focus on his family instead. It was on the thirtieth operation on a woman named Anarcha that he succeeded. The rest is history. James Marion Sims, M.D. *Persistence.*

Courage should permeate not only what we do as physicians, but also the entire doctor-patient relationship. One moral philosopher calls courage "a virtue for physicians in addition to the excellences of competence and compassion and a virtue for patients in addition to the excellences of compliance and gratitude."[4] But reflecting further on the monuments to Hayne and Sims, one picks up a common word—more powerful than any we have discussed so far. And it is here, Dr. Jowers, that our views can be reconciled. The word is of course *love.*

In Hayne's case, the saying comes from scripture: "Greater love hath no man than this that he lay down his life for his friends" (John 15:13). In Sims's case, it's attributed to Hippocrates: "Where the love of man is there also is love of the art." Love—first among the theological virtues—thus embraces both competence and compassion. In the last analysis, it is the main thing, perhaps the only thing, we have to offer. As physicians or as anything else.

Thank you, Reverend Baroody, for stimulating these musings. And thank you, Dr. Jowers, for your objections. And if any of you readers out there disagree with either of us, let's hear from you!

References

1. Walton DN. *Courage: A Philosophical Investigation.* Berkeley: University of California Press; 1986.
2. Bryan CS. Eulogy written in a country churchyard (editorial). *J SC Med Assoc* 1988; 84: 94-95.
3. Servan-Schreiber J-L. *The Return of Courage.* Reading, Massachusetts: Addison-Wesley Publishing Company; 1987: 82.
4. Shelp EE. Courage: A neglected virtue in the patient-physician relationship. *Soc Sci Med* 1984; 18: 351-360.

The Duties of Patients: A Distant Mirror

J SC Med Assoc 1998; 94: 79-80

*The patient, who believes in a kind and all-merciful Provi-
dence, and possesses an unshakable fortitude and strong vital
energy and who is laid up with a curable form of disease, and
is not greedy, and who further commands all the necessary
articles at his disposal, and firmly adheres to the advice of his
physician, is a patient of the proper or commendable type.*
— Sushruta-Samhitá, ? fifth century B.C.E.

Excerpts of the Code of Medical Ethics adopted by the American Medical Association in 1847 and endorsed by the South
Carolina Medical Association at its first meeting in 1848 appear
in this issue. A large portion of this document would be considered "etiquette" rather than "ethics" as the latter discipline
is now understood. Yet many of the issues are timeless. They
reflect not only the highest ideals of medicine as a beneficent
calling but also the nuances of how flawed human beings relate to each other during encounters freighted with peril and
uncertainty.

Of special interest is the section on "the duties of physicians
in regard to Consultations" (section 1, article 4). Consultations
back then were a far cry from what we know today. Physicians
usually had similar training; there were no formal residencies
or fellowships. Therefore, today's usual reason for consultation — the need to obtain an opinion from a physician in another
specialty — did not apply. Egos were on the line. Consultations
were carried out by prior arrangement in the presence of the attending physician, who took the lead in demonstrating the history and physical examination to the consultant. The consultant
then questioned and examined the patient, and the two physicians retired "to a private place for deliberation." These discussions were to be kept strictly confidential. The consultant's
opinion was then presented to the patient in the presence of

the attending physician. Formal rules governed the resolution of differences of opinion. Reading between the lines, we sense the uneasiness captured in the mot that "a consultant is someone who doesn't answer the question but steals your patient." Reputations were at stake.

Also of interest is the section on "obligations of patients to their physicians." How one might enforce such obligations, then or now, is left unclear. However, this section offers what might be called a "flip side" to the Samaritan contract—the need for the care recipient (patient) to respect the rights and needs of the caregiver (health care provider). An update of this section might read somewhat as follows:

• Check out your doctor's qualifications. Did he complete an approved residency? Is she board certified? In medicine, the authors noted, "the world ought not to suppose that knowledge is intuitive."

• Check out your doctor's local reputation. Is medicine his main interest or does his life revolve mainly around his hobbies and social standing? The authors recommended a physician "whose habits of life are regular, and who is not devoted to company, pleasure, or to any pursuit incompatible with his professional obligations."

• Don't be reluctant to consult your doctor about seemingly-minor problems. The authors observed that trivial signs might in fact be "the forming stage of violent diseases." This desideratum translates into the desirability of a good relationship with one's primary care physician.

• Tell your doctor what you think is causing the problem. The patient "should never be afraid of thus making his physician his friend and adviser." Trust your doctor to maintain confidentiality. If you're concerned about confidentiality, tell her that, too, since she can't do her best unless she knows what you know.

• Be concise. Remember that your doctor is on a schedule and that he has other patients waiting. Thus, "a patient should never weary his physician with a tedious detail of events or matters not appertaining to his disease." Think about what you want to say in advance and try to give your doctor an edited version.

• Follow your doctor's prescriptions and advice to the letter.

Doctors call this "compliance." The "Sig:" on their prescription forms literally means "take that." If you have reason to doubt the wisdom of your doctor's prescriptions or advice, be frank and negotiate with her. Don't try to fool your doctor.

• Don't self-medicate without your doctor's knowledge. A surprisingly large portion of medical problems, including life-threatening conditions, stems from taking over-the-counter drugs or wares gathered from health food stores or "alternative medicine" advisers. The authors of the 1847 code advised patients to "never allow themselves to be persuaded to take any medicine whatever, that may be recommended to them by the self-constituted doctors and doctresses, who are so frequently met with, and who pretend to possess infallible remedies for the cure of every disease."

• Don't "doctor-shop" without your doctor's knowledge. Serious problems can arise when patients receive prescriptions and advice from different physicians without their knowledge. The authors urged the "great importance that physicians should act in concert; for, although their modes of treatment may be attended with equal success when employed singly, yet conjointly they are very likely to be productive of disastrous results." Also, beware of drug interactions.

• If you decide to leave your doctor for another doctor let him know this. If freely asked, your doctor will probably tell you that he knows he's not the best doctor for everybody. You always have the perfect right to choose someone else. But remember that she probably cares about you (whatever you might think!), and therefore "justice and common courtesy require" that you tell your doctor why you're dismissing him.

• When possible and practical, be considerate about when and where you consult your doctor. It's best to start early in the morning by calling her secretary and asking when she's available. Remember that your doctor is usually on a tight schedule. And, since he's human too, avoid calling "unnecessarily during the hours devoted to meals or sleep."

• Express appreciation. Doctors, like everyone else, relish sincere positive feedback. Even in a world grown cynical, most doctors like to believe that theirs is a higher calling, that they see medicine as a way to serve their fellow humans beyond their self-interests. Therefore the patient "should, after his recovery, entertain a just and enduring sense of the value of the services rendered him by his physician: for these are of such a character, that no mere pecuniary acknowledgment can repay or cancel them."

Good advice, indeed! And should we physicians not similarly respect the rights of those in other walks of life? Whatever their shortcomings, our forebears certainly knew the ramifications of the Golden Rule!

Y2K.4. Virtues and Values

J SC Med Assoc 2000; 96: 276-279.

The philosopher's school, sirs, is a physician's consulting room.
　　　　　　　　　　　—Epictetus

For the first time in medical history, self-interest has been given legal and moral legitimation and profit has been turned into a professional virtue. These trends are making the physician into a businessperson, an entrepreneur, a proletarian, a gatekeeper, and a bureaucrat. Never has there been more confusion about who and what it is to be a physician.
　　　　—Edmund D. Pellegrino and David C. Thomasma[1]

To resume our meditations on medicine in the new millennium, will the profession survive as we have known it? I'm optimistic that the medical profession can and will survive, indeed that it will soon be stronger than ever. However, this will require collective action and a renewed sense of identity. What is missing, what needs to be restored, is agreement on a common set of principles. Call it what you will: code, credo, manifesto, or — better still but use it carefully and advisedly — virtue.

The jeremiad of the recently-retired that "I entered a profession and I left a business" is hardly new. People in many walks of life have been saying this for centuries. What is new for medicine in the United States is the massive intrusion of third-party payment systems and large-scale bureaucracies. Yet what is also new, I submit, is a small but definite groundswell of enthusiasm for returning to certain basic principles or virtues.

There is, to be sure, a widespread opinion that virtue is an outmoded concept in today's society. The philosopher Alasdair McIntyre suggests that we've made the virtues obsolete, that we've lost our concept of morality, and that we would do well to focus on duties, goals, or rights rather than virtues.[2] Physicians, attorneys, businesspeople, and just about everyone else can easily argue that virtues and ethics are fine in theory but impossible to follow in a competitive, free-market, and highly bureaucratic society. Yet there are signs that people are thinking about virtue again, if perhaps not by that name.

"Virtue" generally means "moral excellence or righteousness," but it is a highly-charged word to be used hesitantly if at all in everyday conversation. Originally derived from the Latin *virtus*, which meant "manliness" or "valor," the meaning of virtue has mutated over time and indeed there is a massive body of literature known as virtue theory. Pellegrino and Thomasma divide the history of virtue into four periods:
• The classical-medieval period, during which virtue was central to all moral philosophies.
• The post-medieval and modern period, during which other systems of moral philosophies emerged with the result that virtue, although still important, was reshaped.
• The positivist-analytical period, during which both ethics and also traditional normative (rule-based) ethics declined; and
• The present, in which efforts are being made to resuscitate virtue as a basis for behavior.

Some Landmarks in the History of Virtue Theory

Author	Date	Synopsis
Homer	Ninth century B.C.E.	Holds virtues to be those qualities that enable an individual to fulfill his or her social role (for example, to excel at war [Odysseus] or homemaking [Penelope]).
Sophists	Fifth century B.C.E.	Teach that virtues can be explained by reason alone; that they are essential to the use of power; and that they can be taught.
Plato	427?-327? B.C.E.	Defines four virtues (now the cardinal virtues): wisdom (prudence), justice, temperance, and fortitude (courage). Views virtue as knowledge (*Episteme*) of the excellence (*aretê*) inherent to the good life.
Aristotle	384-322 B.C.E.	Suggests that virtues are means between opposite extremes, and can be equated with character. Believes that virtues can be taught. Distinguishes between the intellectual and the moral virtues.
Stoics	308 B.C.E. through the second century C.E.	View virtues as conformity with the laws of nature. Emphasize benevolence and duty. Take the position that virtue is its own reward — not just a means to power and the good life.
Saint Paul	5?-67? C.E.	Posits (in 1 Corinthians 13:13) what are later called the "theological" virtues: faith, hope, and charity (love).
Saint Ambrose of Milan	339?-397	Becomes the first to call the Greek virtues the cardinal virtues (from cardo, "hinge") and suggests three Christian virtues: fear of God, love of God, and resemblance to God.

Author	Date	Synopsis
William of Auxerre	1150?-1231	Calls Plato's four virtues "the cardinal virtues" and becomes the first to call faith, hope, and charity (love) "the theological virtues."
Saint Thomas Aquinas	1225-1274	Characterizes the cardinal virtues as mental habits that can be acquired by acting repeatedly in the same way (*habitus acquisitus*) and the theological virtues as traits acquired by grace (*habitus infusus*). Ranks wisdom (prudence) the highest of the former and love the highest of the latter.
Machiavelli	1469-1527	Expresses cynicism about the survival value of virtue. Considers proper virtue to be primarily *viri* (manliness), an expression of power rather than a disposition to act according to what is right and good.
Thomas Hobbes	1588-1679	Denigrates the virtues as taught by Judaism and Christianity as the virtues of slaves and emasculated weaklings.
Benjamin Franklin	1706-1790	Carries out a self-improvement program based on daily monitoring of 17 virtues, selected from among the various lists of virtues available to him.
Ayn Rand	1905-1982	Exalts selfishness as a virtue; opines that altruism is actually dangerous.
G.E.M. (Elizabeth) Anscombe	1919-2001	In 1958, points out the limits of ethics founded solely on duty (deontology) and results (consequentialism), urging that virtue, character, and the emotions must be taken into account.

Author	Date	Synopsis
Alasdair MacIntyre	Contemporary	In 1981, publishes *After Virtue* in which he distinguishes between inner goods and external goods. Virtuous practices constitute inner goods reflecting an end (*telos*) that transcends particular practices.
Bernard Williams	Contemporary	In 1985, publishes *Ethics and the Limits of Philosophy* in which he argues that ethics — as a wider subject than morality (which is concerned primarily with rules) — must take into account psychological considerations such as emotions.
Numerous contemporary philosophers and psychologists		Debate the substance and meaning of virtue theory, often from the perspective of Aristotle, Nietzche, or other philosophers.

Let us briefly review some highlights of this checkered history (Table).

Certain pre-Socratic philosophers known as Sophists spoke of *aretê* necessary for worldly success and claimed that they could teach it. Aretê had many nuances; it could mean virtue as a moral concept but could also mean excellence in anything, manliness, fame, success, or even divine power. Plato, in *The Republic* and elsewhere, had a great deal to say about the virtues of which he recognized four: wisdom (prudence), justice, temperance, and courage (fortitude).

Aristotle equated virtue with character and, like the sophists, held that virtue can indeed be taught in the sense that it is a habit that can be developed with practice. Dating back to Homer, all of the major Greek philosophers and writers viewed the virtues as a set of qualities that help the individual discharge his or her role in society. Their virtues are sometimes called "masculine" as they promote such heroic ideals as courage and patriotism.

Enter Christianity. St. Paul (1 Corinthians 13:13) spoke of faith, hope, and love (or charity) — virtues that are sometimes called "feminine," promoting the gentler side of humanity. Compassion as a virtue was embraced by the later Stoic philosophers, who influenced one Scribonius Largus, a Roman of the first century A.D. (or C.E.) who may have been a physician. Scribonius vigorously promoted a then-obscure document now known as the Hippocratic Oath; he was possibly the first to call medicine a profession as opposed to a trade; and he insisted that medicine required not only technical competence but also sympathy (*misericordia*) and humane feeling (*humanitas*).[3,4] The twin pillars of love of humanity (*philanthropia*) and love of technology (*philotechnia*) became firmly-entrenched in medicine's self-image.

Later philosophers affirmed the concept of two complimentary sets of virtues. William of Auxerre (1150?-1231) was apparently the first to call St. Paul's virtues (faith, hope, and love) the "theological virtues" and Plato's virtues (wisdom, justice, temperance, and courage) the "cardinal virtues." Thomas Aquinas proposed that the cardinal virtues are mental habits that can be acquired by acting repeatedly in the same way (*habitus aquistus*) while the theological virtues are acquired through divine grace (*habitus infusus*). Aquinas taught that love (or charity) ranks highest among the theological virtues, while wisdom (or prudence) ranks highest among the cardinal virtues. Love and wisdom bring order to their counterparts. Love, compassion, or charity (call it whichever you like) informs the cardinal virtues and is essential to the practice of medicine.

So far, so good. Isn't this just a long way of saying what most of us told the medical school Admissions Committee: "I like science and I want to help people"? Problems enter when one starts to question the relevance of these virtues to worldly success.

Machievelli argued that his prince could not be virtuous and powerful at the same time in a world where other princes are not virtuous. Taking up that line of reasoning in the twentieth century, Ayn Rand exalted the virtue of selfishness and this idea has taken hold in much of society. We honor power and wealth, not goodness. Serious, important, and influential moral philosophers such as Robert Veatch and H. Tristram Englehardt argue that rules are more relevant than virtues in an era characterized by (1) high technology and (2) the frequent brief convergence of the lives of doctors and patients mainly because of their shared interest in technology. Enter rules, exit virtues.

Why, then, am I optimistic about the virtues in medicine? Here are three reasons.

First, there is growing emphasis at multiple levels on such topics as listening skills, ethics, professionalism, and sensitivity to the human condition. These topics now receive more time in medical schools, more space in medical journals, more attention at meetings. And a common term for these topics is "virtue" in the Aristotelian sense of ingrained habits. The "good doctor" does not necessarily have all the right answers to thorny ethical dilemmas, but he or she will consistently hold dear such basic values as human rights, equality, and freedom.[5] Medical schools increasingly emphasize these values under the rubric of "professionalism" and underscore the importance of appropriate role models.[6]

Second, more and more women are entering medicine. Inevitably, this will infuse into medical education and practice what is commonly called "feminist psychology."[7] To be a successful physician, one will need to become, among other things, a better listener. There will be more and more dialogue about virtues pertaining to medicine,[8] and we will understand them better.

Finally, I believe that we will come to appreciate more and more the importance of viewing medicine as a moral community. Our potential is huge and largely-untapped. Pellegrino and Thomasma comment:

Without in any way depreciating what is being done by many conscientious individual physicians and their organizations, the full spectrum of our obligations as a moral community are yet to be fulfilled. Medicine has yet to use the tremendous moral power it possesses for good. To do so, it must act collectively in certain ways.[9]

Act collectively! Does this sound familiar?

References

1. Pellegrino ED, Thomasma DC. *The Virtues in Medical Practice.* New York: Oxford University Press; 1993: 154.

2. McIntyre, A. *After Virtue: A Study in Moral Theory.* 2nd ed., Notre Dame, Indiana: University of Notre Dame Press; 1984: 2.

3. Ferngren GB, Admundsen DW. Virtue and health/medicine in pre-Christian antiquity. In: Shelp EE., ed. *Virtue and Medicine: Explorations in the Character of Medicine.* Dordrecht, The Netherlands: D. Riedel; 1985: 3-22.

4. Pellegrino ED, Pellegrino AA. Humanism and ethics in Roman medicine: Translation and commentary on a text of Scribonius Largus. In: Barondess JA, Roland CG, ed. *The Persisting Osler-II. Selected Transactions of the American Osler Society 1981-1990.* Malabar, Florida: Krieger, 1994: 21-34.

5. Shelton, W. Can virtue be taught? *Acad Med* 1999; 74: 671-674.

6. Kopelman LM. Values and virtues: How should they be taught? *Acad Med* 1999; 74: 1307-1310

7. Gilligan C. *In a Different Voice: Psychological Theory and Women's Development.* Cambridge, Massachusetts: Harvard University Press; 1982.

8. Beauchamp TL, Childress, JF. *Principles of Biomedical Ethics.* 4th ed., New York: Oxford University Press; 1994.

9. Pellegrino ED, Thomasma DC. *The Virtues in Medical Practice.* New York: Oxford University Press; 1993: 45.

Medicine and the Seven Basic Virtues
I. Introduction

J SC Med Assoc 2005; 101: 280-284

*The modern world, obsessed with liberty, has slain virtue,
leaving us morally bereft, in a world of darkness.*
— Amitai Etzioni

For nearly 20 years I've harbored a harmless obsession: To teach everyone within earshot what I call "the seven basic virtues." Patient readers of *The Journal* possibly recall a story I told on myself in the April 1990 issue concerning a game of Trivial Pursuit® with my wife, Donna. She usually wins. I can get most of the way around the board but when it comes to questions in the Entertainment category I'm helpless, having spent most of my adult life as a nerd. On that particular evening, however, I was within one answer of a stunning upset. Donna read the question: "What are the three cardinal virtues?" I knew the cardinal virtues cold. I'd recently read a monograph on them by the German theologian Josef Pieper. Yet I suspected the answer on the reverse side of the card might be wrong, since there are four cardinal virtues, not three. It was. The card gave: "Faith, hope, charity." Those, my friends, are not the cardinal virtues.

Since that game of Trivial Pursuit, I've asked many people including occasional large audiences to name the cardinal virtues. Few can. Even learned theologians, historians, and philosophers (unless they happen to be especially interested in virtue theory) fumble. A gentleman from New Orleans once got it right and told me that most of his fellow citizens know them because they're inscribed around the base of an enormous monument in Metarie Cemetery that greets visitors approaching the Crescent City on Interstate 10. I therefore asked my New Orleans friends Bo and Julia Sanders to photograph the monument for me, which they did — fortuitously on my birthday, January 15, 2005. The gentleman who knew the answer had evidently not been to the cemetery recently, for the monument's base contains only the surname of the deceased, "Moriarty." It seems that a Mr. Daniel Moriarty and his departed (and much older) wife had been snubbed by New Orleans Society. Mr. Moriarty had the 85-foot-tall monument (possibly the tallest private monument in the United States) built in her memory so that she would tower over everybody else. According to the New Orleans Bureau of Tourism, Mr. Moriarty asked for statues of "the four graces" to adorn the monument's base. When told that there were only three of them he insisted on a fourth. Thus, Mr. Moriarty and also the New Orleans Bureau of Tourism got it wrong.

Here's the correct answer. The four cardinal virtues are prudence (wisdom), justice, temperance, and fortitude (courage). They were first elaborated by Plato in *The Republic*. The other three—faith, hope, and charity (love)—come from St. Paul (1 Corinthians 13:13) and are commonly known as the theological virtues or, as I prefer to call them, the transcendent virtues. A few generations back, I suspect that most people could name the cardinal virtues. Now, just about nobody knows them.

The reader might ask, why focus on these particular seven virtues? The question whether the essential virtues are few or many is an old one, dating back at least to Plato's dialogue, *Meno*, in which a character by that name challenges Socrates on this issue. Through the years, many have sided with Meno. Benjamin Franklin, for example, selected for his self-improvement project 17 virtues from lists circulating during the eighteenth century. William J. Bennett's *The Book of Virtues*, a recent best seller, lists 10 virtues starting with self-discipline.[1] André Comte-Sponville's *A Small Treatise on the Great Virtues*, another best seller, lists 18 virtues starting with politeness.[2] Most recently, however, two leaders of the positive psychology movement, Christopher Peterson and Martin E. P. Seligman, conclude that across all cultures and political persuasions there are six clearly recognizable clusters of character strengths. These are: wisdom and knowledge (read: prudence [wisdom]), justice, temperance, courage, transcendence (read: faith and hope), and humanity (read: love).[3] Thus, we come full circle. We have seven basic virtues, as enumerated by Plato and St. Paul, now substantiated by scholars working under

184

the imprimatur of the American Psychological Association. Today there is much talk about "values," especially "family values." What do we mean by "values," and how do they differ from "virtues"? For the purpose of this and subsequent editorials, I offer the following short definitions of some highly nuanced words:

• *Virtues*: Excellences that enable us to achieve what is good for society and for oneself.

• *Values*: Determinations of what constitutes the good, informed by virtues.

• *Morals*: Determinations of what constitutes right and wrong, informed by values.

• *Ethics*: Disciplined reasoning about right and wrong in problem cases, informed by virtues, values, and morals.

In recent decades there has been a surge of interest among professional philosophers and psychologists in a field of inquiry known as virtue theory. "Virtue ethics" is usually seen as a supplement to the two prevailing ethical theories: deontology (Kantianism), based on duties and rules; and consequentialism (for example, utilitarianism), based on sensitivity to specific situations. My purpose in this series of editorials is to offer some perspectives on how these seven basic virtues — wisdom, justice, temperance, courage, faith, hope, and love — apply to the practice of medicine.

References

1. Bennett, WJ. *The Book of Virtues: A Treasury of Great Moral Stories.* New York: Simon & Schuster; 1993.
2. Comte-Sponville A. *A Small Treatise on the Great Virtues: The Uses of Philosophy in Everyday Life.* New York: Henry Holt and Company; 1996.
3. Peterson C, Seligman MEP. *Character Strengths and Virtues: A Handbook and Classification.* New York: Oxford University Press; 2004.

Medicine and the Seven Basic Virtues
II. Prudence (Practical Wisdom)

J SC Med Assoc 2005; 101: 329-331

On the day that Jeannette Mangels, our managing editor, reminded me that this editorial was overdue, my first patient was a teenager accompanied by an understandably anxious mother. While vacationing two months earlier, the young woman had sustained an extensive laceration caused by a boat propeller. A month later she underwent excision of necrotic tissue with skin grafting to the affected lower extremity. A culture revealed *Vibrio alginolyticus*. My examination confirmed that the wound had been expertly treated; she was for all intents and purposes cured. However, the mother had a list of questions. How could we be sure that there were no more *Vibrio alginolyticus* organisms in her tissue? How could we be sure that the problem would not recur? How could we be sure that she would not lose her leg?

Having never before encountered *Vibrio alginolyticus*, I checked it out in the latest infectious diseases textbook and also did a MEDLINE search. This organism causes serious problems for various marine animals but is much less pathogenic for humans than its cousins, *Vibrio vulnificus* and *Vibrio parahemoyticus*. I found only two case reports of its causing necrotizing fasciitis in humans. Neither report emanated from the United States and both were in rather obscure journals. As it turned out, the mother already knew all this. She'd done a computer search herself. Indeed, she'd found on the Web photographs of the two patients described in the medical literature. I looked again at her list of questions. Obviously, I had no way to prove that every last *Vibrio alginolyticus* organism had vanished from her daughter's body. What I had to offer — my epistemic authority in this matter — was not based on information but rather on perspective. I could offer clinical judgment. Wisdom.

"Prudence" was once synonymous with "wisdom," which explains its prominence in the virtue vocabulary. From its Latin root, *providencia*, prudence literally means foresight, "to see ahead," to anticipate the consequences of our actions or inactions. Prudence has three components: (1) to gather the facts, (2) to reason based on information from the facts, and (3) to outline a plan of action that serves a good purpose. Prudence (wisdom) is essential to the other virtues because it informs them as to the right course of action. Without it, justice endorses cruelty, temperance promotes fanaticism, courage invites foolhardiness, faith fosters intolerance, hope lacks guidance, and love courts disaster. Plato and most other philosophers have ranked prudence or practical wisdom first among the cardinal virtues because only the prudent person can be just, temperate, and wise. Moreover, we are good only to the extent that we are prudent and wise. As Samuel L. Clemens (Mark Twain) put it, "Always do right. This will gratify some people and astonish the rest."

By "prudence" today we often mean avoidance of unnecessary risks and dangers. In this limited sense, prudence is for humans what instinct seems to be for animals. However, the word "prudence" has all but disappeared from most people's moral vocabulary because of such Victorian connotations as "timid," "overly cautious," and "not much fun to be around." About the only people who use it regularly are stockbrokers, who invoke the Prudent Man Standard for managing other people's money. Here's my own working distinction between "prudence" as this word is now used and other forms of wisdom: It pays to be prudent, but not wise, in one's own estimation. Prudence correlates with observable traits that are within our control and self-appraisal. These include being organized, thorough, conscientious, practical, and deliberate—all highly desirable for the practice of medicine. However, observers other than we ourselves are better positioned to determine, on the basis of long-term consequences, whether our decisions, judgments, or advice rendered in the face of uncertainty represent "wisdom."

Plato identified three categories of wisdom. These were:

- *Sophia* — the wisdom of philosophers and others who spend

187

much of their time contemplating the truth ("philosophy" literally means love of this type of wisdom).

• *Phronesis*—the practical wisdom of the statesman and the lawgiver, a type of wisdom that, resisting the urges of the passions and the deceptions of the senses, seeks a prudent course of action.

• *Episteme*—the wisdom of scientists and others who study the nature of things and the principles that govern them.

Here, we are concerned mainly with the second of these categories (phronesis) because it applies to all of us, not just philosophers and scientists. Aristotle discussed phronesis, as he did the other virtues, as a middle course between two extremes. On the one hand, we must oppose impulsive surrender to appetites and desires when these conflict with long-term best interests. On the other hand, we must oppose over cautiousness, "paralysis by analysis." Wisdom, as distinct from factual knowledge, entails making sound and beneficial judgments in the presence of uncertainty.

A website maintained by the American Psychological Association defines wisdom as "expertise in the fundamental pragmatics of life." To be a virtue in the strict sense, however, wisdom is incompatible with cunning, guile, plotting, insidiousness, wiliness, sneakiness, trickery, and other synonyms for self-interested scheming. This observation goes against the grain of much conventional wisdom about how to get ahead in the world. Machiavelli advised his prince: "You must realize this: that a prince, and especially a new prince, cannot observe all those things which give men a reputation for virtue, because in order to maintain his state he is often forced to act in defiance of good faith of charity, of kindness, of religion.... He should not deviate from what is good, if that is possible, but he should know how to do evil, if that is necessary."[1] A recent book entitled *The 48 Laws of Power* written in the spirit of Machiavelli includes the following chapter titles: "Get others to do the work for you, but always take the credit," "Play a sucker to catch a sucker—seem dumber than your mark," "Discover each man's thumbscrew," and "Strike the shepherd and the sheep will scatter."[2] I suspect that the incompatibility of true goodness

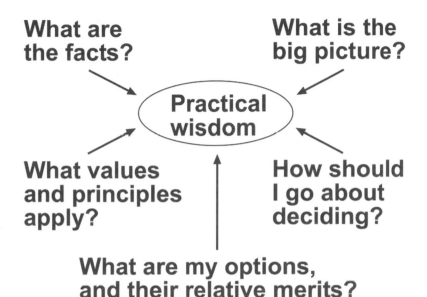

What are the facts?

What is the big picture?

Practical wisdom

What values and principles apply?

How should I go about deciding?

What are my options, and their relative merits?

Wisdom criteria for making a difficult decision in the face of uncertainty. It is proposed that the soundness of the decision usually depends on the extent to which these five questions are addressed (after Baltes and Smith[3]).

with commonly used ways to get the better of others explains, at least in part, the expression, "Virtue is its own reward." Wisdom as a virtue in medicine demands that we manage conflicts of interest and obligation. Wisdom as a virtue in medicine demands that we strive constantly to put the patient's interest above our own.

Can wisdom be quantified? The short answer is no. However, two Berlin psychologists, who define wisdom as "good judgment and advice about important but uncertain areas of life," suggest that wisdom can be evaluated by a family of five types of knowledge criteria (Figure). These are: (1) rich factual knowledge, both general and specific, about the conditions of life and its variations; (2) rich procedural knowledge, both general and specific, about how to go about finding advice and making judgments; (3) rich knowledge about the various contexts and about the relationships between them; (4) rich knowledge about the differences between competing values, goals, and priorities that come into play; and (5) knowledge about the relative unpredictability of various courses of action."[3] Wisdom in the practice of medicine requires good judgment that takes into account not only the relevant science but also the healing powers of nature and the healing powers of the physician's personality.[4]

How can we best foster wisdom in an era of technology-drive consumerism in which patient expectations and market forces often conspire to treat medical services like any other commodity? I offer three suggestions, none of them original.

First, *frame the scenario*. Strive to consider each clinical encounter within the context of the patient's entire life situation. Strive to honor the patient by acknowledging his or her individual worth, his or her contributions to society. Strive to see the big picture. Ask, "What is the very worst thing this could be?" Ask also, "Is this problem acute, or does it permit sorting things out with Tincture of Time?" If the answer to the latter question is yes, consider close follow-up as an alternative to ordering every conceivable laboratory test, imaging study, or invasive procedure.

Second, *think and document your thought process*. I especially like a charting format employed by my hospital's emergency room. The physicians are asked to document their thought processes under the header, "Medical Decision Making." All of us are vulnerable to missing the correct diagnosis on account of faulty reasoning. A recent reviewer lists five pitfalls:[5]

• Judging by recalling past or similar cases ("availability heuristic"), which can be corrected by bringing legitimate statistics to bear ("When you hear hoof beats in a barnyard, think of horses, not zebras").

• Relying on first impressions ("anchoring heuristic"), which can be corrected by looking for new data or by asking yourself for your own second opinion ("If this patient should die unexpectedly, what would be the likely cause of death"?).

• Being swayed by subtle wording ("framing effects"), which can be corrected by examining the case from different perspectives ("Let's play devil's advocate here...").

• Being unduly influenced by authority or technology ("blind obedience"), which can be corrected by keeping in mind the possibility that all authorities and technologies are fallible.

• Taking a narrow-minded approach ("premature closure"), which can be corrected by returning to the problem when your mind is refreshed, time permitting ("What is the one diagnosis I don't want to miss here?").

Evolving areas include the extent to which we should include and document ethical reasoning and emotional reasoning in our clinical decision making.

Finally, *cultivate humility*. We recall that Socrates claimed to be wise only to the extent that he at least knew that he knew little or nothing for sure.

Let's return to the case with which we started. I explained to the mother that I was 99.99% confident that her daughter was rid of *Vibrio parahemolyticus*. I told them that if it came back I wanted to be among the first to hear about it. I explained to them my opinion that they'd received expert care. I tried to empathize with them for all they'd been through. I also empathized with the daughter about being in the seventh grade, telling her that it's difficult for everybody but that she'd get through it just fine. I told her she could be anything she wanted to be including a long distance runner. Were they satisfied with the consultation? Did I come across as wise? I'll never know.

References

1. Machiavelli, N. *The Prince*. George Bull, translator, London: Penguin Books; 1981: 101.
2. Greene, R. *The 48 Laws of Power*. New York: Penguin Books; 2000.
3. Baltes PB, Smith J. Toward a psychology of wisdom and its ontogenesis." In Sternberg RJ, ed. *Wisdom: Its Nature, Origins, and Development*. Cambridge: Cambridge University Press; 1990: 87-120.
4. Szawarski Z. Wisdom and the art of healing. *Medicine, Health Care & Philosophy* 2004; 7: 185-193.
5. Redelmeier DA. The cognitive psychology of missed diagnoses. *Ann Intern Med* 2005; 142: 115-120.

Medicine and the Seven Basic Virtues. III. Justice

J SC Med Assoc 2005; 101: 388-390

During the 1980s and early 1990s, the HIV/AIDS epidemic thrust my cohort of infectious diseases specialists onto center stage. There were relatively few of us—we were the first wave of physicians to sit for the board examination in this newly recognized subspecialty—and we had much in common. Most of us were in our thirties or early forties when the epidemic struck. We fancied ourselves as idealists (we had, after all, chosen a relatively low paying subspecialty), but in truth most of us did not want to preside over the deaths of patients with long, drawn-out illnesses. We did not want to be oncologists making daily rounds on cancer patients. We did not want to be nephrologists spending hours in dialysis units. We did not want to be pulmonologists with their lobbies full of "pink puffers" and "blue bloaters." We wanted to be pure consultants, doctors' doctors. We wanted to be called in for difficult problems, make brilliant diagnoses, and then give the patients back to the referring physicians. HIV/AIDs changed our practice patterns and indeed our lives. We found ourselves caring for promising young people doomed to early deaths. We made house calls. We dealt with disturbing emotional issues. We tried to reassure the public. As the patients kept on coming and dying, most of us suffered burnout. Some of us went broke. Others changed jobs. I took an administrative position and reduced the size of my clinical practice.

Looking back, we were privileged to live through what amounted to a truncated history of medicine, compressed between 1981 and 1996. In 1981, when the first cases occurred, we were clueless. As my medical school classmate Donna Mildvan (the first to describe AIDS in New York City) put it, we were thrown back to medieval times. In 1996, when highly active antiretroviral therapy (HAART) became available, we could suddenly treat the disease successfully using the latest tools of molecular biology. With a single blood sample, measuring the patient's CD4 lymphocyte count and HIV-1 viral load, we could stage the disease better than oncologists can stage malignancies even after exploratory surgery. By sequencing the genome of the patient's virus, we could determine exactly which drugs to use. The disease had become "medicalized." During those early years, my self-doubts revolved around whether I was giving my patients sufficient empathy and compassion. It's Sunday afternoon—should I play golf or watch a football game on television, or should I drive 30 miles to a neighboring town to visit one of my patients whom I'll probably never see again? Today, my self-doubts revolve mainly around whether I'm using the best combinations of drugs. This summer, all 15 of my private patients on therapy for HIV, some of whom I've followed as far back as 1987, were living normal lives with high CD4 counts and undetectable viral loads. Incredible![1]

In 1993, I wrote a grant for Ryan White Title II funding for HIV/AIDS patients in central South Carolina, thus launching the Midlands Care Consortium. Undetectable viral loads are the exception rather than the rule among the 1,000-odd patients who now attend this clinic. Why? Federal and state funding makes HAART available for them. Theoretically, they should therefore do just as well as my private office patients. The problem lies beyond the clinic walls, beyond the reach of molecular biology and the new drugs. To sum it up in a single word, the problem is "socioeconomic." The demography of HIV/AIDS in South Carolina, as elsewhere, has changed dramatically. Newly-infected patients are typically poor, sometimes homeless. They've had very tough lives. Kathryn Whetten of Duke University, who has written an engaging book entitled *"You're the First One I've Told": New Faces of HIV in the South*,[2] points out that most of these patients have endured conditions that are almost inconceivable to us, the privileged. Her initial data indicate that 7% grew up with one or both parents in prison, 10% had been in foster care, 17% had seen a family member killed or maimed in a crime, 43% had seen someone killed or seriously injured, and most had some combination of inadequate housing, inadequate employment, and inadequate transportation. Thus, while HIV/AIDS holds center stage in the lives of the patients seen in private practices, for the disadvantaged it's usually "just one more dang thing to deal with."

I recently heard from a visiting professor a fine definition of social justice: "vigilance against systematic disadvantage." So many people in our society, including most of the patients in our Ryan White clinic, suffer from what the professor calls "densely woven patterns of systematic disadvantage." What exactly do we mean by "justice"? Is ours a "just" society?

Justice among the four cardinal virtues is unique in that it is a good thing by itself, not just a means toward something else. The other three—prudence (wisdom), temperance, and courage—are worthwhile only as handmaidens to other desirable goods. Justice is intrinsically good because it insists on fairness between and among individuals who, left to their own devices, usually behave selfishly. Aristotle called justice "the greatest of the virtues," adding that "neither evening nor morning star" is so wonderful. Cicero suggested, "Good men are so called chiefly from their justice." Yet perfect justice however prized in theory proves elusive in practice. The great trial lawyer Clarence Darrow said, "There is no such thing as justice—in or out of court." Whenever my children, when they were young, complained that something was unfair, I told them: "Life's not fair. Robins eat worms—that's unfair to the worms."

In medicine, justice is unique in that it's included both among the four cardinal virtues and also among the four principles of medical ethics as put forth by Beauchamp and Childress (the others being beneficence, nonmaleficence, and autonomy). Our legal system takes as its premise that justice requires continual refinement—hence, the accretion of law based on layer upon layer of legislative and judicial decisions. Also, we consider ourselves liberals, moderates, or conservatives based largely on our opinions of what constitutes justice.

Some claim that we are born with an innate sense of what is "just" or "moral." Others appeal to a "State of Nature" whereby people, left to their own devices, conclude that certain behavioral restrictions are to their own best interests. But how do we extend these notions of justice to those who are not more or less like us? How would we act toward a band of Martians

194

that dropped in friendly and smiling but carrying dangerous-looking weapons? The philosopher Alasdair MacIntyre wrote a book entitled *Whose Justice? Which Rationality?*[3] MacIntyre contends that our ideas about justice are highly dependent on the tradition to which we happen to belong. We are prisoners of the paradigms of our particular cultures.

Three basic types of justice correspond to the three basic relationships of our life together:
• The relationships between individuals (reciprocal, or mutually exchanged justice; also known as compensatory or commutative justice).
• The relationships of individuals to the social whole (legal justice; also known as rectificatory justice)
• The relationships of the social whole to its individuals (distributive justice; also known as ministering justice).

The first of these (reciprocal justice) embraces all that we call the "physician-patient relationship" which has, alas, now morphed into the "physician-patient-society (read: insurance carrier) triad." Reciprocal justice impels us to be honest, to be fair, and to practice the Golden Rule or, even better, the Platinum Rule (Do unto others as they themselves would like to be treated).

The second category (legal justice) embraces the rules, regulations, and legal remedies that apply to medical practice, reference being made to a recent editorial in these pages.[4]

The third type is the most problematic. How can we best assure that everyone not only has access to optimum health care but also benefits from it? Clearly, and as illustrated by so many patients with HIV/AIDS in South Carolina today, this problem transcends the practice of medicine.

Just allocation of health care resources is problematic especially in the United States and, unfortunately, largely overlooked by group practice arrangements and by health plans.[5] Nonetheless, we spend more per capita on health care than any other nation in the world and it's rare for even the poorest citizens to be deprived of life-saving interventions, at least in acute situations. Yet sober reflection suggests that we as a society tend to throw money at health care without commensurate benefit to individual lives. In my three-plus decades of practice in Columbia, S.C., I've been impressed that, year after year, the construction cranes hover around the hospital complexes more than anywhere else. Social critics suggest we've made our hospitals temples of excellence in an otherwise failed society. In my humble opinion, the cranes should cluster mainly around the public schools, not the hospitals. We should do everything possible to improve everyone's standard of living, their ability to enjoy and contribute to life, their good citizenship, and healthy lifestyles. Dating back to the Old Testament prophets, sages have held that the gap between rich and poor constitutes the best measure of the extent to which a society is just. Recent data suggest that current preoccupation with "evidence-based medicine" diverts our attention away from the social and cultural determinants of health, directing us instead to technical matters that may be of little relevance to the disenfranchised.[6]

Individually, there's not much we can do about these overarching inequities that so badly affect our patients. Collectively — well, I remain sufficiently idealistic to believe that we as physicians can indeed make a difference. In a prosperous society that is also a just one, a rising tide raises all boats. Organized medicine has a distinguished, if imperfect, history of promoting justice in health care, and we should do everything within our power to advance this cause.

References

1. Bryan CS. HIV/AIDS and bioethics: Historical perspective, personal retrospective. *Health Care Analysis* 2002; 10: 5-18.
2. Whetten-Goldstein K. *"You're the First One I've Told": New Faces of HIV in the South.* New Brunswick, New Jersey: Rutgers University Press; 2002.
3. MacIntyre A. *Whose Justice? Which Rationality?* Notre Dame, Indiana: University of Notre Dame Press; 1988.
4. Bryan CS. Advancing medical professionalism. V. The social contract, and why tort reform is essential. *J SC Med Assoc* 2005; 101: 47-49.
5. Berkman ND, Wynia MK, Churchill LR. Gaps, conflicts, and consensus in the ethics statements of professional associations, medical

groups, and health plans. *J Med Ethics* 2004; 30: 395-401.

6. Rogers WA. Evidence based medicine and justice: A framework for looking at the impact of EBM upon vulnerable and disadvantaged groups. *J Med Ethics* 2004; 30: 141-145.

Medicine and the Seven Basic Virtues.
IV. Temperance

J SC Med Assoc 2006; 102: 22-24

Temperance among the cardinal virtues is the most observable. It takes forming an opinion to decide whether someone is wise, just, or courageous. It takes only paying attention to determine that someone abuses potentially dangerous substances, eats to the point of gluttony, talks boorishly without listening, behaves promiscuously, disobeys traffic regulations, dresses ostentatiously, or fails to observe moderation in pursuit of wealth, possessions, amusement, or fame. Moreover, temperance understood as self-control is unique among the cardinal virtues in that its frame of reference consists only of the person in question. However, "temperance," like "prudence," has been trivialized since Victorian times. Temperance has a wider meaning if we understand it as a virtue that helps us steer between behavioral extremes, for example between cowardice and foolhardiness. In everyday usage, we often assign to "temperance" its narrowest meaning, restraint in the use of alcoholic beverages, as epitomized by the Temperance Movement and its most celebrated participant, Carrie Nation.

Among my dearest friends I'm proud to claim Earl F. Nation, a retired urologist now living in Sierra Madre, California who, at the time of this writing, is 95 years of age. Earl is a giant among his colleagues—he's made numerous scholarly contributions, been president of the American Urological Association, and once numbered the rich and famous of Pasadena and Hollywood among his patients—but he is not a large man physically. This observation helps substantiate his claim that he bears no genetic relationship to Carrie Amelia Nation (1846-1911), whose second husband was one of Earl's distant relatives. Nearly six feet tall and weighing somewhere between 170 and 180 pounds, Carrie Nation bursting into a saloon with her hatchet and entourage of angry women must have been a formidable sight indeed. The great heavyweight champion John L. Sullivan once ducked into hiding when Carrie Nation crashed into a bar.

She was born Carry Amelia Moore—"Carrie" was misspelled "Carry" in the family Bible. Her first husband, a physician named Charles Gloyd, was drunk at their wedding and died from alcoholism six months later leaving her pregnant with child. Later, having lost her job and needing a means of support, she married David Nation, a lawyer, minister, and newspaper editor who was nineteen years her senior. They soon discovered they had nothing in common. She became increasingly bitter. As Earl Nation puts it, she "was against alcohol, tobacco, sex, politics, government, the Masonic Lodge, William McKinley, Theodore Roosevelt, and William Jennings Bryan, in approximately that order." Her assaults on saloons began in 1880 in Kansas, where prohibition had been approved by the voters but was not being enforced. She single-handedly destroyed the bar in the Hotel Carey, the most elegant in Wichita, smashing the liquor bottles, a $1500 Venetian mirror, and an enormous nude oil painting of *Cleopatra at the Bath*. Becoming a celebrity overnight, she changed the spelling of her name back to "Carry," believing that as "Carry A. Nation" she had been divinely ordained, "a bulldog running at the feet of Jesus, barking at what He doesn't like." Divorced by Mr. Nation, repeatedly arrested and jailed, she supported herself by lecturing, publishing newspapers entitled *The Smasher's Mail* and *The Hatchet*, selling souvenir hatchets, and writing her autobiography, *The Use and Need of the Life of Carry A. Nation*. She died in 1911. In 1924, the Carry A. Nation Association erected for her grave a monument inscribed, "Faithful to the cause of Prohibition. 'She hath done what she could.'" She would have approved, having once said: "I never saw anything that needed rebuke, exhortation, or warning, but that I felt it was my duty to meddle with it."

The story of Carrie Nation is in some ways risible, but one cannot deny that the Temperance Movement of which she was a part accomplished much good. It is the rare person today who does not know first-hand of a life destroyed by alcohol or other potentially dangerous substances. We should likewise note that the so-called Seven Deadly Sins — pride, greed, envy, anger, lust, gluttony, and sloth — are in the main breaches of temperance. Temperance is a virtue not to be treated lightly.[1]

"Temperance" comes from the Latin *temperantia*, which means "moderation." In classical antiquity there were four broad concepts of temperance, as follows:

• *Sophrosyne*, which, freely translated, meant a "soundness of mind" including psychological well-being.

• *Moderation*, including not only "moderation in all things" but also and more specifically moderation of emotional responses.

• *Temperantia*, understood as a virtue toward a "proper mixture" and thus regulating appetites and desires.

• *Social manner*, including a sense of decorum, seemliness, modesty, balance, and restraint when in the company of others.

Aristotle defined temperance as "a mean with regard to pleasures," adding that the appetites of a temperate person "should harmonize with the rational principle." The Latin verb, *temperare*, means in essence "to dispose various parts into a single unified and ordered whole." We, too, use the verb form in everyday speech: for example, "to temper one's enthusiasm,"

199

or "to temper one's emotions."[1-3]

Most of us understand temperance as self-control—the ability to monitor and manage our emotions, desires, and actions without calling for help. Psychologists studying self-regulation stress the importance of delayed gratification. People with high self-control consistently see the long view, the larger picture. They avoid overindulgences of all sorts because of dangers lurking down the road. Some psychologists offer cybernetic theory as an alternative to self-regulation therapy. In cybernetic theory, one compares oneself against a relevant standard. If one falls short of the standard, one looks for ways to correct the deficiency. These two approaches are clearly complementary.[4]

Concepts advanced by Abraham Maslow, the father of today's humanistic psychology, offer another perspective on temperance. According to Maslow, we have certain basic needs: physical needs, sexual needs, ego needs, esteem needs, and so forth. Maslow calls these "deficit needs," things that need to be satisfied before we can progress up the higher rungs of the ladder. The highest plane, which he calls "being needs," consists of self-actualization, "being all you can be." According to Maslow, few people, far below 5% of the population, ever reach this higher plane of "self-actualization" (Figure 1). To what extent must we satisfy the various lower order needs before moving onward and upward? Maslow agreed with the psychiatrist Viktor Frankl that self-actualization occurs in relationship to the people and circumstances around us as a call to service that transcends self-interests. Frankl and others have expressed this concept as "self-transcendence."[5-6]

The challenge as I see it is to set limits to our deficit needs. Early satisfaction of lower-order needs assures the self-preservation requisite to moving up the needs hierarchy toward self-transcendence. We can argue this point from either a religious perspective (for example, from the Gospels, from the works of St. Augustine and St. Thomas Aquinas, or from the lives and works of ascetics and members of religious orders) or from a secular perspective (from the Stoic philosophers of antiquity to contemporary psychologists). How much is enough?

Making money, amassing wealth, is for better or worse a

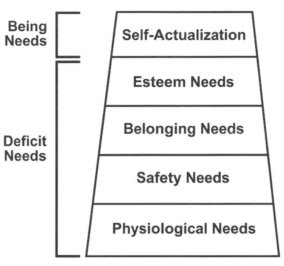

Figure 1. *According to Abraham Maslow's famous needs hierarchy, we must address lower deficits before ascending to the higher "being needs" or self-actualization, a level obtained by few.*

defining feature of our society. Many maintain that we in the United States, lacking any form of hereditary aristocracy, have created a pseudo-aristocracy based on wealth—that is, a plutocracy. Money and possessions establish the value we are inclined to place on others and, sadly, ourselves. Does money buy happiness? A Google search of "income and happiness" yields a large literature on this correlation. Many researchers have asked large numbers of people two questions: (1) "Do you consider yourself very happy, somewhat happy, or not too happy?" (2) "How much money do you make?" Sure enough, high incomes increase the likelihood of reporting "very happy" and reduce the likelihood of reporting "not too happy." However, after an income of about $110,000 a year (2006 dollars), additional income buys little additional happiness (Figure 2). Beyond a certain income level, happiness depends mainly on things money can't buy such as health, family, friends, outside interests, and spiritual enrichment. It depends less on financial statements, high-priced possessions, and lavish lifestyles.[7]

All this being said, what's the significance of the virtue of

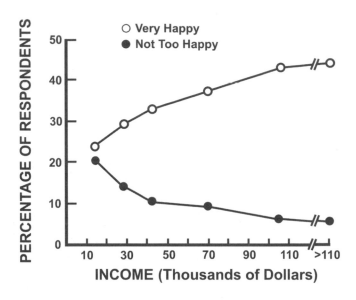

Figure 2. *Correlation between reported annual income and responses to the question, "Do you consider yourself very happy, somewhat happy?" Higher incomes correlate with increased happiness. However, the happiness increments become relatively small beyond an annual income of about $110,000 (based on data from Bok[9], updated to 2006 dollars according to the Consumer Price Index).*

temperance for us physicians? While a full discussion would far exceed the scope of this article,[8] my top three suggestions are as follows.

First, we should value the simple and temperate life. We should set reasonable limits to our deficit needs. We should remember why we chose medicine in the first place: to serve.

Second, we should value temperance as a facilitating virtue between behavioral extremes. We should pay attention, for example, to how we balance technical preoccupation with empathic concern for the patient. We should pay attention to how we balance overaggressiveness with caution (or, in the terms of bioethics, the oft-competing principles of beneficence and nonmaleficence).

Finally, we should help our fellow citizens set reasonable limits on the utilization of medical resources. It's been said that we Americans are "addicted to addiction." It's becoming increasingly and painfully obvious that society simply cannot afford all things for all people. And it's on this final point that the efforts of organized medicine can and indeed should make a difference.

References

1. Pieper J. *The Four Cardinal Virtues*. Notre Dame, Indiana: University of Notre Dame Press; 1966: 145-147
2. Aristotle. *The Nichomachean Ethics*, translated by D. Ross. Oxford: Oxford University Press; 1991: 72-78
3. Carr MF. *Passionate Deliberation: Emotion, Temperance, and the Care Ethic in Clinical Moral Deliberation*. Dordrecht, The Netherlands: Kluwer Academic Publishers; 2001: 15-46.
4. Peterson C, Seligman MEP. *Character Strengths and Virtues: A Handbook and Classification*. New York: Oxford University Press; 2004: 38.
5. Maslow AH. *Motivation and Personality*. Second edition, New York: Harper and Row, 1970.
6. Hoffman E. *The Right to be Human: A Biography of Abraham Maslow*. Los Angeles: Jeremy P. Tarcher, Inc.; 1988: 256.
7. Bryan CS. Medical professionalism and Maslow's needs hierarchy. *Pharos* 2005; 68 (2): 4-10.
8. Pellegrino ED, Thomasma DC. *The Virtues in Medical Practice*. New York: Oxford University Press; 1993: 117-126.
9. Bok D. *The Cost of Talent: How Executives and Professionals are Paid and How it Affects America*. New York: The Free Press; 1993: 230.

Medicine and the Seven Basic Virtues.
V. Courage

J SC Med Assoc 2006; 102: 134-135

Two splendid recent biographies illustrate aspects of courage in the doctor-patient relationship. My friend Michael Bliss of Toronto gives us a richly detailed portrait of Harvey Cushing, founder of neurosurgery. Although Cushing does not come across as an especially likeable man, we marvel at the courage it took to perform more than 2,000 operations for brain tumor with nothing remotely resembling today's CT and MRI scans to show him where to cut—and the courage of the patients to undergo the procedures![1] Walter Bonner, who is variably associated with Charleston, Mt. Pleasant, and his beloved McClellanville, gives us an intimate portrait of the doctor-patient relationship in his chronicle *A Doctor's Toughest Case: A Girl, a Disease, a Medical University*.[2] We marvel at the courage demanded of Bonner and his patient, the late Dianne Lewis, as they strove to stare down systemic lupus erythematosus, the red wolf, back in the 1970s. Yet the call for courage in medicine today transcends the doctor-patient dyad as portrayed by Bliss and Bonner. Increasingly, we are challenged to do the right thing in a complicated corporate environment, an environment in which conventional wisdom (that is, "common sense") often urges us to back down, to compromise our principles. Let's first say a word about courage as it's understood by philosophers.

Courage among the cardinal virtues is the most universally admired. It's the stuff of myths and legends, the inspiration for the best stories. Courage denotes acting in the face of vulnerability, putting us at risk in an area that matters such as life, health, reputation, or socioeconomic well-being. Sir Winston Churchill, probably paraphrasing Samuel Johnson, ranked courage first among the cardinal virtues because it makes the others possible. Courage serves the other cardinal virtues (wisdom, justice, and temperance) like a pivot or hinge. However, courage gains its status as a virtue only when informed by prudence and justice. Courage also requires temperance, to steer between the extremes of rash bravery (foolhardiness) and reluctance to act (cowardice).

If courage is indeed the most universally admired cardinal virtue, why do most virtue theorists rank it behind prudence, justice, and even temperance? I find at least four explanations. First, courage is difficult to define. All attempts to define courage from Plato to the present have drawn harsh critics. Second, moral philosophers have traditionally placed most of their emphasis on duty. Courageous actions are problematic for philosophers because they are by definition above and beyond the call of duty. Third, we sometimes see courageous actions performed by people who in other respects don't seem especially virtuous. Finally, cultural context conditions our recognition of courage and its opposite, cowardice. For example, the fifteen 9/11 hijackers were called cowards by many Americans but courageous heroes by their supporters.

Plato rendered one of the earliest accounts of courage, separating valor from rashness. In one of his dialogues he quotes Socrates as having said that "thoughtful courage is a quality possessed by a few," whereas "rashness and boldness, and fearlessness which has no foresight, are very common qualities." It is for this reason that St. Thomas Aquinas and others considered prudence (practical wisdom) the first among the cardinal virtues, with courage (fortitude) subordinate to it. It is immediately apparent, however, that both prudence and courage are essential to whatever we do. To use a simple example, prudence tells us to get out of bed each morning but it's courage that enables us to do it. Thus, the French philosopher André Comte-Sponville says: "All virtue is a form of courage and all virtue is a form of prudence."[3]

My favorite definition of courage is that of the Canadian philosopher Douglas N. Walton, who defines it essentially as the overcoming of obstacles by both moral and practical reasoning to achieve a socially desirable goal.[4] Moral reasoning requires altruism as its facilitating virtue, while practical reasoning requires persistence. We determine what needs to be done and calculate that the potential gains warrant the risk to ourselves through moral reasoning, facilitated by altruism. We decide how to do it and resolve to keep up our efforts despite potential pain and setbacks through practical reasoning, facilitated by persistence. "Courage" comes from the Latin *cor* meaning "heart." "Fortitude" figures heavily as a synonym for courage in virtue talk because "courage" was not in common usage when Thomas Aquinas classified the virtues during the thirteenth century. "Fortitude" comes from the Latin *fortus*, which means "strong" or "powerful." However, neither courage nor fortitude presumes overwhelming strength or power. We can exercise courage and fortitude only when we are vulnerable in one or more areas of well-being. These include health and physical security, serenity (peace of mind), and financial or social standing. Most people agree that the willingness to die for a just cause constitutes the ultimate test of courage.

Walton's definition of courage resonates with the three principal types of courage: *physical courage* (overcoming fear of injury or death in order to benefit others or oneself), *moral courage* (overcoming the risk of losing one's job, prestige, privacy, or friends in order to maintain one's ethical integrity and authenticity), and *psychological courage* (overcoming one's own inner demons in order to confront a bad situation, habit, or illness). Medicine has always required physical courage. The HIV/AIDS pandemic and the more recent outbreaks of SARS (severe acute respiratory syndrome) remind us that we sometimes risk death during routine patient care. Medicine has always required psychological courage to render service to distressed fellow humans especially when we don't have all the answers. However, it's my impression—shared by many others—that medicine increasingly requires substantial moral courage to stand up for what's best for others, not only our patients but also our fellow physicians and other health care workers, in an era in which traditional professional values are assailed from many directions.

As physicians we commonly find ourselves deciding not only "what's best for this patient" but also "what's best for my organization," be it a group practice, a hospital-based practice, or society at large. In 1993, Drs. Edmund Pellegrino and David

Thomasma wrote:

> To act courageously in … an environment of "corporate
> medicine" will become more and more difficult. There is
> increasing demand for physicians who are "team play-
> ers," people who can function well in the environment
> of HMOs and corporate structures. Being a team player
> does not necessarily preclude acting with courage. Yet it
> does diminish the likelihood that individual physicians
> … will speak out courageously about inequities or on
> behalf of patients when the necessity arises.[5]

Numerous examples could be cited, but the one that I find most distressing is the pressure to give in to "groupthink," whereby members of a group place greater value on solidarity, unanimity, and their own self-righteousness than on objective appraisal of the available data. How else can we explain the fierce rivalries bordering on hatred that erupt all too frequently between competing physician groups and competing hospitals, especially in larger communities? How else can we explain the apparent paucity of peacemakers among us? Courage, like the other cardinal virtues, contains many dimensions but at its core consists of serving others despite personal risks. George Bernard Shaw wrote: "It is courage, courage, courage that raises the blood of life to crimson splendor." Or, as Dad put it: "Son, just do the right thing and don't worry about it."

References

1. Bliss M. *Harvey Cushing: A Life in Surgery*. Toronto: University of Toronto Press; 2005.
2. Bonner W. *A Doctor's Toughest Case: A Girl, a Disease, a Medical University*. Charleston, South Carolina: History Press; 2005.
3. Comte-Sponville A. *A Small Treatise on the Great Virtues: The Uses of Philosophy in Everyday Life*. New York: Henry Holt and Company; 1996: 50.
4. Walton DN. *Courage: A Philosophical Investigation*. Berkeley: University of California Press; 1986.
5. Pellegrino ED, Thomasma DC. *The Virtues in Medical Practice*. New York: Oxford University Press; 1993: 112 n.

Medicine and the Seven Basic Virtues. VI. Faith

J SC Med Assoc 2006; 102: 348-349

Having previously considered the four cardinal virtues (wisdom, justice, temperance, and courage), we now take up the three transcendent (theological) virtues: faith, hope, and love. Writing about the transcendent virtues in a secular setting is somewhat risky. When Sir William Osler wrote that "nothing is more wonderful than faith," he could just as well have said that "nothing is more controversial." My purpose in writing sketchy accounts of faith, hope, and love is to demonstrate how general frameworks for understanding these virtues might apply to the daily practice of medicine.

Faith among the transcendent virtues receives first mention because it is after all the principal subject of religious thought and doctrine. "Faith" is most commonly understood as a synonym for "belief." St. Paul famously defined faith as "the substance of things hoped for, the evidence of things not seen" (Hebrews 11:1). A physician-scientist of my acquaintance expresses the same idea more cynically: "Faith is belief without data." I have lived my adult life convinced that "faith" and "belief" are by no means identical. In brief, "faith" embraces belief but is a much larger and more complicated construct. A mature faith system, at least in my own partial understanding, includes belief, doubt, awareness of the transcendent, responsible relationships with one's fellow humans, and, above all, an abiding trust that things will eventually work out for the best (Figure).

My favorite definition of faith, indeed my favorite definition of any kind, is this one given in 1920 by a theologian and biblical scholar named Kirsopp Lake. Lake wrote: "Faith is not belief in spite of evidence, but life in scorn of consequence—a courageous trust in the great purpose of all things and pressing forward to finish the work which is in sight, whatever the price may be."[1] The notion that faith engages and holds in tension both belief and doubt was, however, stated most clearly by the great theologian Paul Tillich. Defining faith as a state

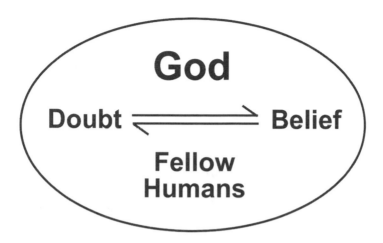

My concept of a "faith system" as opposed to a "belief system." Faith is understood not only as ultimate concern toward God (or the Ground of Being) and personal destiny (the threat of non-being) but also as "preliminary concerns" toward fellow humans. Put differently, faith relates to (1) the transcendent, expressing trust in the great purpose of all things, and (2) the here-and-now, guiding actions aimed toward making the world a better, safer place for one's own time and for future generations.

of "ultimate concern," Tillich wrote: "If faith is understood as belief that something is true, doubt is incompatible with the act of faith. If faith is understood as being ultimately concerned, doubt is a necessary element in it. It is a consequence of the risk of faith."[2] The opposite of religious faith, Tillich suggests, is not doubt but rather indifference to the dilemma of what it means to be a finite human being.

Let us now consider faith in the secular sense. What do we mean by patients' "faith in doctors" or "faith in modern medicine"? What do we mean by our own faith that what we're doing for patients is in their best interests? Referring to the figure, it would seem obvious that we must (1) have some reason to believe that we're doing the right thing; (2) maintain at least a measure of doubt, a healthy-minded, ever-questioning attitude of mature skepticism; and (3) relate all that we do not only to our fellow human beings in the here-and-now but also, at an abstract level, to trust in "the great purpose of all things."

Edmund D. Pellegrino and David C. Thomasma clarify the relationship of faith to medicine as follows:

Faith orients the healer to the way in which the practice of healing becomes charitable healing.... Faith keeps before the healer his or her ultimate end and that of the patient. Faith restrains the hubris technology so easily engenders in today's physician or nurse.... Faith restores hope, even in the face of an incurable illness, not because cure of the illness is less a good but because faith promises more than cure.

They add: "Faith is also the spiritual compass we need in the face of the moral and ethical dilemmas of modern medical practice."[3]

In the remaining editorials in this series, we'll explore theoretical constructs of hope and love as they apply to medical practice. Let's conclude briefly by exploring how medical practice can — at least for some of us, some of the time — offer glimpses of the transcendent.

The psychologists who launched in 2000 the Values in Action Classification Project now include under "strengths of transcendence" such traits as aesthetic appreciation, awe, gratitude, humor (of the subtle, self-effacing variety), playfulness, purpose, and wonder.[4,5] Such traits enable us to rise above (transcend) the here-and-now trials and tribulations of our daily existence, our *quid pro quo* services for others, our petty concerns and conceits. The psychologist Abraham Maslow, although himself an atheist, described how such traits, and especially awe, facilitate what he called peak experiences. Aspects of peak experiences include:

• Perceptions that help us transcend our own egos and self-interests.

• Perceptions that the world is good, desirable, and beautiful despite suffering and evil.

• Perceptions that we should become more accepting of others, more willing to listen, and more loving.

Maslow's research led him to conclude that people differ widely in the extent to which they are open to peak experiences.

He concluded that great religious figures such as Moses, Jesus, Arjuna, and Mohammed were "peakers."[6] Medical practice in any specialty affords abundant opportunities for peak experiences. The challenge, at least in my experience is to rise above the hurly-burly of excruciating time pressures, paperwork hassles, beepers, cell phones, and other distractions in order to smell the roses, to realize how fortunate we are to study medicine and to apply what we've learned for the benefit of fellow humans.

References

1. Lake K. *Landmarks in the History of Christianity*. London: MacMillan and Company; 1920: 96.
2. Tillich P. *The Dynamics of Faith*. New York: Harper & Row, Publishers, Inc.; 1957: 1-29.
3. Pellegrino ED, Thomasma DC. The virtue of faith. Chapter 3 in Pellegrino ED, Thomasma DC. *The Christian Virtues in Medical Practice*. Washington, D.C.: Georgetown University Press; 1996: 42-55.
4. Seligman MEP, Peterson 2003. Positive clinical psychology. Chapter 21 in Aspinwall LG, Staudinger UM, eds. *A Psychology of Human Strengths: Fundamental Questions and Future Directions for a Positive Psychology*. Washington, DC: American Psychological Association; 2003: 305-317.
5. Peterson C, Seligman MEP. *Character Strengths and Virtues: A Handbook and Classification*. New York: Oxford University Press; 2004.
6. Maslow AH. *Religions, Values, and Peak-Experiences*. New York: Penguin Compass; 1976: 16-17.

Medicine and the Seven Basic Virtues. VII. Hope

J SC Med Assoc 2007; 103: 21-22

Has any virtue through the ages helped more patients than hope? Galen (second century A.D.) opined: "Confidence and hope do more good than physic." Robert Burton (1577-1640) chimed: "Hope and Patience are two sovereign remedies for all ... the softest cushions to lean on in adversity." The layman Samuel Taylor Coleridge (1772-1834) wrote: "He is the best physician who is the best inspirer of hope." William Osler said: "Gain the confidence of a patient and inspire him with hope, and the battle is half won." Yet what do we mean by "hope"? How does "hope" differ from "optimism"? Is it possible to capture "hope" in quasi-scientific terms?

Hope among the three transcendent virtues (the others being faith and love) and indeed among all seven of the virtues we've been reviewing (as a reminder, the cardinal virtues are wisdom, justice, temperance, and courage) is at first blush the most suspect, the subject of many disparaging remarks through the years. Plato called it "a foolish counselor," Euripedes "a curse upon humanity," Francis Bacon "a good breakfast, but a bad supper." Benjamin Franklin alleged, "He that lives on hope will die fasting." The theologian Paul Tillich was more cautiously optimistic: "Hope is easy for the foolish, but hard for the wise. Everyone can lose himself into foolish hope, but genuine hope is something rare and great." Hope in the spiritual sense is usually considered a divine gift; hence, "We hope and pray that ..." Hope in the secular sense, psychologists increasingly agree, has a sound basis only when accompanied by clear goals and strategies.

"Hope" comes from an old Anglo-Saxon word, *hopa*, meaning "expectation." Here's the most useful definition I've found: Hope represents goal-directed thinking under conditions in which the probability of achieving one's goals is intermediate—that is, approaching neither 100% nor zero.[1] If the likeli-

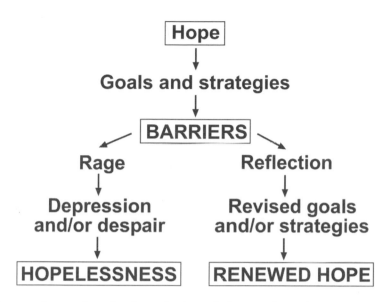

```
        ┌──────┐
        │ Hope │
        └──────┘
           ↓
   Goals and strategies
           ↓
      ┌──────────┐
    ↙ │ BARRIERS │ ↘
      └──────────┘
   Rage              Reflection
    ↓                    ↓
 Depression         Revised goals
 and/or despair     and/or strategies
    ↓                    ↓
┌──────────────┐   ┌──────────────┐
│ HOPELESSNESS │   │ RENEWED HOPE │
└──────────────┘   └──────────────┘
```

Hope understood as the formulation of clear goals and strategies, re-quiring both willpower and "waypower." Seemingly insurmountable barriers demand revision of goals and/or strategies if hope is to be renewed (based on concepts developed by Snyder[1,2]).

hood that an action will produce the desired result approaches 100% — that is, it's a sure thing — one does not need hope. If on the other hand the likelihood that an action will produce the de-sired result approaches zero — that is, it's literally "hopeless" — hope is counterproductive. We'd be better off accepting the in-evitable or setting another goal. And that's exactly what the late C.R. ("Rick") Snyder, who taught psychology at the University of Kansas, captured in his operational account of hope.

According to Snyder, hope is best understood as the imple-mentation of clear goals and strategies through the combined use of willpower and what he calls "waypower" (Figure). Hope, Snyder contends, is "a specific way of thinking about oneself." People with high scores on a "hope scale" tend to set clear goals, to be task-oriented, to anticipate problems, and — mark this well — to revise their goals and/or strategies when they en-counter barriers. When we encounter seemingly insurmount-able barriers to important goals, most of us tend to rant and rage. We then develop some combination of hostility, depression, and despair. High-hope persons make a habit of reflecting on the problem, then revising their goals and/or strategies. This conclusion reflects the old saw that "where there's a will there's a way," but Snyder contends there's more to it than that.[2]

High-hope people, according to Snyder, diversify their hope portfolios. Compared to low-hope people, they set more goals and in more different areas of life. When they encounter major barriers, they change focus and direction. Like successful field generals and head coaches, they know when and how to cut their losses and build on what seems to be working. High-hope people also know how to plan, plan, plan. They are highly specific about their aims.

Snyder's account holds obvious relevance to patient care. The physician should help the patient set clear goals, then outline a plan for achieving those goals. Sometimes the goal is clear-cut and the plan a simple one. Often, especially in primary care, the goal is nebulous. Of the patient with multiple vague complaints I sometimes ask: "If I were a magician and could solve *one* problem for you, what would you want it to be?" Visualizing a clear goal becomes problematic for patients with serious illnesses for which there is no readily apparent cure. What constitutes the appropriate goals of care? Are the patient's expectations realistic? If not, how should we work with him or her to set more realistic goals? I often take comfort from an old motto that reads: "To cure—sometimes; to improve—often; to comfort—always." This motto takes on special meaning for me with the patient with multiorgan failure including respiratory failure requiring mechanical ventilation. I often ask to what extent our state motto, *Dum spiro spero* ("While I breathe, I hope") should apply to patients on respirators and with little prospect for ever breathing again on their own. Snyder's account of hope gives us permission, in a sense, to help the patient and his/her family work toward a desirable end of life. As the great surgeon Ambrose Paré (1517?-1590) put it, "Always give the patient hope, even when death seems at hand."

"Optimism," unlike "hope," is a relative newcomer to the English vocabulary. It was popularized during the 1770s to denote a reasoned judgment that good would prevail over evil despite the possibility of suffering. "Hope" and "optimism" have a great deal in common, including increased likelihood of physical and mental health, good social relationships, and achievement in just about any area. However, hope as we have defined it requires clear goals whereas optimism does not. Also, hope represents an Aristotelian mean between despair (unwarranted pessimism) and presumption (unwarranted optimism).[3] The psychologist Martin Seligman popularized the concept of "learned optimism" as "non-negative thinking." The optimist is inclined to see a setback as temporary but a success as permanent. The optimist is inclined to attribute a setback to a specific circumstance, but sees success as enhancing all of life. The optimist attributes a setback to external factors beyond his or her control, but attributes a success to his or her prowess. The pessimist does exactly the reverse of all of these.[4] It behooves us to bring to the examining room or bedside both hope and optimism, but these desiderata are not exactly the same.

Is hope deficient in the world today? Many people would say yes. Can physicians make a difference? I say yes, provided we're willing to work collectively. In a world torn and divided in so many ways, the benefits of medicine constitute one area in which all people can agree. As Osler put it, "Linked together by the strong bonds of community of interests, the profession of medicine forms a remarkable world-unit in the progressive evolution of which there is a fuller hope for humanity than in any other direction." Let's make a difference!

References

1. Snyder CR. *The Psychology of Hope: You Can Get There From Here.* New York: The Free Press; 1994: 6.
2. Snyder CR. *Handbook of Hope: Theory, Measures, & Applications.* San Diego, California: Academic Press; 2000: 9, 25-50.
3. Pellegrino ED, Thomasma DC. *The Christian Virtues in Medical Practice.* Washington, D.C.: Georgetown University Press; 1996: 65.
4. Seligman MEP. *Learned Optimism.* New York: Alfred A. Knopf; 1991: 44-49, 207-234.

Medicine and the Seven Basic Virtues. VIII. Love

J SC Med Assoc 2007; 103: 74-75

Educators dichotomize the medical school curriculum into the preclinical years given largely to the intricacies of the basic sciences and the clinical years given largely to learning the ropes of patient care. Wags call these respectively the "pre-cynical years" and the "cynical years." Preclinical students persevere through the grueling months of anatomy, biochemistry, and the like supported by a vague notion that they'll rescue humanity from pain and suffering. Then they hit the wards. They encounter patient after patient with incurable end-stage diseases. They encounter seemingly insoluble social problems. They work alongside residents who feel pressured to get patients out of the hospital. They encounter patients who seem unappreciative or even hostile. Educators call this process of enculturation the "hidden curriculum."

Recently, a third-year student made the following insightful observation: "I always thought being compassionate and respectful would be the easy part of being a doctor and gaining the large amount of knowledge would be the hard part. I have realized it is the exact opposite." Norman Cousins, observing students and physicians-in-training at the University of California at Los Angeles, similarly concluded that over time the "hard" subjects of the medical curriculum become soft while the "soft" subjects become hard. How difficult it sometimes seems to care — that is, to *really* care.

How can we preserve the idealism of preclinical students? How can we preserve (or recapture) such idealism ourselves? Educators ponder this problem. Studies suggest that the students most resistant to becoming cynical are usually those who bring to the wards tenaciously-held values and attitudes derived elsewhere. Some of these students are deeply spiritual. Some are blessed with unusually sunny dispositions. Some have the innate ability to size up quickly what they can and cannot

Competence and Caring: The Twin Pillars of Medicine		
Hippocratic maxim	**Today's term**	**Key virtues**
Love of humanity (*philanthropia*)	Caring	Love; also, faith and hope
Love of the art (*philotechnia*)	Competence	Practical wisdom; also, justice, temperance, and courage

do to make a difference in people's lives and to act accordingly. Although clinical experience tempers the idealism of most students, nearly all of them manage to graduate with a quiet resolve to honor what they told the curriculum committee, some variation on the theme that "I like science and I want to help people." And they do.

Some years ago, I wrote in these pages and elsewhere: "In a sense, benevolent competence *is* compassion, whereas compassion without competence is fraud." Although pilloried for this simple pronouncement in the prestigious *New England Journal of Medicine*, I stand my ground. Competence, as the pioneering clinical ethicist Edmund Pellegrino has written, is the physician's first and foremost obligation. Competence comprises what the physician, as opposed to a family member or friend, uniquely brings to the bedside. *Everyone* (not just physicians) should strive to be the very best at what he or she specifically professes to be able to do in exchange for monetary compensation. Yet it is imperative that competence be benevolent. Competence and caring, you see, are the twin pillars of medicine (Table). Here's the punch line: Prudence (practical wisdom) is the key virtue for competence; love is the key virtue for caring. Wisdom ranks foremost among the cardinal virtues and love ranks similarly among the transcendent virtues.

Indeed, most of us would agree that love ranks highest among all the virtues. Love, most great religious leaders have taught, is the great leaven of life. St. Paul, author of what we now call the transcendent (or theological) virtues, crowned love the greatest by far and thus it has remained in Christianity. The great Jewish sage Hillel the Elder, a contemporary of Jesus of Nazareth and who like Jesus insisted that love matters more than the law, was once challenged to recite the entire Torah while standing on one foot. He replied in effect: "Love the Lord with all your heart and love your neighbor as yourself. That is the entire Torah. All the rest is commentary."

It is often suggested that in medicine we function under the Samaritan Contract. We accept as our calling, indeed we pledge under oath, to help the stranger in distress. Recent writers distinguish between the "minimally decent Samaritan," the "good Samaritan," and the "splendid Samaritan." Caring, you see, is a graded construct. Previously in these pages I've grouped four "caring" terms in ascending order of difficulty as follows: *beneficence* ("active kindness"), *empathy* ("in-feeling," understanding intellectually how another feels), *sympathy* ("like-feeling," experiencing at least to some extent emotions similar to another's), and *compassion* ("to suffer-with," to become a fellow sufferer). Most contemporary usage trivializes the meaning of "compassion" in the strict sense implied by its etymology. However, we can formulate in concrete terms what we mean in medicine by "compassion." Examples include rendering service for which one is unpaid or inadequately paid, rendering service when one would rather be doing something else, rendering service at one's own emotional risk, and rendering service at one's own physical risk including the potential to acquire a life-threatening disease. All clinical situations call for competence and caring (at some level). But if we are to assert our claims that medicine represents a higher calling, we must demonstrate, at least from time to time and when the occasion calls for it, compassion in the strict sense of this much abused noun. Compassionate care constitutes what I've elsewhere called "higher professionalism," defined briefly as service that clearly transcends self-interest. Philosophers through the ages have of course belabored these distinctions.

"Love" comes from an old Anglo-Saxon word, *lufu* or *lufe*, which may be why English and German seem to be the only Western languages with only one word for love's diverse meanings. Speakers of the various Romance languages enjoy a much richer love vocabulary than we do (perhaps that's why we call them "Romance languages"). The ancient Greeks commonly spoke of *eros*, *agape*, and *philia*. Eros and *agape* correspond roughly with what C.S. Lewis called "need love" and "gift love" and what Abraham Maslow called "deficit love" and "being love." Most of us most of the time love in expectation of some benefit for ourselves — at the very least, to be appreciated. And that's okay. It's been suggested that love is the only investment we can make that consistently returns a 30% dividend! The theologian Reinhold Niebhur suggested that "love … is only *agape* in its purest and most unadulterated form, which means in a form which is known in human experience only in rare moments of evangelical fervor or crisis heroism."

For most of us most of the time, *agape* remains an ideal, not a reality, but nevertheless an ideal that defines us as physicians, heirs to the Hippocratic ideal that "where there is love for humanity, there also is love for medicine." Today, when we can do so much for our patients, when we are blessed (and cursed) with so many seductive technologies, and when patients increasingly view medicine as a commodity to be bought and sold like any other, caring well beyond the call of duty sometimes seems increasingly difficult.

The more I think about it, the more I realize the profundity of what the student wrote. "I always thought being compassionate and respectful would be the easy part of being a doctor and gaining the large amount of knowledge would be the hard part. I have realized it is the exact opposite." How true!

Medicine and the Seven Basic Virtues.
IX. Summing Up

J SC Med Assoc 2007; 103: 135-137

In mid-April I was eagerly anticipating the annual meeting of the American College of Physicians in San Diego, California. I'd been invited two years earlier to deliver the Nicholas E. Davies Memorial Scholar Award Lecture, probably the biggest honor I'd ever received. For my text I'd chosen the opening paragraph to the first nine editions of *Harrison's Principles of Internal Medicine*, which inspired several generations of medical students and which reads as follows:

> No greater opportunity, responsibility, or obligation can fall to the lot of a human being than to become a physician. In the care of the suffering he needs technical skill, scientific knowledge, and human understanding. He who uses these with courage, with humility, and with wisdom will provide a unique service for his fellow man, and will build an *enduring edifice of character* within himself. The physician should ask of his destiny no more than this; he should be content with no less (*emphasis added*).[1]

Since 1950, when these ennobling words first appeared, much has happened to erode the high confidence of Western civilization and, more specifically, of American physicians. The sociologist Elliott A. Krause concluded from his study of major professions in the United States, Britain, France, Italy, and Germany that between 1930 and 1990 the American medical profession constituted the most extreme case of rise and fall.[2] For the Davies lecture I planned to discuss in the context of today's medical profession three questions traceable to Greek antiquity: What do we mean by "character"? Can character be taught? Does character suffice for happiness? Hence my title: "To 'build an enduring edifice of character': Why and How for Today's Physicians?" I'd worked hard on the lecture and could hardly

220

wait to give it.

The trip was not to be all work. I was especially looking forward to playing the South Course at Torrey Pines, chosen for next year's U.S. Open for its scenery and difficulty, with a friend from Kentucky. However, my golf game was in its usual state of neglect. To that end I'd planned to spend the last Friday afternoon on the practice range. As I was leaving the office the telephone rang. "A patient has just been admitted with periorbital and facial cellulitis and they want you to see her." As the only available infectious disease consultant, I knew I had to go but the question was when. Wouldn't it be okay to phone the ward, make sure that appropriate cultures and antibiotics had been ordered, and show up several hours later? Or should I go right now, forgetting about my swing plane and tempo? Then spoke the inner voice. "Aren't you getting ready to stand up before a large audience and talk about 'character'? Aren't you being a bit hypocritical? And what about that short definition of 'a professional' — 'a pro is someone who always does his or her best job even when he or she doesn't feel like it'?"

I therefore did exactly what I'm sure that you, gentle reader, would have done. I went. The patient, a retired nurse, had marked inflammation of the left side of her face and especially of the left periorbital tissues. She was in pain but did not look toxic. I checked out the latest antibiotic recommendations and, before leaving the hospital, reviewed the CT scan with the radiologist to make sure that she did not have cavernous sinus thrombosis.

In these editorials, we've reviewed the four cardinal virtues—wisdom, justice, temperance, and courage—and the three transcendent (theological) virtues, faith, hope, and love. We've reviewed how wisdom and love are, respectively, the preeminent virtues for competence and caring, the twin pillars of medicine. And we've reviewed how love, at least at some level, should always inform wisdom to assure that our actions are benevolent, that our patients' needs supercede our own. How does all this relate to the project of building character?

Character consists of being virtuous and/or consistently acting in a virtuous way. Virtues are the components of char-

acter. Thus, the definitions of "character" and "virtue" recipro-
cate. Philosophers can spend weeks arguing what we mean by
such things as "character," "virtue," "morality," and "ethics,"
but, to repeat the working definitions from the first editorial in
this series, I proffer the following:
• *Virtues* are excellences that enable us to achieve what is good
for society and for oneself.
• *Values* (or principles) are determinations of what constitutes
the good, informed by virtues.
• *Morals* are determinations of what constitutes right and wrong,
informed by virtues and values.
• *Ethics* are determinations of how best to act (that is, disciplined
reasoning about right and wrong in problem cases), informed
by morals, values, and virtues.

Virtues, then, are the essential building blocks for the project of striving to be a good human being, a person of character.
The seven basic virtues reviewed here can be viewed as "primary colors" for ethical behavior. They can be mixed to yield
other desirable traits or "subvirtues." Thus, as one advocate
for this position notes: "Love plus faith yields loyalty. Courage
plus prudence yields enterprise. Temperance plus justice yields
humility. Justice, courage, and faith yields honesty."[3]

Tinsley R. Harrison and his colleagues in that memorable
opening paragraph hint that building character constitutes (1) a
lifelong project that (2) requires engagement in one or another
line of work that (3) poses conflicts between competing desiderata. "Character," as I see it, represents the cumulative effect
of making difficult choices in tough situations. And the task of
building character is never complete. I try to remind myself,
"You're only as good as your last case."

Looking back on my own odyssey, I recognize two attempts over the past 10 years to summarize character building
in a single figure. In the first I defined "character" as congruity between benevolent principles, goals, and actions (Figure
1).[4] We consider someone a "person of character" when his
or her actions are benevolent and consistent—that is, predictable and thereby reflecting certain principles—even though we
might not endorse that person's definition of "the good" on a

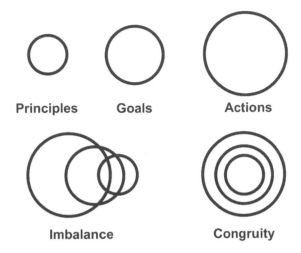

Figure 1. *"Character" can be defined as congruity between princi-*
ples, goals, and actions. One way to achieve such congruity is to keep
in writing a system of time management whereby principles inform
goals and goals inform actions.

liberal-to-conservative spectrum of priorities. One approach to achieving such congruity is to keep a system of time management based on written principles, goals, and action steps. My second attempt consists of a framework for situational character analysis based on ethical reflection (Figure 2). We consider someone to be a "person of character" when they seem to do the right thing in tough situations, again and again. The Roman historian Plutarch defined character as "long-standing habit" and the Victorian novelist Charles Reade offered this prescription: "Sow an act, and you reap a habit. Sow a habit and you reap a character. Sow a character and you reap a destiny." Aristotle said much the same thing about virtue.

Many physicians would maintain that the project of building character is made increasingly difficult by today's conditions of medical practice. These include excruciating time pressures, the demands of third party payers, and inadequate reimbursement for time spent listening to patients as opposed to doing things to them. And building character requires a certain amount of autonomy, since this process hinges on the freedom to make

A FRAMEWORK FOR SITUATIONAL
CHARACTER ANALYSIS

FACTS (SCENARIO)	VIRTUES AND VALUES
1. 2. 3.	1. 2. 3.
ETHICAL FRAMEWORKS	CHOICES AND ACTIONS
1. 2. 3.	1. 2. 3.

Figure 2. *Since "character" represents the cumulative effects of choices made in difficult situations, building character can be facilitated by keeping in writing a journal whereby one reviews choices and actions made in difficult situations. What were the facts? What virtues and values applied? What were the relevant ethical frameworks (for example, rule-based frameworks [deontology] or results-based frameworks [consequentialism])? What choices did I make and what did I do? How might I have done it differently?*

tough decisions in the first place. It behooves us to present to the public, as one profession, the case for practicing our art and science as indeed it should be practiced, in environments that nurture the doctor-patient relationship. It is difficult to be virtuous in an environment that devalues virtuous behaviors. The claim by various philosophers that virtuous behavior is much more situation-dependent than we'd like to think finds support in a body of experimental evidence.[5] In one classic experiment, seminarians who were told that they were running ahead of schedule for their next appointment were much more likely to help a stranger slumped in a doorway than were those who were told they were running a bit late.[6] As physicians, we're subject to the same behavioral shortcomings as everyone else.

Let's return to the simple story with which began, a story

typifying tensions over priorities faced by every physician every day of his or her practice. Did my decision to head for the ward rather than the practice range affect the outcome? No. Medicine is not only a jealous mistress; she's also a cruel one. The cellulitis improved but by the third hospital day the patient met criteria for streptococcal toxic shock syndrome, perhaps the second case of that syndrome as a complication of periorbital cellulitis.[7] She responded briefly to intravenous immune globulin but died the morning I left for San Diego. I told the story briefly in the Davies lecture, which seemed to go well. I butchered Torrey Pines, but felt better about myself than if I'd broken the course record currently held by Tiger Woods.

References

1. The Editors. Approach to the patient. In: Harrison TR, Beeson PB, Thorn GW, Resnik WH, and Wintrobe MM, eds. *Principles of Internal Medicine*. Philadelphia: The Blakiston Company; 1950: 1.

2. Krause EA. *Death of the Guilds: Professions, States, and the Advance of Capitalism, 1930 to the Present*. New Haven: Yale University Press; 1996: 36.

3. McCloskey DN. *The Bourgeois Virtues: Ethics for an Age of Commerce*. Chicago: The University of Chicago Press; 2006: 361.

4. Bryan CS. *Osler: Inspirations from a Great Physician*. New York: Oxford University Press; 1997: 217-218

5. Doris JM. *Lack of Character: Personality and Moral Behavior*. Cambridge: Cambridge University Press; 2002.

6. Darley JM, Batson CD. From Jerusalem to Jericho: A study of situational and dispositional variables in helping behavior. *J Pers Soc Psychol* 1973; 27: 100-108.

7. Meyer MA. Streptococcal toxic shock syndrome complicating preseptal cellulitis. *Am J Opthalmol* 1997; 123: 841-843.

Medical Education

Personality and Medical Students

J SC Med Assoc 1978; 74: 260-261.

The functions of few committees rival in importance those that decide who will be our future physicians. The paper by Sutker, Newberry, and Bradham in this issue of *The Journal* makes a potentially important contribution to the literature on how medical school admission committees might function more objectively.

Although the authors indicate that "efforts to predict medical student or physician success with certain nonintellectual variables such as personality characteristics" are relatively recent, the underlying concepts are old. Over a century ago, Sir James Paget, a British surgeon, traced the careers of 1000 of his former pupils. Twenty-three achieved distinguished success, 66 achieved considerable success, 507 achieved fair success, 66 failed entirely, 96 left the profession, 87 died within twelve years of commencing practice, and 41 died during pupilage. Paget commented that "the personal character, the very nature, the will" must be strong if the student were to survive and achieve success during medical school and later professional life.

Recently a similar study was made of 1337 medical students at the Johns Hopkins University School of Medicine.[1] It was determined that 3.1 percent of the graduates, and alarmingly 11.2 percent of the non-graduates, died prematurely. Incipient mental illness and emotional disturbance appeared to have contributed substantially to academic failure, poor performance during and after medical school, and premature death. The author concluded that "psychological stamina is of vital importance to the entering medical student if he or she is to reach the goal of becoming a sound physician," and that "poor self-image, damaged self-esteem and covert depression, anger, and fear take their toll when certain students undergo the pressures of medical school."

How do undergraduate students who gain entrance to medical schools differ from their peers both during college and at long-term follow-up? Over 30 years ago, a prospective study of 268 college sophomores was begun at a leading Eastern university.[2] Of these 268 men, 47 attended medical school and 46 graduated. These 47 men were compared with a group of 79 men who sought other careers and who were matched socioeconomically for control purposes.

Bad marriage or divorce characterized 47 percent of the physicians, compared to 32 percent of the controls. Excessive or high use of drugs characterized 36 percent of the physicians, compared to 22 percent of controls. Of the physicians, 34 percent had seen a psychiatrist for 10 or more visits, compared to 19 percent of the controls. All of these findings were significant ($p < 0.01$).

Apologists for physicians offer several explanations. Bad marriages reflect the long hours and the demands of patients; medical practice drains one's emotional resources, leaving little for spouse and family. Drug abuse reflects physicians' ready familiarity with and access to agents that might help one cope, temporarily, with fatigue that threatens occupational efficiency. Psychiatric visits reflect awareness; physicians may recognize their symptoms earlier than most people. Nevertheless, there is another viewpoint—and here, the observations by Sutker and colleagues gain relevance.

This viewpoint holds that physicians— those who competed successfully during college for entry into medical school— tend to be high achievers and that lurking behind their high achievements are dark forces (most notably, low self-esteem) that ultimately doom them to maladjustment. Possessing a type A personality may be useful for earning a high mark in organic chemistry but eventually leads to the serious syndrome of "overwork," recently defined as "working beyond one's endurance and recuperative capacities," "a hazard in certain personality types engaged in open-ended occupations."[3] Thus, the ability of objective parameters, even if "nonintellectual," to predict the problems of such individuals early would be useful to the individual, to the medical school, and to society.

However, some of the conclusions of Sutker and colleagues seem alarming. They noted that reliance on personality variables alone enabled better prediction of medical student performance during the clinical years than did the results of conventional objective tests. They also noted that specific personality traits seemed to correlate with success. "Tendencies toward exhibitionism, aggressiveness, autonomy, aloofness, need for achievement, and personal dominance were more characteristic of students who were highly successful in terms of clinical performance." Would you want your own doctor to have all of these traits?

The authors note carefully that additional research is needed. Much anecdotal support for their observations could, of course, be gleaned from published and unpublished observations. Sixty-three years ago, an editorial entitled "Personality and Practice" appeared in these pages, the author noting the following:

> The astonishing way in which some men, who left medical schools with seemingly the least possible acquaintance with medicine, suddenly spring into practice, usually seems unaccountable ... To the more earnest and thorough students, it seems puzzling that the superficial should succeed so well. There is one explanation that covers it all. The success is due to the peculiar personality of the practitioner ... This personal touch, this psychic appeal to the patient and his friends, is not to be neglected by the scientific; it is a part of the practice of medicine ... a part [which] should not be overlooked....[4]

And more recently, another editorialist wrote in these pages:

> The pressures of modern living and modern practice are causing very unpleasant effects upon our doctors. They display too much impatience, too much irritability, too little self control, and too little of the "milk of human kindness." To be a good physician, someone has said, one must be a fool and a kind man.[5]

"Nothing," said the late Charlie Chaplin, "transcends personality." The observations of Sutker and colleagues suggest that this holds for performance during medical school, as in other aspects of life. Nevertheless, one must share the sentiments of the recent British writer who noted that "one of the great attractions of the medical profession is that it can assimilate such a diverse range of personality types."[6] Not all patients would necessarily prefer that their physician manifest the tendencies that seem to characterize the high performers in the study reported in this issue. There is room for diversity, and hopefully such diversity will increase with the increasing numbers of young physicians.

References

1. Thomas CB. What becomes of medical students: The dark side. *Johns Hopkins Med J* 1976; 38: 185-195.
2. Vaillant GE, Sobowale NC, McArthur C. Some psychologic vulnerabilities of physicians. *New Engl J Med* 1972; 287: 372-375.
3. Rhoads JM. Overwork. *JAMA* 1977; 237: 2615-2618.
4. Personality and practice (unsigned). *J SC Med Assoc* 1915; 11: 301.
5. Guess JD. The organization man of medicine. *J SC Med Assoc* 1960; 61: 351-356.
6. Bennet G. If I were dean. *Lancet* 1978; 1: 86-87.

Bedside Body Language

J SC Med Assoc 1980; 76: 144-145

Franklin Roosevelt had it. John Kennedy had it in spades. Fiorello LaGuardia had it not only in English but also in other languages, and it helped him reign over the polyglot city of New York. Lyndon Johnson and Richard Nixon tried hard but never quite got the hang of it. Adlai Stevenson, George Mc-Govern, Eugene McCarthy, and Arthur Goldberg never learned it, either, demonstrating that without it even the brightest men are unlikely to win elections.

The recognition that many and perhaps most persons judge a speaker more by watching his movements than by listening to his words makes body language a powerful instrument for politicians. The importance of body language to physicians has received much less attention. In the following editorial, psychologist David Adams explores the current state of the art.

Photographs suggest that the great physicians of the past, such as Sir William Osler often had it instinctively. Photographs of Osler, for instance, usually illustrate what psychologists today would call "effective posture." This may have been one way by which Osler inspired great confidence during his daily rounds without spending large amounts of time with individual patients. He was usually able to exit gracefully without allowing what he called "the floodgates of talk" to open. Other physicians might spend more time but inspire less confidence. I've been told that the great surgeon Alfred Blalock nearly always gave patients the impression that he'd spent lots of time with them when in fact his visits were relatively brief. He always sat down and conveyed with his Southern drawl and relaxed posture that he was in no hurry whatsoever.

The message seems to be that while a lucky few come by effective body language naturally, all of us can improve through practice and self-awareness. Certain postures such as barricading the arms on the chest (Left panel of figure, next page; observe how often physicians do this when they talk to each other!) or

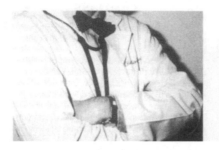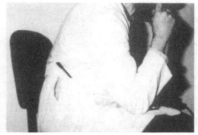

(Left) "I'm in charge here" and/or "I may be somewhat defensive." (Right) "I'm concerned, and I really want to hear what you have to say." The position on the left is an example of "closed" body language whereas that on the right is "open."

clasping the hands behind the occiput, elbows splayed out like wings (observe how often administrators do this behind their big desks!) convey defensive "power" body language. It may be preferable to relax the upper extremities—arms dangling freely by the sides. Sitting down and leaning slightly forward (Figure, right panel) conveys obvious interest in the patient. That this is the usual posture of effective salesmen should come as no surprise.

A residency director in another state recently reported that his trainees were "more productive" if they were placed in examining rooms with no place for them to sit down. Without chairs they were less comfortable and made quicker exits. One must ask, however, whether this policy makes for better medicine. I doubt it. Several years ago, Dr. Edmund Taylor wrote a provocative editorial in *The Recorder* of the Columbia Medical Society about the importance of sitting at the bedside, however briefly, as Alfred Blalock and other great physicians have done. Effective bedside body language should convey the notion that the doctor is both relaxed and concerned. We are fortunate that psychologists such as Dr. Adams are now providing data on this subject.

Found: A Point on the Compass

J SC Med Assoc 1980; 76: 442-443

In the minds of many, the deaths of men like Dr. Vince Moseley (1912-1980) symbolize the passing of an era. The golden age that seems to be in jeopardy is that of the "Oslerian tradition" in internal medicine.[1] This tradition found its embodiment in well-rounded internists like Dr. Moseley who, rather than retreating to one or another subspecialty, demonstrated broad competence across the discipline. Diagnosis now seems to hinge more often on laboratory or radiographic procedures than on the well-reasoned opinion of a master clinician.

Among the Oslerian aphorisms is the famous "four points on the compass" — inspection, palpation, percussion, and auscultation. These are still taught to medical students. But it must be admitted that one of them, percussion, has been de-emphasized in recent years. We have been taught that this method is an unreliable way to estimate heart size. Although still used to evaluate the lung fields, it's not unusual to find it omitted. Speaking only as one physician, I have to admit that I've found percussion to be of less value than the other points on the compass, except perhaps to determine whether the diaphragm moves. And I've always had difficulty sensing with the pleximeter finger all that's described in the older textbooks of physical diagnosis.

Recently, Dr. John Guarino of the Veterans Administration Medical Center in Boise, Idaho, described in *The Lancet* a novel method for percussing the chest that he's used for more than 25 years. Dr. Guarino relies neither on the note made by the percussion finger striking the pleximeter finger nor on the sensations obtained by the pleximeter finger. Instead, he listens to the chest with the diaphragm of the stethoscope. He taps the manubrium of the sternum lightly with one finger while moving the stethoscope around the lung fields and comparing the notes transmitted to different areas. Dr. Guarino reports that he can detect lesions less than two centimeters in diameter with his method.[2]

Having tried his method, I'm happy to report that it works! It's remarkably simple and time-saving, and seems to be—as Dr. Guarino alleges—much more sensitive than the usual way to percuss the chest. What a delight to find, in this day of the computerized scan, powerful new methods of physical diagnosis! Optimistically, one hopes that there will always be a place for physicians made in the old mold, who, like Dr. Vince Moseley, practice listening to patients, recording careful histories, performing detailed physical examinations, and exercising clinical judgment.

References

1. Regelson W. The weakening of the Oslerian tradition: The changing emphasis in departments of medicine. *JAMA* 1978; 239: 317-319.
2. Guarino JR. Ausculatory percussion of the chest. *Lancet* 1980; 1: 1332-1334.

Editorial Note: Although some recent observers have questioned the validity of Dr. Guarino's observations, the larger point (and the reason to include this short essay in this collection) is the need to resist today's tendency to dispense with much of the physical examination, and hence the human touch. There is now a tendency to submit physical findings to the same objective standards (such as sensitivity, specificity, positive predictive value, and negative predictive value) that we demand of laboratory tests. Unfortunately, physical findings are notoriously vulnerable to interobserver variability.

Should Philosophy be Required in the Premedical Curriculum?

J SC Med Assoc 1981; 77: 94-95

In this issue of *The Journal* our president-elect, Dr. William Hunter, and Professor William Maker of Clemson University discuss the need for an adequate liberal arts curriculum for undergraduate premedical students. This hardly constitutes a new concern, having been aired many times by many observers through the years. However, Drs. Hunter and Maker take a surprising turn midway through their essay by arguing that philosophy is an especially crucial subject for would-be physicians. They develop the theme that formal study of philosophy improves one's capacity for critical, reflective thought. This capacity is necessary both for making difficult judgment decisions in clinical practice and for serving one's community in non-medical capacities.

We need not be reminded of the extent to which differences in philosophies determine the great conflicts in the world. The extent to which philosophies influence our decisions in daily medical practice can, however, be easily overlooked. One can argue that medicine and philosophy have always been closely interrelated. Both medicine and philosophy as we know them, Drs. Hunter and Maker observe, originated in ancient Greece. The Hippocratic Oath, taken for centuries as a timeless standard for medical practice, dramatizes this relationship.

Examination of the Hippocratic Oath reveals that several medical practices — such as euthanasia, abortion, and surgery including surgery for stone — are specifically prohibited. These restrictions run counter to orthodox medicine in ancient Greece. Euthanasia was encouraged in certain situations; abortion was recommended by the greatest gynecologist of antiquity, Soranus, when the mother's life was endangered; surgery, when indicated, was not discouraged. There is very little evidence to suggest that the Hippocratic Oath was written by Hippocrates

237

or his followers. The late historian Ludwig Edelstein made a strong case that the Oath was written by Pythagorean philosophers, not Hippocratic physicians.[1]

Although we seldom mention the Pythagoreans in the same breath with which we mention certain other Greek philosophers — such as Socrates, Plato, Aristotle, the Stoics, and the Epicureans — their perspectives on the relationship of medicine to philosophy is worth examining. The Hippocratic Oath contains the statement that "in purity and holiness I will guard my life and my art." Pythagoras taught that philosophy purifies and frees the mind; purity is achieved by quiet self-examination. Medicine and science, on the one hand, and philosophy and religion, on the other, are virtually inseparable in the Pythagorean world view. Thus, the Oath expresses specific religious, philosophical, and medical tenets consistent with a Pythagorean manifesto.[1]

The relationship of medicine to philosophy in the ancient world was often complicated,[2] and I resist the temptation to opine on the nature of this relationship today. Supporting the case made by Drs. Hunter and Maker, I suggest that there are two compelling reasons for premedical students to concentrate on philosophy (or, alternatively, on religion studied in a philosophical way). The first is to provide a basis for later restraint in the unreflective use of technology, a problem frequently aired within our own ranks.[3] The development of rational, philosophical thought patterns offers a welcome antidote. The second reason is to provide a basis for avoiding emotional unrest and spiritual malaise — pitfalls of demanding scientific occupations[4] that can be prevented, at least in part, by cultivating a philosophical worldview. The ancients emphasized the need for systematic cultivation of these desiderata, predicated on instruction. We cannot assume that our future colleagues will acquire such desirable attributes completely on their own.

References

1. Edelstein L. *The Hippocratic Oath: Text, Translation and Interpretation.* Supplements to the Bulletin of the History of Medicine, No. 1. Balti-

more: The Johns Hopkins Press; 1943.

2. Edelstein L. The relation of ancient philosophy to medicine. *Bull Hist Med* 1952; 25: 299-316.

3. Genkins, C, Matta RJ: Procedures after acute myocardial infarction (letter to the editor), *N Engl J Med* 1950; 303: 1534.

4. Friedman M: The modification of type A behavior in post-infarction patients. *Am Heart J* 1979; 97: 551-560.

Preparation for Medical School: What Have we Learned, and What Can we do Differently?

J SC Med Assoc 1983; 79: 407-408

The fact is that only the most competent and confident pre-medical students can plan a rational college experience, given their impressions of the competition for admission to medical school. How much better it would be if students were to know by the end of their second year of college that they were (or were not) admitted to medical school.

—Robert H. Ebert[1]

In this issue of *The Journal,* Dr. Robert M. Sade and Ms. Carol Lancaster of The Medical University of South Carolina observe that the choice of undergraduate major for students entering the College of Medicine between 1978 and 1980 bore little relationship to performance in medical school. Undergraduates who concentrated in the liberal arts tended to have broader interests and to be more articulate and adaptable than the science majors. The end-point for pre-medical education, they suggest, should be enthusiasm for learning, not a large body of memorized scientific facts. Undergraduates aspiring to medical school should major in whatever interests them most.

Dr. Sade and Ms. Lancaster reemphasize old conclusions. In 1911, for example, President A. Lawrence Lowell of Harvard likewise studied the relationship of undergraduate major to medical school performance. Lowell compared students who majored in literature and language, natural science, history and political science, and philosophy and mathematics and found that a remarkably similar number of persons in each group went on to earn honors in medical school. He concluded that "natural science in college is certainly not a markedly better preparation for the study of medicine than other subjects."

The pre-med syndrome, traced by college officials to the early 1970s, lends urgency to this message.[2] Signs and symptoms of the pre-med syndrome include aggressiveness, anxiety, cynicism, and narrow-minded pursuit of grades. And it may be contagious. Lewis Thomas, observing that the competitiveness of pre-medical students affects other undergraduates, wrote that "the influence of the modern medical school on liberal arts education in this country over the last decade has been baleful and malign, nothing less."[3] Thomas predicted that unless the situation is radically changed, "all the joy of going to college will have been destroyed, not just for the growing majority of undergraduate students who draw breath only to become doctors, but for everyone else." Today's college students have been characterized as highly competitive and determined to succeed at all costs, whatever the fate of their society may be; as someone put it, they wish to "go first class on the *Titanic*."

There is a somewhat depressing ring to the continued cries and exhortations that a broad liberal arts education is desirable for students who contemplate medical school. Gert H. Brieger, a medical historian who is writing the first comprehensive history of pre-medical education in the United States, suggests:

The various so-called problems of pre-medical education and admission to medical schools have been identified and described for many decades. Repeated conferences, surveys, and other studies are witness to the fact that we are a wealthy society. We keep on spending money to talk, to write, to plan changes, but few improvements of lasting value have resulted."[4] Noting that today's educators often merely echo the same complaints voiced around the turn of the century, Brieger asks: "Who is not speaking clearly, and who is not listening? Are we simply living a lie?" He argues that what is needed is a general education for medicine.

Brieger goes on to suggest that the medical university, while representing the optimum site for graduate medical education and research, may not be the best environment for undergraduate medical education. Although medical schools should ideally be places where students study and teachers teach, we all know that this is usually a vast oversimplification. Medical school faculty members often, perhaps usually, find their graduate students — the Ph.D. candidates for the basic sciences faculty, the residents and fellows for the clinical faculty — more fun to teach than the undergraduates. We speak of undergraduate medical education, yet we insist on teaching medical students in graduate schools. Is this to the students' detriment?

Blending the ideas expressed by Dr. Ebert, Dr. Sade and Ms. Lancaster, President Lowell, Dr. Thomas, and Dr. Brieger, one might propose the following:

• Undergraduate students should be admitted to medical school at the end of their sophomore years.

• The next four years of study should combine the biologic sciences with the liberal arts. If physicians are to be broadly-educated persons, why should formal instruction in the liberal arts arbitrarily cease upon admission to medical school? Would not the simultaneous study of literature or philosophy be a welcome and enriching diversion to the study of anatomy and biochemistry? A college diploma would be awarded at the end of the second year of medical school.

• The final two years of medical school would emphasize the clinical sciences with electives spent in traditional tertiary care settings. A thesis would be required for graduation.

Does this sound ridiculous? Perhaps. Our collective thoughts about premedical education and about the "physician as an educated person"[5] tend to change in Hegelian cycles, coming back to the same starting point. One finds, for instance, SCMA president Dr. John T. Darby telling his South Carolina colleagues as far back as 1873 that "our Medical Schools should be fewer, our courses longer, our teachers stronger, if we would elevate our profession."[6] Darby's address presaged the famous Flexner Report of 1910, which indeed resulted in fewer medical schools with more rigorous instruction and more strenuous requirements for admission. But perhaps we've gone too far. Perhaps we've lost sight of the primary purpose of education: to foster life-long enthusiasm for learning and to encourage the learners to think.

References

1. Ebert RH. Can the education of the physician be made more rational? *N Engl J Med* 1981; 305: 2343-2346.
2. "What's Wrong with Pre-Meds?" *Newsweek*, 1 March 1982.
3. Thomas L. How to fix the pre-medical curriculum. *N Engl J Med* 1978; 298: 1180-1181.
4. Brieger GH. "Fit to study medicine": Notes for a history of premedical education in America. *Bull Hist Med* 1983; 47:1-21.
5. Rhoads PS. Premedical students, admissions committee and "the physician as an educated person." *JAMA* 1982; 247: 2671-2673.
6. Darby JT. The progress of medicine and surgery in the past five decades (annual address by the president of the medical association). *Transactions of the South Carolina Medical Association, Annual Session, 1873*. Charleston, SC: Edward Perry, Printer; 1873: 36.

Second Schools: Second Thoughts

J SC Med Assoc 1984; 80: 217-218.

Nearly a century and a half ago, Daniel Drake, a pioneer American medical educator, observed that "the establishment of medical schools is a prolific source of discord in the profession." In the history of medical education in South Carolina, there have been three periods during which two medical schools coexisted in our state: 1832 to 1838; 1867 to 1876; and 1977 to the present. It would be an understatement to say that a measure of discord has characterized each of these periods.

What is now the Medical University of South Carolina (MUSC) in Charleston began in 1824 through the efforts of several individuals, especially Dr. Thomas Cooper, president of what is now the University of South Carolina (USC) in Columbia, and certain prominent members of the Charleston-based Medical Society of South Carolina. It was not long before conflict arose over whether the faculty itself or the Board of Trustees of the Medical Society should control faculty appointments. In 1832 an embittered faculty resigned *en masse* and began a second, competing school, destined to become the dominant institution. Dr. Samuel Henry Dickson, now remembered as a pioneer medical educator in South Carolina, observed that "in vain have we been assailed with all the weapons of malignant warfare; and the ultimate amount of advantage gained by the persevering hostility against us, has been merely to rest from us for a time the results of the well-known munificence of the Legislature, and ... (caused) an unkind and partisan blow to be struck at us...."[1] The judgment of history, rendered by the late Dr. Joseph I. Waring, is that the ensuing "period of strife and recrimination ... evoked numerous public statements that did little to elevate the dignity of the medical profession.[2]

What should be remembered as the first University of South Carolina School of Medicine in Columbia opened in October 1867 after its establishment by the trustees of the university during the Federal occupation. Facilities and funding were meager. The first class of eight students enrolled with no entrance requirements[4] whatsoever. Despite these humble beginnings, the faculty of the Medical College of the State of South Carolina in Charleston took note and petitioned the legislature that "the proposed plan is unnecessary and uncalled for, because the State already possesses one Medical College, advantageously located in a large and prosperous city.... The measure (of a second medical school) ... is impolitic and detrimental because ... a second medical school is not needed, and the creation of one could not fail to prove detrimental by injuring that already existing ... It would prove greatly detrimental to the interests of the state, ... imposing upon the people, already impoverished, uncalled for oppressive taxation to sustain an institution in no respect needed....[3] The school in Columbia never thrived and ceased to function entirely in 1876.

The history of medical education in the United States abounds with calls to close medical schools due to impending physician surpluses. Indeed, the thought has been expressed that in any state at any time in history, at least 51% of practicing physicians would vote to close down one or more schools. Physicians are, of course, hardly unique in this regard; it is likely that persons in most occupations would do the same. In the years before the Flexner report, calls to close medical schools were almost routine.

In recent years, the second University of South Carolina School of Medicine in Columbia has become something of a *cause célèbre*. Recalling Benjamin Franklin's observation that men's opinions and philosophies, even in times of war, nearly always reflect their self-interests, it is hardly surprising that non-partisan viewpoints within South Carolina have been few and far between. At this point in our history, it might be worthwhile to review again four major conclusions rendered two years ago by a committee of outside consultants and expressed in the Lee Report:[4] (1) MUSC has made enormous strides toward becoming a nationally recognized research institution and tertiary care medical center. (2) The fledgling school at USC has performed quite well on a limited budget. It has become a significant resource for South Carolinians. (3) Problems identified at MUSC tend to reflect impaired institutional morale, whereas those identified at USC tend to reflect uncertainty about the institutional mission. (4) Taxpayers would be "best served by cooperation between the two schools ... (which is) highly desirable, publicly called for, and (possible) on a broad basis."

In this time of diminishing resources, it appears that nearly all medical schools will face increasingly stiff competition for research monies.[5,6] The president of the University of Connecticut, reviewing the prognosis for academic medical centers, concludes that "cooperative efforts between institutions will (in the future) be not only desirable but also required for fiscal viability."[7] In what ways can the two schools now coexisting within South Carolina cooperate to the maximum benefit of the state's citizens and physicians? This question, and the question of the separate functions of the two schools, might be best posed in terms of the three functions of medical schools: teaching, research, and service.

As to teaching, to what extent does enrollment of both undergraduate medical students and also of residents and fellows reflect primarily the needs of the state rather than the needs of the schools? And to what extent are the continuing education needs of the state's physicians being met by the faculties within our borders?

As to research, to what extent do the schools undertake ventures, either separately or cooperatively, seeking to identify health problems unique to South Carolinians? And to what extent do the faculties convey to the state's practicing physicians the flavor and excitement of being on the cutting edge of new medical knowledge?

As to service, to what extent do the schools provide effective primary and secondary medical care for selected patient populations and effective tertiary care for all citizens? And to what extent do these services complement rather than compete with services available from private practitioners?

For medical schools everywhere these are perilous times. Dr. Lewis Thomas, an ardent supporter of medical schools, observes: "I have lived most of my professional life in one medical school after another, and have a deep affection and admiration for these institutions, but I can see that some things are wrong with them and are beginning to go wronger still. If I were the president of a major university I would not want to take on a medical school, and if it already had one, I would be lying awake nights trying to figure out ways to get rid of it."[8]

Our history indicates that the issue of "second schools" will be resolved primarily by the social, economic, and political conditions of the times, not by the medical profession. Physicians, then, might serve the state best by focusing primarily not on the issue of the schools' existence, but rather on both schools' responsible fulfillment of their proper and necessary functions.

References

1. *Introductory Lecture Delivered on the Eleventh of November, 1833 by Samuel Henry Dickson, M.D., Professor of Institutes of the Practice of Medicine, in the Medical College in the State of South Carolina, Charleston, SC.* Charleston, SC: J.S. Burgess; 1833.
2. Waring JI. Samuel Henry Dickson (1796-1872). *J Med Educ* 1960; 35: 421-428.
3. *Memorial of the Dean and Faculty of the Medical College of the State of South Carolina, to the Honorable Senate and House of Representatives of the State of South Carolina.* 6 January 1869.
4. Darby TJ. *The progress of medicine and surgery in the past five decades (annual address by the President of the Medical Association, Annual Session, 1875).* Charleston, SC: Edward Perry, printer; 1873: 36.
5. Sutusky JC. Summary of a review of medical education in South Carolina. *J SC Med Assoc* 1983; 78: 279-282.
6. Perry DR, Challoner DR, Oberst RJ. Research advances and resource constraints: Dilemmas facing medical education. *N Engl J Med* 1981; 305: 320-324.
7. Dibaggion JA. A twenty year forecast for academic medical centers (editorial). *N Engl J Med* 1981; 304: 228-230.
8. Thomas L. *The Youngest Science: Notes of a Medicine-Watcher.* New York: The Viking Press; 1973: 175.

Comprehensive Health/Lifestyle Education in the Secondary Schools... An Idea Whose Time Has Come?

J SC Med Assoc 1987; 83: 229

As Dr. Donald Kilgore observes in the preceding editorial, AIDS is not the only unhappy by-product of sexual activity among our high school students.[1] For years, South Carolina has ranked among the leading states in the incidence of sexually transmitted diseases. Worse, approximately 5,000 South Carolina schoolgirls between the ages of 14 and 17, and approximately 100 between the ages of 10 and 13, become pregnant each year. Over 80 percent of those who drop out of school will fail to complete their educations. The projected 10-year public sector cost for each year's cohort of teenage mothers and their first-born babies exceeds $125,000,000.

A bill being drafted for our General Assembly to amend the code of laws of 1976 would increase the extent of comprehensive health education in South Carolina. This bill would again mandate comprehensive health education between kindergarten and the eighth grade. The draft stipulates that "at least one time during the four years of grades 9-12, each student must receive instruction in reproductive health education and, at the discretion of the local board, instruction in family life education or pregnancy prevention education." The bill would leave considerable discretion to local school boards, who could choose their own instructional materials "addressing the subject of reproductive health education, family life education, and pregnancy prevention education."

The drafted bill provides that "health education for students in grades 9-12 may be given as part of an existing course or as a special course." This may be a step in the right direction, but hardly seems strong enough. At present, fewer than five percent of our secondary school students are receiving any type of health education course. Is there not a compelling need for our

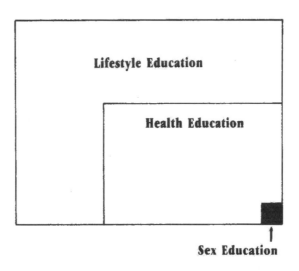

Sex Education

Although health education is an important component of lifestyle education, the latter curriculum should also include other topics (for example, frameworks for making ethical and moral decisions). Sex education should include both health education and also other components of the lifestyle education curriculum. Note that sex education, although important, is a relatively small part of the lifestyle education curriculum – despite publicity to the contrary.

educators to formulate a comprehensive curriculum?

For years, the SCMA has strongly advocated for comprehensive health education in our schools (one recalls, for instance, that this was the major theme of Dr. Harrison Peeples's presidency). Sex education should be taught as part and parcel of a comprehensive program in health education. Further, as Dr. Kilgore suggests, students need to receive a framework within which to make moral and ethical decisions. Therefore, why not teach health education only as part and parcel of a comprehensive program of lifestyle education (Figure)?

It has been clearly demonstrated that school health education promotes healthy behavior.[2] As Dr. Kilgore points out, it has not been shown that education about the anatomy, physiology, and complications of sex promotes promiscuity (for the record, one poll of sexual activity according to occupation indicates that physicians — who know all about the technical aspects of these matters — have the poorest sex lives; firemen have the best). We must not allow the emotionally-charged issue of sex education to divert the public's attention from the broad need for education about healthy lifestyles. We must encourage our legislators to pass a stronger bill. We must assist our educators in the drafting of an appropriate broad-based curriculum.

References

1. Kilgore DG. Sex education — a path with pitfalls (editorial). *J SC Med Assoc* 1987; 83: 226-228.
2. The effectiveness of school health education. *Morbidity and Mortality Weekly Report* 1986; 35: 593-594.

Whither Academic Health Centers?

J SC Med Assoc 1994; 90: 295-297

Ten years ago, Dr. Allen H. Johnson of the Medical University of South Carolina gave us an editorial on "The Quandary of Teaching Hospitals." Reflecting on the challenge then posed by per-case prospective payment and by a recommendation that Medicare no longer underwrite medical education, he concluded that

> teaching hospitals, particularly those associated with medical schools, face a number of problems; the solutions seem obscure ... the challenge in this transition is to

develop and support planning which will nurture and preserve excellence in health and medical education.[1]

Recently, Dr. Johnson reread his editorial and suggested that I write one on the new challenge to teaching hospitals: health care reform and managed competition. The following thoughts are meant to be generic, with no particular hospital or locality in mind. And, as always, letters-to-the-editor are welcomed and encouraged.

It is trendy nowadays to speak of "academic health centers" rather than "teaching hospitals." What exactly *is* an academic health center? A current technical definition is "an allopathic or osteopathic medical school, one or more affiliated teaching hospitals, and, usually, one or more other schools or programs in the health professions." By this definition, South Carolina would have two academic health centers (MUSC in Charleston and USC in Columbia). A stricter definition includes only those schools with their own tertiary care hospitals, in which case South Carolina has but one (MUSC). A looser definition includes all hospitals with residency programs, in which case South Carolina has at least seven. But by any of these definitions, one can generalize that academic health centers "own" the current problem (survival in the age of managed competition) to the extent that they depend upon practice revenues for operation.

The bottom line is the perception that academic health centers will be forced to compete (if they are not already competing) with everyone else for managed care contracts. Some form of universal entitlement to health care services seems inevitable, and in such a system efficiency will be mandated. It is widely perceived that our country's major academic health centers cannot survive in this environment without some kind of special recognition and compensation. There is little or no evidence that insurance companies are sympathetic to the reality that clinical practice is less efficient at academic centers. Still, as two reviewers recently put it, "In times of fundamental social change, institutions face both mortal threats and unparalleled opportunities."[2] The integrity of the medical profession—our sense of unity, our collective sense of self-esteem as professionals — hinges in part upon how this scenario plays out.

To some extent, the problem for academic health centers is that they have been entirely too successful. A century ago, there were hardly any full-time faculty members in the clinical departments of United States medical schools. The growth of full-time faculties was promoted by the Rockefeller Foundation, institutionalized by the Flexner Report, and accelerated by the National Institutes of Health. After World War II, full-time faculties grew almost exponentially. What was formerly charity care became profitable for academic health centers under Medicare and Medicaid, whose provisions recognized the additional costs incurred in teaching settings. Put simply, today's quandary for academic health centers was brought about by a truism of American life: Government giveth and government taketh away.

One opinion holds that academic health centers will not survive unless the public sector lends financial support to their missions. Each third party payer might be required to contribute to an "all payer pool of funds." By the year 2000, it is estimated that 1.5 billion dollars would be required to maintain the infrastructure of America's medical schools; 7.3 billion dollars for direct medical education costs; and 13 billion dollars for indirect medical education costs. What should the public expect in turn? Here are some desiderata:

• Greater accountability of academic health centers to their constituencies.

• Emphasis on networks rather than fiefdoms, which may require responsible downsizing.

• Research in the relevant areas of health care provision: cost, access, and quality.

• Supportive and reciprocal relationships between academic health care centers and private practitioners.

The last of these deserves further comment.

An issue-of-the-day (again, I speak generically) concerns the relationship of "public" and "private" medicine. As it evolved in the United States, "public" medicine associated with training programs became synonymous with academic health centers. Typically, such centers have provided primary and secondary

251

medical care for the indigent poor and tertiary care by referral from private practitioners. This is changing. Thousands of former trainees—now specialists, subspecialists, and sub-subspecialists—ply their mentors' trades in private hospitals thereby reducing referrals to academic health centers. Universal access to health insurance empowers the indigent poor to seek health care from the private sector. Competition from the private sector has already eroded the patient base of some academic health centers on the West Coast. The directions of health care reform will profoundly affect the relationship between academic physicians and physicians in private practice. And, as Dr. Johnson wrote a decade ago, "The solutions seem obscure."

What can, or should be done?

First, some kind of allowance should be made for academic health centers under any program for health care reform that emanates from Washington. Quality medical education and research requires subsidization. Most academic health centers probably need to downsize in at least some areas, but few deserve to die on the vine.

Second, the public is entitled to accountability. Academic health centers should be willing to commit to new paradigms.[3] They should spearhead efforts to develop practice guidelines; to streamline procedures and technologies; to conduct research on cost-effectiveness and quality; to promote relevant continuing education geared to real-life situations; and to lead Americans in debate concerning the limits we are willing to accept and/or impose upon health care delivery.

Third, new models of medical education should be vigorously pursued. We should reconsider the merits of having "the town wear the gown" as was formerly the case. Academic health centers burgeoned in an era in which it was possible for individuals to excel in teaching, in patient care, and in basic research. The "triple threat" physician-researcher-educator is today a vanishing breed. Mechanisms should be explored whereby practicing physicians are adequately trained and adequately rewarded for teaching medical students and residents.

Finally, we should continue to emphasize that we are, in the last analysis, one profession, committed to high standards in the public interest. We are bracing for a brave new world fraught with the potential for increasing divisiveness. The best safeguard against this happening is to be willing to talk to one another and to encourage involvement, participation, and dialogue in our relevant medical organizations.

References

1. Johnson AH. The quandary for teaching hospitals. *J SC Med Assoc* 1984; 80: 507-508.
2. Blumenthal D, Meyer GS. The future of the academic medical center under health care reform. *N Engl J Med* 1993; 329: 1812-1814.
3. Barondess JA. The academic health center and the public agenda: Whose three legged stool? *Ann Intern Med* 1991; 115: 962-967.

Just Thinking

J SC Med Assoc 1996; 92: 280-282

What is the hardest task in the world? To think.
—Emerson

Browsing through Bartlett's *Familiar Quotations*, I came across the following attributed to Robert Louis Stevenson: "Do you know what the Governor of South Carolina said to the Governor of North Carolina? It's a long time between drinks, observed that powerful thinker."[1] I bristled at yet another slur on the intelligence of Southerners in general and of South Carolinians in particular. Why should Stevenson, or anyone else for that matter, single out the Governor of South Carolina? And certainly the expression "It's a long time between drinks" is intelligence-neutral. On further reflection, I choose to be charitable toward Stevenson's unfortunate remark, to take it as a more generalized comment on how few of us really think. And how few of us think well!

The Chicago philosopher Allan Bloom, in *The Closing of the American Mind,* suggests that our society to its great detriment rewards performers rather than thinkers.[2] We pay billions to watch basketball players, opera singers, actors and actresses — really, just about anyone who performs well. We respect those who think — columnists, justices, humanities professors, and the like — but we pay them relatively poorly. This criticism also resounds within medicine and is reflected by higher reimbursement rates for technical skills than for cognitive activities. But the purpose of this editorial is not to lament these truisms; it's likely that most societies have, at least in the short run, paid performers better than thinkers. Rather, the purpose is to suggest that we try to think clearly and well about where medicine is going and what we can do about it, and that we must think collectively.

We are prisoners of our paradigms. We must think hard if we are to change them. Francis Bacon (1561-1626), who often receives credit for what came to be known as the inductive method of reasoning, listed four components of clear thinking: observation, experimentation, reasoning, and generalization. He added the caveats that we must control our observations, neutralize bias, and exercise extreme caution when we draw conclusions. Bacon's reflections encapsulate what we now call the scientific method, yet they transcend science. What, to pose a central issue, do we mean by "the profession of medicine?" There is nothing unique to medicine about trying to help other people in matters relating to their health. There is nothing unique to medicine about our science, which increasingly belongs to biology as a whole. It seems inevitable that our identity as a profession will be a major twenty-first century theme.

The educational literature contains a great deal of debate about what it means to think cirtically.[3] There is no universally agreed-upon definition of critical thinking. However, we can recognize it when it occurs by certain features such as the following:

• Identifying and challenging assumptions, including awareness of the contextual basis of assumptions.

• Exploring and imagining alternatives, including a deliberate, reflective skepticism of passed-down dogma and "universal truth."

• Alternating phases of action and analysis; we do what we are trained to do (act) yet step back and reflect from time to time on why we act (analyze).

• Challenging assumptions, especially after "trigger events" that prompt discomfort or perplexity.

• Realizing that the things that happen to us as individuals — both good and bad — nearly always reflect wider social phenomena.

Critical thinking cannot be taught in the classroom setting, although good teachers know how to challenge their learners. Critical thinking is not an entirely rational activity. It is person-specific. No method for enhancing it works for everyone. Yet it is a necessary activity, crucial for personal effectiveness in our jobs, our personal relationships, and our contributions to society.

The essence of critical thinking is to identify and challenge assumptions, and then to imagine and explore alternatives. To think critically ourselves, the most pressing task is to reflect on a problem and then test new approaches or solutions. To encourage critical thinking in others, the most important skill is attentive listening — again, an active, energy-requiring process. Critical thinking carries risks. It requires that we challenge both psychological and cultural assumptions. Indeed we must weigh the risks because the consequences of critical thinking can be both positive and negative. Yet not to think critically also incurs risks; namely, someone else may do our thinking for us!

Critical thinking about the medical profession must address two key questions: What do we *do* as physicians? What *are* we as physicians? With regard to the former, we would like to think that we are in excellent shape. To an increasing extent our collective literature and presumably our private thoughts reflect such hard questions as sensitivity, specificity, positive and negative predictive values, risk-benefit ratios, and cost analyses. But again, we are prisoners of the paradigms of our era. How will future generations judge us? The late Lewis Thomas once made a striking statement: "It was discovered, sometime in the 1830s, that the greater part of medicine was nonsense."[4] What will future historians, with hindsight steeped in technologies that we have not even conceived—say about us? I suspect that most physicians reflect on a daily basis (sometimes almost unconsciously as a way of life) on the real wisdom of what they do. Lester S. King, the distinguished former senior editor of *JAMA*, observed that "the modern riot of technology has given rise to linguistic usage that obscures clear thinking."[5] Put simply, are we as good as we think we are?

As a profession, we must ask who we are, what we stand for, and what is best not only for ourselves but also for society. What should we do differently? How should we do it? Whose help should we enlist, and on what basis? Unfortunately, the isolated, rugged individualism that historically characterizes physicians can be a powerful impediment to addressing questions that must be answered collectively. Fortunately, an increasing volume of literature exists on various methods for collective thinking. These include:

• *Brainstorming* (encouraging participants to think of as many ideas as they can, with no criticism aloud).

• *Envisioning alternative futures* (speculating on how things might turn out.)

• *Developing preferred scenarios* (that is, concrete descriptions of what we desire in the future).

• *Imaging alternatives* through "right brain" aesthetic triggers (such as poetry, fantasy, drawing, photography, songwriting, and drama); and

• *Futures invention* (a technique involving the questioning of the validity of futures created for us by others).[3]

The latter technique would seem especially valuable as a collective enterprise. What should be our specific goals? How can we measure the goals? What will be the positive and negative consequences of achieving our goals? How might the goals be modified? Using skilled group facilitators, it is possible to construct scenarios and to write individual and collective futures histories. The essence of all of these activities, of course, is that collectively we must be proactive rather than reactive. We must remember that—in contrast to the law and the ministry—there is nothing about medicine that ensures its survival as a profession as opposed to a mere activity.

The discerning reader will glean from all of this many questions and few clear-cut answers. We must think, we must think about what it means to think, and we must do our thinking collectively. Let us not allow future historians to say about us what Robert Louis Stevenson said about the Governor of South Carolina. Even if it has been a long time between drinks!

References

1. Kaplan J. ed. *Bartlett's Familiar Quotations*. Sixteenth edition, Boston: Little Brown and Company; 1992: 562.
2. Bloom A. *The Closing of the American Mind*. New York: Simon and Schuster; 1987.
3. Brookfield SD. *Developing Critical Thinkers: Challenging Adults to Explore Alternative Ways of Thinking and Acting*. San Francisco: Josey-Bass; 1987.
4. Thomas L. *The Medusa and the Snail*. New York: Viking; 1979: 159-160.
5. King LS. *Medical Thinking: A Historical Preface*. Princeton, New Jersey: Princeton University Press; 1982: 59.

Reflections on the SMA-1
(A.K.A., The Medical History)

J SC Med Assoc 1997; 93: 387-389

These thoughts about the medical history are based on 30 years of reflection and are offered here because of the increasing extent to which our written work is scrutinized by others.

— CSB

A tongue-in-cheek aphorism of unknown attribution holds, "When all else fails, take a history." A refinement is to ask, "What did the SMA-1 show?" I call the history the SMA-1 and the physical examination the SMA-2 — ideally, neither should be preceded by any other tests! In presenting here some personal preferences for the history, I don't wish to imply that there's only one way to do it. Indeed, I marvel at one colleague's ability to construct a pathophysiologically-based problem list, at another's ability to capture the essence of a case with a few terse phrases. Each physician should work out and take pride in an individual style. Here's my abbreviated version of Strunk and White's *Elements of Style* as applied to the SMA-1.

1. **Introduce the patient** by name and record number. Thereafter, just say "he" or "she." Who else but the patient? Who else but Mrs. Brown?

2. Frame the scenario in a **lead paragraph** — ideally, a single long sentence — that includes the chief complaint and its duration and whets the reader's appetite for more. Your task is to make your patient seem like the most interesting human being in South Carolina, for you are this person's advocate. Recall Rudyard Kipling's famous ditty: "I kept six honest serving men/They taught me all I knew/Their names are What and Where/ and Why and How and When and Who." Like a good newspaper reporter, you should try to answer all of these questions in the opening paragraph. Is there anything distinctly

newsworthy about your patient? If so, include it (for example: "This is the first admission to this hospital, and indeed the first lifetime hospitalization, for this 96-year-old still-active farmer.") Here's a fuller example (based on a tongue-in-cheek hypothetical case):

> This is the 17th Mecca Medical Center admission for this 59-year-old divorced (X3) white male house painter who carries previous diagnoses of alcoholism, biopsy-proven Laennec's cirrhosis, and esophageal varices, who was last discharged 6 weeks ago after an episode of endoscopically-documented variceal bleeding, and who is now admitted by way of the emergency room to which he was brought early this morning by friends with a chief complaint of "vomiting up bright red blood" which began at 3 A.M. today in the course of an all-night poker game.

Note here the literary device of "who carries previous diagnoses of" or "whose previous diagnoses include." Revealing the key elements of the patient's previous diagnoses enables the reader to begin forming hypotheses about what's wrong with the patient. You should of course justify each of these diagnoses in the body of your workup or, in the event of incomplete data, with something like "presumed" or "according to the patient" or "according to the most recent discharge summary."

3. The **present illness** should be segmented into a series of relatively short paragraphs. You should write like Hemingway, not Faulkner. You should begin each paragraph with a participial phrase indicating time in relation to today's date. Remember that future readers will have no frame of reference for "last Wednesday" or "October 17" unless they happen to be idiot savants. There are two approaches: Start with the most recent event and work backwards, or start with the first event and work forwards. I don't think it matters, but don't forget to ask, "When was the last time you were in your usual good health (or baseline health)?" Try to avoid medical terminology unless your patient uses it or unless you make it clear that the

terms came from the old records. For example:

> *At 3 AM this morning,* he was in his usual state of poor health when, while holding three aces and two kings in a game of five-card stud, he suddenly began to vomit bright red blood ...
>
> *Twelve years ago (1985; see old records),* he had his first episode of hematemesis ...

Be generous about what you include in the present illness, bringing in relevant portions of the past history, review of systems, family history, and social history. The present illness should contain most if not all of the information relevant to formulating a hypothesis about what's wrong with the patient.

4. Start **the past medical history** with a statement about the patient's general health—ideally, his or her verbatim response to your question, "How has your health been *most* of your life, except for the problem bothering you now?" This is the lifetime equivalent of the "chief complaint." Properly done, it conveys a great deal of information. Contrast, for example, the patient who exclaims "Perfect!" with the one who laments that "I've been sickly most of my life, and my mother says that even as a baby I got everything that came around." The former patient may be a stoic; the latter may have a somatization disorder. After cataloguing her acute infectious diseases, hospitalizations, operations, immunizations, and present medications, be sure to include under "allergies" whether she has ever taken penicillin-type drugs. If she reports a drug allergy, state when it occurred and exactly what happened. Remember that "NKA" won't help the future reader very much during an emergency.

5. Don't skimp on the **review of systems**, especially since auditors are now indicating that they plan to take your thoroughness here quite seriously. The components are straightforward and known to all physicians, but I'd like to emphasize two categories that are often neglected: sleep and weight. What are his sleep patterns, and does he snore loudly? What is her all-time maximum (non-pregnant) weight? What did she weigh at high school graduation? What did she weigh a year ago, and

what does she weigh now?

6. Make the **family history** concise unless it's really interesting and relevant. Indicate what the parents and any siblings may have died from and at what ages. Try to include heart disease, diabetes, and cancer, and any diseases that might bear on the present illness.

7. Make the **social history** a distinct portrait of the patient and his lifestyle, and—ideally—a celebration of his uniqueness. How far did she go in school? Where has she lived? Tell about occupations, marriages, children, and hobbies. Mention any special accomplishments. What does he do during a typical day? And of course mention use of tobacco, alcohol, and any illicit drugs.

8. The **physical examination** should not be a dissertation on normal external anatomy, but neither should it be skimpy. Remember that "WNL" means "we never looked." I especially cringe at "HEENT: WNL," since it's a rare person who doesn't have some imperfection above the clavicles—a fleck of calcium on the right tympanic membrane, arcus corneae, slight deviation of the nasal septum to the left, or a torus palatinus deformity. Likewise, you should nearly always find some abnormality on the skin in anyone past early childhood. Avoid diagnostic terms unless the abnormality is relatively trivial and the diagnosis reasonably obvious. Even then it's best to use modifiers such as "consistent with" (for example, "hypopigmented macules on the upper chest consistent with tinea versicolor").

9. The **impression** or **problem list** should reflect the depth and accuracy of your thinking about the case. Remember that a "problem" is any abnormality identified by the history, the physical examination, or further studies defined to its fullest extent but no further. Problems are not "rule outs." I strongly encourage such phrases as "etiology uncertain" or "cause undetermined (suspected this or that)," for they indicate intellectual honesty. My preference is to group problems if it seems logical to do so, to lump rather than to split. And I try to suggest possible etiologic relationships and the interrelationship of various problems whenever possible. In listing problems and their "sub-problems," you should not be fettered by strict di-

agnostic terminology. Make the problem list read like a kind of Table of Contents to the patient's history. Feel free to list as sub-problems such things as the patient's last cardiac ejection fraction as determined by echocardiograpy or the date of the patient's last colonoscopy. Here's a problem list for our hypothetical patient:

PROBLEMS:
1. Acute hematemesis, cause undetermined, suspected secondary to (2. b.)
2. Laennec's cirrhosis, biopsy-proven, secondary to (3), complicated by
    (a) ascites
    (b) esophageal varices, endoscopically-verified
    (c) elevated BUN and creatinine — suspect early hepatorenal syndrome, consider other possible causes
    (d) previous episode of hepatic encephalopathy, resolved, now on maintenance lactulose
3. Alcoholism by history, related to (4)
4. Suboptimal social situation.

Note here the attempt to keep the number of active problems relatively small and therefore manageable.

10. Write a brief **formulation** or **discussion** in which you summarize your thinking about the patient. This is your chance to show your knowledge of medicine, your grasp of the differential diagnosis and the likely outcome. Make it clear that you've considered unusual possibilities ("zebras," we call them), and why you've elected not to pursue these aggressively at this time. Mentioning such possibilities may be extremely helpful later on should the outcome be unfavorable or the case come to litigation. A well-reasoned and well-documented clinical judgment nearly always suffices to establish that you've met and even exceeded the proverbial "standard of care." This is also your chance to document, however briefly, that you've delved into the medical literature seeking evidence-based knowledge to bear on the current problem. For example:

Formulation: This unfortunate man with known cirrhosis presents with massive hematemesis probably caused by his varices, as was the case on his last hospitalization. The sudden onset without vomiting argues against a Mallory-Weiss tear; lack of recent use of alcohol, NSAIDs, or other corrosive drugs argues against gastritis, and the normal stomach and duodenum on his recent endoscopy makes peptic ulcer unlikely. We plan to control the bleeding by sclerotherapy or banding (for a recent meta-analysis of the literature, see *Blood and Guts* 1997; 6: 14-28). If he survives the acute illness, we should again enlist the help of Social Services to see whether a living arrangement more satisfactory than his present boarding home can be found. His present condition is serious, and his long-term prognosis is poor.

11. Outline your **plan** succinctly and systematically, making liberal use of such phrases as "studies as per order sheet."
12. **Sign** your work with pride!

Editorial Note Written 10 Years Later: Calling the medical history the "SMA-1" was, to my knowledge, begun by my good friend Dr. Charles V. (Bo) Sanders, longtime chair of the Department of Medicine at Louisiana State University School of Medicine in New Orleans. He coined "SMA-1" after the then-popular term "SMA-7" for a panel of chemical determinations (blood or plasma glucose, blood urea nitrogen, serum creatinine, serum sodium, serum potassium, serum chloride, and serum carbon dioxide combining power). This term has since been replaced by the "basic metabolic panel." Beginning in 2006, I've spent two hours reviewing this material with each group of five or six third-year medical students rotating through our internal medicine service. I remind them that clear, concise, and thoughtful writing and speaking remains important to the physician's professional identity.

Physical Diagnosis and the Technological Imperative

J SC Med Assoc 2001; 97: 259-261

Doctor, I wanna know *exactly* what's wrong with me!" The patient before me had been referred for evaluation of chronic cough. Five minutes into the history I was reasonably certain that the answer would be gastroesophageal reflux disease (GERD) and that the next step should be a therapeutic trial of a proton pump inhibitor. I was also reasonably certain that this approach would not satisfy her. I therefore obtained a 24-hour esophageal pH study which, sure enough, showed acid reflux that correlated with her symptom diary. "Doctor," she beamed, "you knew exactly what was wrong with me!" I also knew that I had practiced cost-ineffective medicine, allowing myself to be bullied by that widespread societal phenomenon, the technological imperative.

Last month's issue of *The Journal* contained a paean to Dr. Peter C. Gazes of the Medical University of South Carolina. Dr. N. B. Baroody was especially complimentary of Dr. Gazes' prowess at physical diagnosis. To see a master clinician such as Dr. Gazes honored appropriately during his lifetime is gratifying indeed, and we note with pride that a research institute at MUSC now bears this eminent cardiologist's name. Dr. Baroody did not mention his mentor's famous sense of humor. I've mused over one of his quips: "The electrocardiogram sent my children to college and my wife through Niemann-Marcus. I suspect that the echocardiogram will do my trainees even better!"[1] Reimbursement rates favor procedures. Newer technologies threaten to place master physical diagnosticians on the endangered species list. I'm often impressed that today's average echocardiography technician can within a few minutes glean more information about the heart's inner workings that all but the finest physical diagnosticians, such as Dr. Gazes and Dr. J. O'Neal Humphries of the University of South Carolina School of Medicine in Columbia. And I'm sometimes saddened that the echocardiogram has deprived me of what I used to consider the greatest bedside thrill in medicine: being the first to hear a murmur of mitral stenosis ("a sound resembling an oxcart rumbling over a distant wooden bridge"). Will physical diagnosis become largely obsolete?

Dr. Joseph Sapira, author of an incredibly entertaining yet thorough textbook on physical diagnosis, believes that a revolution in academic medicine began around the year 1968 "when the intellectual approach to diagnosis and its attendant techniques of clinical examination fell into disrespect, superseded by an inappropriately exclusive reliance on dogma and modern technological devices."[2] The year 1968 also marked the beginning of my career in internal medicine. I've been increasingly amazed by the impact of the technological imperative on so much of what we think, say, and do. Reimbursement rates aside, there is much to be said for the newer approaches. Noninvasive procedures such as CT, MRI, and ultrasound make medicine increasingly humane, decreasing as they do the need to poke and probe the body with needles and other sharp instruments. These innovations are in some ways the twentieth-century counterpart to the nineteenth-century's introduction of anesthesia. Downsides to the technological imperative include (1) spiraling costs, due in part to consumer demand; (2) less emphasis on thinking our way through various diagnostic possibilities; and (3) adding distance between the patient and his/her primary care physician.

Is it possible to compare the accuracy of physical diagnosis with that of technologically advanced procedures? Dr. Faith Fitzgerald lists five barriers to such comparisons:[3]

• Unreliability of method. Who did the physical examination? Who interpreted the results of the technological procedure?

• Rapid evolution of technology. Frequent improvements in machines and devices make it difficult to conduct accurate prospective studies, and to compare the results of new studies with those of previously published ones.

• The time, expense, and ease of diagnosis. If a brain lesion can be demonstrated by a CT scan within 30 minutes, is this not preferable to an hour or more of an accomplished neurologist's time?

• Quality control. Do we really know a good physical finding when we encounter it?

• Clinical significance of findings. The newer technology, compared with physical diagnosis, is more likely to yield "incidentalomas" — unexpected findings of uncertain significance which may, however, propel the unwitting physician and his/her patient down a primrose path or "diagnostic cascade" with its potential for morbidity and even mortality.

Despite such barriers, many researchers now submit findings from physical examination to rigorous analysis. For a given finding, what are the sensitivity, specificity, positive predictive value, negative predictive value, and likelihood ratio? These questions now drive a movement for teaching evidence-based physical diagnosis.[4] *The Journal of the American Medical Association* has since 1993 featured a series entitled "the rational clinical examination," designed to help us make the best of bedside physical diagnosis. Certain life-threatening lesions — for example, sphenoid sinusitis, epidural abscess, and abdominal aortic aneurysm — demand imaging procedures. However, most of the time we can get along quite well, at least in the outpatient setting, with the medical history (which according to various experts still provides up 80 to 90 percent of useful diagnostic information), the physical examination, and a few highly selected tests or procedures.

Every now and then the medical literature serves up a new bedside test, an approach to diagnosis that is useful, cost-effective, and even life-saving. The most recent example to catch my attention is the *jolt test*, or jolt accentuation of headache, for the diagnosis of meningitis in patients with fever and headache. The patient is asked to rotate his/her head laterally at a frequency of two to three times per second (Figure). Accentuation of the headache constitutes a positive response. Originally described by two Japanese investigators,[5] jolt accentuation of headache was found to have a sensitivity of 100 percent, a specificity of 54 percent, a positive likelihood ratio of 2.2, and a negative likelihood ratio of zero for the diagnosis of meningitis in patients

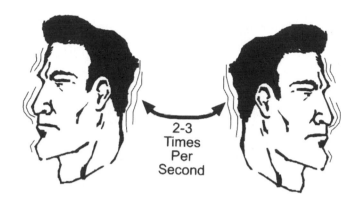

2-3
Times
Per
Second

The jolt test for accentuation of headache consists of rotating the head laterally at a frequency of 2 to 3 times per second. Experience suggests that this simple measure carries a high sensitivity (100%) but low specificity (54%) for the presence of meningitis.

presenting with fever and headache.[6] Put differently, the absence of jolt accentuation of headache allows one to state confidently that meningitis is extremely unlikely. The presence of jolt accentuation, especially if accompanied by other symptoms and signs such as nausea, vomiting, and stiff neck, suggests the need for lumbar puncture or, at the very least, for close observation and careful follow-up.

My friend Bruce Fye of the Mayo Clinic, who has recently published a definitive history of American cardiology, wonders aloud how much longer the stethoscope will remain the preeminent symbol of the medical profession. Will the stethoscope soon go the way of the leech and the urine specimen glass? What will take its place? All we know for certain is that the technology at our disposal will get better and better. It's up to us to determine the value and cost-effectiveness of our own eyes, ears, touch, and even smell.

"Doctor, I wanna know *exactly* what's wrong with me!"

Note and References

1. In repeating this tongue-in-cheek quip, I am, of course, in no way critical of Doctor Gazes, who exemplifies our best traditions. I sometimes jest that acne put me through college, my father having been a dermatologist.
2. Sapira JD. *The Art and Science of Bedside Diagnosis*. Baltimore: Williams & Wilkins; 1990: xiii.
3. Fitzgerald FT. Physical diagnosis versus technology: A review. *West J Med* 1990; 152: 377-382.
4. Fagan MJ, Griffith RA. An evidence-based physical diagnosis curriculum for third-year medicine clerks. *Acad Med* 2000; 75: 528-529.
5. Uchihara J, Tsukagoshi H. Jolt accentuation of headache: The most sensitive sign of CSF pleocytosis. *Headache* 1991; 31: 167-171.
6. Altia J, Hatala R, Cook JJ, et al. Does this adult patient have meningitis? *JAMA* 1999; 282: 175-181.

Editorial Note: This editorial was written during my preparation of a textbook (Bryan CS, ed. *Infectious Diseases in Primary Care*. Philadelphia: W.B. Saunders Company, 2002). To quote from the introduction:

> Special emphasis is given to emergencies because of the recognition that primary care clinicians, compared with their hospital-based counterparts, are at a huge disadvantage. Primary care clinicians often see patients who harbor life-threatening infections, but before the telltale symptoms and signs have appeared. Yet primary care clinicians are under increasing pressure to maintain crammed schedules and to be "cost-effective," with parsimonious use of laboratory tests and imaging studies.

When patients who later turn out to have acute meningitis are first seen, headache and stiff neck are frequently less prominent than nausea and vomiting—hence, the fairly common misdiagnosis of "gastroenteritis". Therefore, the jolt test struck me as a potential helpful and time-efficient addition to the physician's diagnostic armamentarium.

Public Health and the HIV/AIDS Epidemic

Immunization Against Swine Influenza: A Major Challenge for South Carolina Physicians

J SC Med Assoc 1976; 72: 303-304

Much of the story is in the name: human influenza A virus, A New Jersey (Hsw1N1). The nomenclature tells us, first, that this virus is of the type (A) apt to cause epidemics or pandemics, and that it was isolated from humans in New Jersey during this bicentennial year. But the key is in the parentheses — "(Hsw1N1)." These symbols tell us that this virus has a hemagglutinin antigen (H) and a neuraminidase antigen (N) quite unlike those of the Hong Kong viruses (H3N2) that have been prevalent since 1968. Therefore, the population has little or no immunity, and the stage is set for a major pandemic.

The South Carolina Medical Association has made its commitment to assist in the swine flu immunization program. The scope of this program is without precedent, and we can anticipate many problems. The specific details are, at the time of this writing, still being formulated. The two articles that follow, written on short notice for *The Journal*, deal with the need for massive immunization and the tentative plans for providing it.

Dr. Bernard Lourie's article summarizes what is known about the molecular epidemiology of the influenza virus.[1] From the historic consequences of antigenic shift (Table 1 in Dr. Lourie's article), the decision to proceed with mass immunization would seem to rest on solid grounds,[2] even if a few dissenting voices have been heard in the scientific community. Dr. Richard Parker's article emphasizes the limited Federal assistance (11 cents per citizen) for the actual administration of the vaccine in South Carolina, and outlines the need for substantial assistance from physicians and from voluntary organizations.

The public will need reassurance that the new virus will not cause anything they've not previously experienced. Although there may be a greater tendency for serious disease among young persons compared with other recent strains,[2] swine in-

271

fluenza—if it occurs—will be the "same old flu," which has been called "an unvarying disease (three-day fever) caused by a varying virus."[1] It is the quantitative aspect—the possibility of a pandemic—that concerns us. The public will need to know that the traditional high-risk groups (the aged, those with chronic heart or lung disease, and so forth) should be immunized not only against the swine influenza virus but also against the recently-prevalent A/Victoria/75 (H3N2) strain, still of epidemic potential. And they need to appreciate that, while the recognition of an epidemic or pandemic of influenza A is straightforward, the precise diagnosis in an individual patient is not. We must warn them against blaming any respiratory illness next winter on the failure of the Swine flu vaccine, just as we must be cautious not to assume that any illness closely following immunization is due to the inoculation.

References

1. Kilbourne ED. The molecular epidemiology of influenza. *J Infect Dis* 1973; 127: 478-487.
2. Weinstein L. Influenza—1918, a revisit? (editorial). *N Engl J Med* 1976; 294: 1058-1060.
3. Influenza Vaccine Preliminary Statement. Center for Disease Control: *Morbidity and Mortality Weekly Weekly Report* 1976; 25 (June 4): 165.

Editorial Note Written 31 years Later: The swine flu pandemic never materialized and some would consider the immunization campaign to have been a colossal mistake. However, we learned a lot and I still feel that it was the best decision based on the available facts. Preparation for potential influenza pandemics continues to be highly problematic and fraught with political and ethical overtones.

Physicians and the Environment

J SC Med Assoc 1978; 74: 35-36

The very last sequence of "Li'l Abner," which appeared in the comics section of our newspapers on November 13, 1977, pertains to our topic. Fearless Fosdick grapples with a flock of ferocious vultures, sent over by the Environmental Protection Agency to rid a lady's farm of spiders. How, next, will she get rid of the vultures? The genius at the Environmental Protection Agency proposes to send over some vulture-eating jackals ... then, to get rid of the jackals, he'll send over some man-eating tigers, then ....

Disgusted, the lady proclaims that she'll sell the farm and move to Tibet, where hopefully there are no such geniuses in "their Environmental Protection Agency." Finally, in the very last frame, as Al Capp bade farewell to his devoted readers of 43 years, Fosdick shoots another vulture and says of the Tibetans: "I doubt the poor souls even have an environmental protection agency."

Environmentalists, like the rest of us, tend to take themselves too seriously. Yet we cannot afford to ignore those things that threaten the ecosystems of our fragile planet. We physicians, steeped in cause-and-effect interpretations of biologic systems, should appreciate the issues at least as well and perhaps better than most people. We may have mixed feelings about the survival of the red-cockaded woodpecker versus the need for lumber, or the survival of the loggerhead sea turtle versus the need for seaside resorts and good shellfish, but it's hard to believe that chemicals in our waters that cause defective ovulation in ospreys do not likewise cause harmful, if subtle, effects in *Homo sapiens*. Many issues of our time have heavy meanings not only for individual humans, but also for humans as a species. Physicians, from their immediate experiences, can appreciate the implications of both minor and major alterations of our most precious possession, the gene pool.

A summary of a major symposium on the public health

consequences of outer continental shelf development appears in this issue of *The Journal*. The need for fuel is obvious, and the reader will note that the participants in the symposium do not debate whether the shelf should be exploited. Rather, they discuss the on-shore consequences of this development, helping us brace for the inevitable future shock. The coastal wetlands of South Carolina contain 27 percent of the salt marsh of the entire Eastern seaboard, and provide the biologic beginnings of much of what we associate with "the good life." Already, Drs. McKellar, Turner, and Brantley note, some areas along our coast have an unacceptable level of air pollution, and data suggest that a single oil refinery might increase the death rate by 55 per 100,000 population. The relationships between the environment and *Homo sapiens* become inextricable, and it is a truism, again, to conclude that "the relationship between oil refineries and health in South Carolina is a critical issue."

Practicing physicians and the Department of Health and Environmental Control have not always agreed over some issues, as Dr. Harrison Peeples discusses in his editorial, above. However, we should have little quarrel with efforts of DHEC in environmental control. The unique role of private physicians is the care of individual patients; the unique role of public health is the care of populations. The triumphs of public health are triumphs for populations, the disasters are disasters for populations. The issues that concern Dr. Peeples' committee are issues mainly of health of individuals. Few, if any, of these issues deal with environmental control.

Environmentalists have been heard to complain that DHEC has, in recent years, placed too much emphasis on the issues of the health of individuals and too little emphasis on the issues of the environment. They complain that appointments to the DHEC Board have gone mainly to industrialists (or more recently, to oral surgeons) rather than to persons with proven qualifications in environmental matters. We suggest that the problems posed by conflicts over the drug formulary, the nurse midwife program, and the EPSDT screening program—to name a few—will seem small, even petty, in the eyes of future generations. Their lasting concern will be with what our generation did about the environmental issues of our day.

Our environment is indeed fragile. Physicians, with strong beliefs in cause-and-effect, should support a more active Department of Health and *Environmental Control* (*emphasis added*).

AIDS in South Carolina

J SC Med Assoc 1983; 78: 452-453

The report in June 1981 of five previously healthy men who developed *Pneumocystis carinii* pneumonia proved to be the harbinger of one of the most significant epidemics of this century. Reported in this month's issue of *The Journal* is a similar case, which to our knowledge is the first published case of the acquired immune deficiency syndrome from South Carolina. As of June 20, 1983, physicians and health departments in the United States had reported 1,641 cases of AIDS to the Center for Disease Control.[1] Three confirmed and nine suspected cases had become apparent within South Carolina, of whom nine had died; all but one of the patients were males between ages nine and forty-two, most were either homosexuals or intravenous drug abusers, and nine of the twelve patients had died.[2] Concern that AIDS might spread beyond its present "4-H" Club

(Haitians, homosexuals, hemophiliacs, and heroin abusers) makes AIDS the most widely feared disease in recent memory. Swine influenza, legionellosis, and the toxic-shock syndrome pale by comparison.

The South Carolina Department of Health and Environmental Control has declared AIDS a reportable disease. Physicians, therefore, should know the abbreviated case definition: the occurrence of a disease that is at least moderately predictive of a defect in cell-mediated immunity in a patient without known cause for diminished host resistance (such as corticosteroid therapy, neoplasia, known immune deficiency state, or advanced age). Cases fitting this definition should be reported to the DHEC Bureau of Disease Control or to county health departments. Only by such reporting can the real, rather than the imagined, threat of AIDS be monitored.

It is worth remembering that the epidemiologist's broad working definitions of various disorders, designed with the aim of collecting data in order to solve group problems, often differ from the clinician's more precise definitions, designed with the aim of helping one sick person get well. The official case definition of AIDS, for example, makes no mention of tests of T-lymphocyte function. That some patients have already begun to appear in physician's offices asking for "the test for AIDS" (determination of the ratio of T helper to T suppressor lymphocytes) suggests that a brief review of one aspect of the immune system may be appropriate.

Mature lymphocytes consist primarily of T cells (for thymus-derived), which confer cell-mediated immunity, and B cells (for bone marrow-derived) which confer humoral immunity. Specialized techniques demonstrate that, normally, approximately 80 percent of circulating lymphocytes are T cells and 10 to 15 percent are B cells (the remainder are known as null cells). The T lymphocytes regulate B lymphocyte function by an intricate system of checks and balances. "Helper" T cells enable B lymphocytes to proliferate, to differentiate into plasma cells, and to thus make specific immunoglobulins (antibodies). "Suppressor" T lymphocytes hold in the reins, so to speak, by inhibiting the proliferation of both T helper cells and of B cells.

Normally T helper cells outnumber T suppressor cells in peripheral blood. In AIDS, the ratio is reversed.

The essential nature of AIDS appears to be paralysis of effector T lymphocytes. The cause of this paralysis remains a mystery. Initial observations suggested that repeated, heavy exposure to an agent such as the DNA cytomegalovirus might "switch off" cell-mediated immunity. However, increasing reports of the acquisition of AIDS by seemingly "innocent" persons, such as newborn infants by way of blood transfusion, and the similarity of the epidemiology of AIDS to the epidemiology of hepatitis B[3] point to the possibility that a viral agent may cause AIDS through a single exposure. The present front runner is the recently-discovered human T-cell leukemia virus — an RNA retrovirus which by means of a remarkable enzyme known as reverse transcriptase can produce a DNA copy of its RNA genome.[4,5] Although this virus has been isolated from T-lymphocytes from several patients with AIDS, many questions remain unanswered.

In the meantime, what should practicing physicians tell their inquiring patients about AIDS? A primer for patients might read as follows:

(1) There is no diagnostic test for AIDS. Reversed T helper/suppressor ratios can be found in apparently normal persons, especially those who have received frequent blood transfusions,[6] and we simply don't know the risk that such persons will eventually develop AIDS.

(2) In ambulatory medical practice, possible early clues to AIDS include unexplained weight loss, generalized lymphadenopathy, oral candidiasis without obvious predisposing cause (such as broad-spectrum antibiotic therapy), or nonhealing herpetic ulcerations. If neither these nor the disorders shown in the Table (*Note to reader*: The table is omitted here, as the list of AIDS-defining conditions has changed and has also become common knowledge) are present, and if the absolute peripheral blood lymphocyte count (obtained by multiplying the total white blood count by the percentage of lymphocytes) exceeds 1500 per cmm, AIDS is highly unlikely.

(3) AIDS remains rare within South Carolina. At least four of

the 12 confirmed or suspected cases were probably acquired elsewhere.

(4) The Red Cross screens blood donors for possible membership among the high-risk groups for AIDS. Further, the voluntary nature of most blood donations in South Carolina makes transmission of AIDS unlikely.

(5) The hepatitis B vaccine appears to be safe. Extremely close monitoring of the possibility that the vaccine could transmit AIDS has been completely unrevealing, and we should remember that the vaccine is subjected to three separate procedures capable of inactivating all known viruses. Physicians should recommend the vaccine to patients at high risk of hepatitis B, such as male homosexuals. Health care workers with frequent blood exposures should also consider the vaccine.

(6) The rapid elucidation of the epidemiology, pathophysiology, and possible etiology of AIDS attests to the ability of today's medical and scientific communities to identify and solve problems of public importance.

But lest we become too reassured, let us reflect upon another report in this month's issue. That AIDS is the *acquired* immune deficiency syndrome reminds us of the existence of the *congenital* immune deficiencies. In this issue of *The Journal*, Dr. Burdash and co-workers from the Medical University of South Carolina add to our knowledge of one example among the numerous congenital immune deficiency disorders. It is humbling to realize that the first well-characterized congenital immune deficiency syndrome (Bruton's agammaglobulinemia) was not described until 1952. Eleven years ago, an editorialist in *The Lancet* suggested that the congenital immune deficiency syndromes might ultimately prove to be related to the introduction of antibiotics, which by early treatment of naturally-occurring infections had blunted man's ability to mount an immune response — an ability acquired through untold centuries of co-existence with various pathogens.[7] The recent recognition of AIDS — occurring as it has among the first generation of persons exposed to antibiotics beginning in early childhood — provides further room for speculation. Could AIDS — ultimately — prove to be yet another disease of medical progress?

References

1. *Morbidity and Mortality Weekly Report*, 24 June 1983.
2. Eric R. Brenner, M.D., personal communication.
3. White, GC, Lesesne RR. Hemophilia, hepatitis, and the acquired immunodeficiency syndrome (editorial). *Ann Intern Med* 1983; 98: 403-404.
4. Reitz, MS Jr., Kalyanararnan VS, Robert-Guroff M, et al. Human T-cell leukemia/lymphoma virus: The retrovirus of adult T-cell leukemia/lymphoma. *J Infect Dis* 1983; 147: 399-405.
5. *Morbidity and Mortality Weekly Report* 13 May 1983.
6. Goldsmith JC, Moseley, PL, Monick M et al. T-lymphocyte subpopulation abnormalities in apparently healthy patients with hemophilia. *Ann Intern Med* 1983; 98:294-296.
7. Raeburn JA. Antibiotics and immunodeficiency. *Lancet* 1972; 2: 954-955.

Editorial Note: It's humbling to note how so many paradigms implied and expressed in the above editorial, and even the basic vocabulary, mutated over the subsequent quarter-century! This editorial was written just as the human immunodeficiency virus (currently known as HIV-1) was being established as the cause of AIDS. Within two years there was a diagnostic test. We now commonly speak of "HIV disease" rather than "AIDS", since the diagnosis of "AIDS" remains somewhat arbitrary. (What basic difference is there between a person with a CD4 lymphocyte count of 199 per cmm of blood and a person with a CD4 count of 201, although technically the former has AIDS while the latters does not?) The world "homosexual" has almost disappeared from the daily lexicon, having long been replaced with "gay" and more recently in the medical literature with "men who have sex with men." But distressingly, HIV disease is now quite common in South Carolina, especially among disadvantaged populations.

AIDS Policies

J SC Med Assoc 1987; 83: 332

Future historians should have a field day. Historians of science will ask who deserved credit for isolating the virus, for designing the drugs, and (let us hope) for developing vaccines, and who really deserved the Nobel prizes? Political historians will debate to what extent AIDS, like so many infectious diseases before it, changed the course of history. Social historians will grapple with the impact on society's institutions—and they will measure these institutions in part by their response to the menace. All of these issues will entertain medical historians, who will also want to know how the AIDS epidemic altered medicine as a profession.

Certain signs are on the wall. Consider, for example, the notion that members of a profession differ from laypersons by possession of a body of unique, esoteric information. Not long ago, new information came to us through our little-publicized meetings and journals, couched in our own esoteric vocabulary. Today's laypersons often get new information about AIDS even before the specialist by paying attention to radio, television, or *The Wall Street Journal*. Consider also the notion that a profession is defined by its members' authority. Even our authority to request a laboratory test without first obtaining informed consent is now at issue. Not only do we lack all of the answers; it is highly probable that we've not even asked some of the most pertinent questions.

Among the many phenomena spawned by the epidemic has been the desire of most institutions to formulate "AIDS policies." What precautions should be taken? What persons, if any, should be tested for HIV seropositivity? Who should know the results of such testing? What kinds of education are appropriate? Is quarantine a viable alternative? In this issue, Dr. Jeremy Musher reviews the problems faced by institutions from the perspective of having supervised the formulation of such a policy at a medical school. The "AIDS policy" was concluded to be an ongoing concern, since new information or new legislation might dramatically alter some of its components.

However, one lesson for our species should be the need for each of us to formulate and adhere to our own personal policies. It is unfortunate that most of us never got a short course in assertiveness training in school, since such training teaches the values of personal policies. For example, it is much easier to deal with the unwelcome telephone solicitor who interrupts your evening meal if you can state (as a conditioned reflex): "I'm sorry, but my policy is not to deal with telephone solicitations of any kind. Good luck elsewhere." Policy closes the door, denying the other party the chance to negotiate.

Should we not encourage our children to develop such policies ("My policy is not to use illicit drugs of any kind;" "My policy is not to indulge in sex until I'm married")? Should we not adhere to such policies ourselves ("My policy is to be faithful to my spouse")? And should we not teach the value of such policies to our patients? Would the epidemic have occurred at all had our species insisted upon the old-fashioned virtues?

Although AIDS is new, many of its challenges are not. If the AIDS/HIV epidemic contains even a tiny measure of redeeming value, perhaps it is the rekindling of the question—so often debated by the ancient Greeks and Hebrews but somehow forgotten during our own time—of what it really means to be a good person. And is not such a person, throughout all of the collective wisdom of the ages, ultimately defined by adherence to a set of fundamentally sound personal policies?

Editorial Note: Debates over the ethical issues raised by HIV/AIDS were just heating up when the above editorial was written. The epidemic prompted me to divert more and more of my discretionary reading to ethics and virtue theory.

Ethics and AIDS—One Year Later

J SC Med Assoc 1988; 84: 215-217

At the 1987 annual meeting incoming president Charles B. Duncan announced his intent to establish a standing Ethics Committee. Our 140th annual meeting will showcase this committee's depth and breadth. An entire morning will be given to two AIDS-related debates: (1) Can a physician ethically refuse to treat a patient whose condition is within the physician's realm of competence solely because the patient is seropositive? (2) What is the patient's right to know that his or her physician is seropositive? It should be an interesting morning. These are problems over which honest people of good will can have firmly-held but divergent opinions.

Not long ago, the subject of "AIDS and Ethics" was reviewed by Dr. Albert Jonsen and his colleagues at the University of California.[1] They concluded that "two essential features of sound ethical discussion are as yet absent" in the AIDS epidemic. These are (1) reliable information about the disease and its mode of transmission; and (2) lack of sufficient "prolonged and serious conversations by knowledgeable parties." In my opinion, Dr. Jonsen and his colleagues are wrong on both counts. I suspect that after all is said and done at our annual meeting, SCMA members will hold divergent opinions and that it will be for neither of these reasons.

First, we have excellent information about the transmission of the disease.[2] Sure, there will be many more studies and also anecdotal case reports to define more accurately the risk of transmission from various activities. Nevertheless, especially considering that this disease was not even recognized until 1981, we know an enormous amount about how people get it. Second, there has been no dearth of "prolonged and serious conversations." Innumerable conferences have been held at every conceivable level: local, state, regional, national, international. The problem addressed by Dr. Jonsen and his colleagues, I submit, tells us less about the AIDS epidemic than it does about the nature of ethics.

Ethics is usually defined as the study of standards of conduct and moral judgment (that is, philosophy). It is almost universally acknowledged that our society needs help. *Time* magazine recently reported that more than 90 percent of 1,014 American adults agreed with the statement that morals have deteriorated because parents fail to take responsibility for their children.[3] It seems possible — just possible — that the parents' dilemma in turn reflects the lack of clear directives given by the ethicists themselves. Ethicists grapple with conflicting frameworks of rules and standards. Two decades ago, for example, the noted ethicist Alasdair MacIntyre wrote:

> We cannot expect to find in our society a single set of
> moral concepts ... Conceptual conflict is endemic in our
> situation ... Each of us therefore has to choose both with
> whom we wish to be morally bound and by what ends,
> rules, and virtues we wish to be guided.[4]

If the ethicists cannot agree on standards, how can the rest of us set and enforce any standards among our children or among anyone else, for that matter?

We should empathize with the ethicists. To begin with, there are different ways to go about setting such standards. These are generally considered in three groups: *deontological* ethics, *consequentialist* ethics, and *existential* ethics. Each of these approaches has its strengths and limitations.

Deontological (duty based or rule-based, also sometimes known as Kantian) ethics ultimately derive from the transcendent "ought," classically expressed in the Ten Commandments. Its strength is a clear standard of right and wrong. Its weaknesses are (1) how to derive the standard ("Who makes the rules?") and (2) how to remain sensitive to special situations. *Consequentialist* ethics are generally of two overlapping types: situational and utilitarian. In situational ethics one considers particular circumstances while in utilitarian ethics one considers "the greatest good for the greatest number," as its proponent Jeremy Bentham famously put it. In both types we're left without a clear sense of what is "good," sometimes to the detriment of individual parties. Most physicians probably find it hard to take *existentialist* ethics seriously. Seeking to maximize personal freedom, this approach favors the autonomous fulfillment of personal desires. Almost by definition, it cannot be universalized. Immediately, we begin to see how each of these frameworks could be used in debating AIDS-related issues.

The problem is even more fundamental. The essential disagreement seems to be about the nature of man. Does so-called "natural man" in his native state unfettered by civilization or law have any moral standards whatsoever? It depends on whom you ask. Thomas Aquinas in the thirteenth century said yes. Thomas Hobbes in the seventeenth century said no. It is Hobbes's view that has prevailed. Hence, we are thrown back to the pre-Socratic sophists of ancient Greece. Men are either sheep or wolves, and morality consists only of compromise borne of self-interest. There are no absolute standards. All is value relativism.

Contemporary philosophers sometimes seem unable to tell us the meaning of such things as "morals," "values," and "standards." If they can't agree, how can we? More recently, MacIntyre tells us:

> The most striking feature of contemporary moral utterance is that so much of it is used to express disagreements, and the most striking feature of the debates in which these disagreements are expressed is their interminable character. I do not mean by this just that such debates go on and on — although they do — but also that they apparently can find no terminus. There seems to be no rational way of securing moral agreement in our culture.[5]

It is disconcerting to realize how much of what ought to be decided by moral consensus is in fact decided only by the courts. It is highly likely that the courts, not the ethicists, will settle the major issues now swirling around the AIDS epidemic. Still, we must try. Organizations such as ours, by taking stands, can help. Debates such as those scheduled for this year's annual meeting remind us of the complexities that obfuscate many and perhaps most ethical dilemmas. What, in the final analysis, do we mean by "right" and "wrong"?

References

1. Jonsen AR, Cooke M, Koenig BA. AIDS and ethics. *Issues in Science and Technology* 1986; 2: 56-65.
2. Friedland GH, Klein RS. Transmission of the human immunodeficiency virus. *N Engl J Med 1987*; 317: 1125-1135.
3. "What's Wrong?" *Time*, 5 May 1987.
4. MacIntyre A. *A Short History of Ethics*. New York: MacMillan Publishing Company; 1966: 268.
5. MacIntyre A. *After Virtue*. Second edition. Notre Dame, Indiana: University of Notre Dame Press; 1984:6.

Editorial Note: Years later, Dr. Robert Sade invited me to give the keynote address at a conference on HIV/AIDS and ethics. Reviewing the literature, I concluded that what amounted to an epidemic of papers on this topic peaked around 1990, just before the epidemic itself peaked in the United States (Bryan CS. HIV/AIDS and bioethics: Historical perspective, personal retrospective. *Health Care Analysis* 2002; 10: 5-18). Most of the key issues were indeed resolved by the courts.

Beliefs, Attitudes, and Health Promotion

J SC Med Assoc 1989; 85: 84-85

In this issue, Wheeler and colleagues describe the health promotion beliefs and attitudes identified by a survey of 87 physicians in two South Carolina communities. Most (85%) of the physicians reported that they personally provided information about healthy lifestyles rather than delegating this task to office personnel. Four out of five routinely asked their patients about smoking; two out of three routinely asked about alcohol and other drugs, while fewer than one-half routinely inquired about diet, exercise, or stress. Although most of the respondents considered themselves "somewhat successful" at modifying patients' behavior, fewer than one in ten checked "very successful." Most indicated a need for continuing education courses designed specifically to improve their health promotion skills.

Promoting healthy lifestyles has long ranked among the top priorities of the South Carolina Medical Association. As to our level of activity in this area, we need make no apologies. Health promotion has often dominated the addresses at our meetings, the contents of our seminars, and our legislative agendas. The Health Van is a new concept but not a new point of emphasis. If these comments seem a bit defensive, it is by design rather than accident. The paper by Wheeler and colleagues adds to a large body of literature addressing the beliefs and attitudes of physicians toward health promotion. At times, not all of the conclusions seem entirely realistic.

Consider smoking, for example. Surveys among physicians have clearly identified elimination of smoking as the single most important health behavior needing their attention.[1] No argument. Yet I take umbrage to a conclusion in the *American Journal of Medicine* that "physicians should provide advice about smoking as a regular part of *every* patient visit" (*emphasis added*).[2] While such a conclusion aptly applies to the annual physical examination, it seems entirely unrealistic to expect busy physicians to initiate open-ended conversations about smoking while, say, sewing up lacerations or administering cancer chemotherapy. Everything in its proper time! Most patients would, I suspect, agree. Surveys of patients indicate that they place more priority on receiving appropriate treatment without delay than on some of the things that health educators like to talk about, such as continuity of care and promoting wellness.[3]

There are two issues: (1) What should we do? (2) How should we do it? A reasonable assessment of what health promotion desiderata can be readily accomplished was provided by a questionnaire given to third-year medical students.[4] The students expressed high confidence in the ability of physicians to provide health screening physical examinations, blood pressure control, cancer detection education, family planning, health counseling and education, immunizations, and sexually transmitted disease prevention. However, the students expressed low confidence in the ability of physicians to promote smoking cessation, nutrition counseling and education, and weight reduction. Other surveys indicate that many physicians are ill-equipped to deal with issues related to alcoholism,[5] sexual preferences,[6-7] and thorny family problems.[8] Hence, the observation by Wheeler and colleagues that South Carolina physicians were often unsure of their abilities to have a positive impact on such things as smoking, substance abuse, and stress management is hardly surprising.

As to the second issue, how we should do it, it must be appreciated that there is an important stumbling block: the lack of adequate reimbursement mechanisms. Adequate counseling takes time. Most payment schemes provide little or no allowance for physicians' time devoted to counseling on such matters as smoking cessation and stress management. If health promotion is to be more than the rendering of gratuitous advice, then there must either be adequate reimbursement mechanisms or alternative strategies to one-on-one counseling by physicians.

One strategy is to delegate such counseling to office personnel. A recent survey in Texas indicated that physician's assistants are quite willing to undertake a wider role in health promotion although they, too, are uncertain about their abilities to influence such things as smoking, drinking, and illicit drug use.[9] Another strategy is to organize "wellness programs." Adequate models exist by which physicians can assume leadership in promoting wellness throughout their communities. It is unrealistic to expect that advice given during an annual physical examination will be heeded throughout the year without reinforcement. It is therefore appropriate that such wellness programs require time commitments by patients as well as by physicians.

That most of the physicians surveyed by Wheeler and colleagues were eager to improve their health promotion skills is encouraging. What is needed from educators are more clear-cut demonstrations that our attempts to influence behaviors are indeed successful. Physicians, like most people, are more willing to devote time and energy to those projects that have a reasonable possibility of success.[10] Educators should convince us of the effectiveness of new techniques, just as we explore new ways by which to continue our leadership in promoting health throughout our communities.

References

1. Sobol J, Valente CM, Muncie HL, Jr. et al. Physicians' beliefs about the importance of 25 health promoting behaviors. *Am J Public Health* 1985; 75: 1427-1428.
2. Eraker SA, Becker MH, Strecher VJ, et al. Smoking behavior, cessation techniques, and the health decision model. *Am J Med* 1985; 78: 817-825.
3. Hagman E, Rehnstrom T. Priorities in primary, health care. The views of patients, politicians and health care professionals. *Scand J Prim Health Care* 1985; 3: 197-200.
4. Scott CS, Neighbor WF. Preventive care attitudes of medical students. *Soc Sci Med* 1985; 21: 299-305.
5. Confusione M, Leonard K, Jaffe A. Alcoholism training in a family practice residency. *J Subst Abuse Treat* 1988; 5: 19-22.
6. Smith EM, Johnson SR, Guenther SM. Health care attitudes and experiences during gynecologic care among lesbians and bisexuals. *Am J Public Health* 1983; 75: 1085-1087.
7. Douglas CJ, Kalman CM, Kalman TP. Homophobia among physicians and nurses: An empirical study. *Hosp Community Psychiatry* 1985; 36: 1309-1311.
8. Crouch MA, McCauley J. Family awareness demonstrated by family practice residents: physician behavior and patient opinions. *J Fam Pract* 1985; 20: 281-284.
9. Fasser CE, Mullen PD, Holcomb JD. Health beliefs and behaviors of physician assistants in Texas: Implications for practice and education. *Am J Prev Med* 1988; 4: 208-215.
10. Radovsky L, Barry PP. Tobacco advertisements in physicians' offices: a pilot study of physician attitudes. *Am J Public Health* 1988; 78: 174-175.

HIV, Surgeons, and ... All of Us

J SC Med Assoc 1990; 86: 513-517

Most of the fast-breaking stories of the HIV/AIDS epidemic first surfaced in the CDC's *Morbidity and Mortality Weekly Reports*. Three such stories hold special significance for physicians ... and everyone else.

First there was the back-page story of June 5, 1981, that five gay men in Los Angeles had developed pneumonia due to *Pneumocystis carinii*.[1] This brief report foretold the great pandemic of our times.

Next came the lead story of May 22, 1987, that three health care workers developed HIV infection after contact with patients' blood in the absence of percutaneous injury.[2] The clarion sounded for universal precautions—the need to regard all blood and body fluids as being potentially infectious. To put it bluntly, should we be afraid of each and every patient?

Finally there was the report of July 27, 1990, that a patient apparently became HIV-infected during the extraction of two maxillary third molars by a dentist with AIDS. We have had time neither to digest the significance of this report nor to realize its impact.[3] But again, to put it bluntly, do patients have reason to be afraid of each and every one of *us*?

Let us examine these separate concerns: (1) the risk of HIV-positive patients to health care workers; (2) the risk of HIV-positive health care workers to patients.

RISK OF HIV-POSITIVE PATIENTS TO HEALTH CARE WORKERS

Exposures to patients' blood and body fluids fall into three broad categories: contact exposures to intact skin and mucous membranes, percutaneous exposures as in needlestick injuries, and massive exposures from freak accidents (Table 1) (*Editorial note*: Tables are omitted here, as the information has since become common knowledge). All health care workers are potentially vulnerable to each exposure category. Most of the published reports of HIV seroconversion in the health care setting deal with health care workers other than physicians. Still, surgeons are acknowledged to be at special risk because of the frequency and magnitude of blood exposure in the operating room.

Risks to surgeons: tensions over professional responsibility

In this issue of *The Journal*, Drs. Hebra, Adams, and Holley from the Medical University of South Carolina provide data on HIV-positive patients who underwent surgical procedures at two hospitals in Charleston. Although only two of these patients underwent emergency surgery for trauma, they note that the seroprevalence of HIV is increasing. Hence, all patients undergoing surgery should be considered to be HIV-positive.

Blood exposure is extremely common during surgery. By one estimate, surgeons' gloves are punctured during 25% of procedures, and 10% of these punctures result in skin penetration. In a recent prospective study, 3.5% of operations resulted in puncture wounds or cuts to a surgeon. Risk factors included emergency operation, blood loss greater than 250 mL, and operating room time exceeding one hour.[4]

The risk to a surgeon will depend on the type of procedure and on the prevalence of HIV in the population served. A nationwide study of selected hospitals indicates the range of HIV seroprevalence to be 0.1% to 7.8% of all patients; at one of the sentinel hospitals, 22% of men between ages 25 and 44 were HIV-positive.[5] What is the cumulative risk of a surgeon's acquiring HIV over the course of a career?

Assume that a surgeon performs 360 operative procedures each year, or some 10,000 procedures over a 30-year career. By one estimate, the surgeon's cumulative risk of acquiring HIV is 0.1% if the seroprevalence of HIV in the population served is 0.1% (i.e., one in a thousand), but rises to 10% if the seroprevalence of HIV is 10%.[6] In another study, the lifetime cumulative risk was concluded to exceed 6% for 10% of the surgeons surveyed.[7] One may quarrel with the assumptions but the message is clear: the risk to surgeons (and to other health care workers involved in invasive procedures) must be taken seriously.

Are surgeons morally obligated to perform procedures within their realms of competence on HIV-positive patients? An adequate airing of this issue far exceeds the scope of this editorial. Some argue that our medical heritage dictates that all of us must perform procedures within our competence irrespective of patients' HIV-antibody status.[8] However, closer scrutiny of medical history fails to support this assertion.[9]

The issue has received an ample airing at San Francisco General Hospital due to that institution's high seroprevalence of HIV infection. Tensions arose over the issue of professional responsibility. The chief of medicine held that physicians have the obligation to provide care to HIV-infected patients within their realms of competence. The chief of surgery held that staff surgeons reluctant to perform elective procedures on these patients could be relieved, to a large extent, of such responsibilities.

These positions reflect different frameworks for ethics: the categorical model (chief of medicine) versus the contractual model (chief of surgery).[10] Who is to say which is right? I feel strongly about one point: nonsurgeons (including physicians who do not perform surgery and also the general public) should not legislate to surgeons on these matters. What matters are the policies and perspectives of those who play the game — not those of the spectators. But all of us should encourage reasoned dialogue, for we all have a stake in the conclusions.

Prophylactic AZT (zidovudine; Retrovir) what should be our current practice?

Dr. Hebra and colleagues allude briefly to the use of AZT to prevent HIV infection following exposure. This topic is highly controversial. Prophylactic AZT has not been shown to be effective, nor is the long-term toxicity of AZT well-defined. However, an increasingly widespread body of opinion supports making AZT available in certain circumstances. We should therefore be aware of the rationale and limitations of this non-FDA-approved indication for AZT.[11]

Unfortunately, AZT will not prevent HIV from binding to

and entering target cells, such as the helper (T4 or CD4) lymphocyte. AZT inhibits reverse transcriptase, the enzyme enabling the virus to make a DNA copy of its RNA genome and thus enter the host cell's chromosome. Based on this limitation and also on lessons from animal models of retroviral infection, we must assume that AZT must be given promptly — almost immediately — if it is to be truly effective and prevent HIV from entering the host cell's DNA. It is also intuitively apparent that we must continue AZT for a relatively long time — for example, for four to six weeks. However, the optimum dose and duration of AZT prophylactic therapy are unknown.

Wholesale use of prophylactic AZT should be discouraged. Such therapy clearly represents an unproven halfway technology. However, procedures for prompt institution of prophylactic AZT should be available in order to deal with the problem of "massive" or "deep" exposure of anyone to the blood or body fluids of a known HIV-positive person.

The pros and cons of prophylactic AZT have been aired in an official statement by the Public Health Service.[12] At each institution the issues should be discussed and guidelines formulated.[13] My own recommendations are summarized in Table 2. At the time of this writing, various agencies and institutions (including DHEC and MUSC) are completing formal policies. One can expect some variation from one policy to the next. However, there is basic agreement that AZT must be given as soon as possible — ideally within an hour. My recommendations take into account the theoretical desirability of a loading dose. Informed consent should be obtained. Pregnancy should be excluded since AZT readily crosses the placenta.[14]

I recommend a "starter kit" of 41 capsules (i.e., AZT 100 mg caps, #41, sig: V at once, then II q4h for three days). This allows time for the exposed person to review exactly what happened, to study the issues, to seek opinions, and to decide for himself/ herself under less urgent circumstances. The duration of treatment remains arbitrary. Both 28- and 42- day regimens have been proposed at major institutions. Follow-up testing of HIV antibody status should be obtained at six weeks, three months, six months, nine months, and 12 months after the exposure.

Who will pay for it? Each institution should address this issue. The cost to the pharmacy for the 41-capsule starter kit is about $50. A compromise solution would be for hospitals to offer the starter kit as an employee benefit, and then to share the remaining cost with the exposed person. Cost-sharing would discourage overuse of prophylactic AZT. However, the cost issue should not deter making AZT available in settings where exposure is likely to occur—such as emergency rooms or operating rooms.

We will probably never know the true efficacy of prophylactic post-exposure AZT therapy. Adequate, appropriately controlled prospective studies now seem unlikely. Already, one failure has been reported.[15] However, the benefits of AZT would outweigh the risks if the efficacy were only three to eight percent—provided the exposure is to HIV-positive blood and therapy is begun promptly.[16]

In summary, AZT is being widely recommended for massive or deep exposures to known HIV-positive blood or body fluids, but it must be given promptly after the exposure. Therefore, it behooves all of us to be familiar with the issues and to be prepared to act promptly.

RISKS OF HIV-POSITIVE HEALTH CARE WORKERS TO PATIENTS

Informally, it has been estimated that as many as 5,000 physicians in the United States may be HIV-infected. Should these physicians be limited in their practice in any way, and do their patients have a right to know?

Prior to July 27, 1990, one could hold these questions to be mainly of theoretical interest, since transmission of HIV from a health care worker to a patient had not occurred. It now seems to have happened. Seroconversion was not demonstrated in the dental patient, since a baseline HIV antibody test was not performed. However, the circumstances were suggestive and the viral isolates from the dentist and the patient were quite similar. It seems best to assume that it can happen, and that it did happen.

Despite this report, other data are reassuring. Almost simultaneously, an experience was reported in which a surgeon with AIDS had operated on 2160 patients, of whom 1652 were contacted and 616 tested. Only one of these patients was HIV-positive, and that person was an injecting drug user. It was concluded that "the risks to patients operated on by HIV-infected surgeons are most likely quite low."[17] Assessing these data, an editorialist concluded that HIV-infected surgeons should avoid procedures that are especially high-risk, such as oral surgery, vaginal hysterectomy, and other procedures that require blind, by-feel manipulation of sharp instruments.[18] Otherwise, surgery by an HIV-positive surgeon could be carried out as business-as-usual.

The issues include:
• Should the patient's right-to-know the potential risk—however small that risk may be—outweigh the surgeon's right to confidentiality?
• Should all health care workers, including physicians, be tested for HIV antibodies?
• Should HIV-positive physicians be actively discouraged from performing certain procedures and, if so, how should their activities be monitored?
Already, it has been noted: "If our profession does not effectively grapple with such questions, they will be answered for us in the courts."[19]

The physician-patient interaction carries some inherent risks. It always has, and it always will. With blood-borne diseases such as HIV and hepatitis B, the risks to physicians and other health care workers far exceed the risks to patients. Still, the AIDS/HIV epidemic poses unprecedented, emotionally charged dilemmas to which organized medicine must respond. In Table 3, I have outlined for the sake of discussion some possible agenda items. But the important point is this: we must remain in dialogue both with each other and with the public. It behooves us to reason together during this time of tremendous anxiety and uncertainty.

References

1. *Pneumocystis* pneumonia—Los Angeles. *Morbidity and Mortality Weekly Reports* 1981; 30: 250-252.
2. Update: Human immunodeficiency virus infections in health-care workers exposed to blood of infected patients. *Morbidity and Mortality Weekly Reports* 1987; 36: 285-289.
3. Possible transmission of human immunodeficiency virus to a patient during an invasive dental procedure. *Morbidity and Mortality Weekly Report* 1990; 39: 489-493.
4. Panlilio AL, Perlino CA, Bell DM, et al. Blood exposures during surgical procedures. Proceedings of the 29th Interscience Conference on Antimicrobial Agents and Chemotherapy, Houston, Texas, 17-20 September 1989.
5. St. Louis ME, Rauch KJ, Peterson LR, et al. Seroprevalence rates of human immunodeficiency virus infection at sentinel hospitals in the United States. *N Engl J Med* 323: 213-218, 1990.
6. McKinney WP, Young MJ. The cumulative probability of occupationally-acquired HIV infection: The risks of repeated exposures during a surgical career. *Infect Control Hosp Epidemiol* 1990; 11: 243-247.
7. Lowenfels AB, Wormser GP, Jain R. Frequency of puncture injuries in surgeons and estimated risk of infection. *Arch Intern Med* 1989; 124: 1284-1286.
8. Kim JH, Perfect JR. To help the sick: An historical and ethical essay concerning the refusal to care for patients with AIDS. *Am J Med* 1988; 84: 135-138.
9. Friedlander WJ. On the obligation of physicians to treat AIDS: Is there a historical basis? *Rev Infect Dis* 1990; 12: 191-203.
10. Cooke M. Occupational transmission of HIV: The ethics of physician risk and responsibility. In: Volberding P, Jacobson MA. *AIDS Clinical Review 1990*. New York: Marcel Dekker; 1990: 1-10.
11. Henderson DK, Gerberding JL. Prophylactic zidovudine after occupational exposure to the human immunodeficiency virus, an interim analysis. *J Infect Dis* 1990; 160: 321-327.
12. Public Health Service statement on management of occupational exposure to human immunodeficiency virus, including considerations regarding zidovudine postexposure use. *Morbidity and Mortality Weekly Reports* 1990; 39: No. RR-1.
13. Henderson DK. HIV-1 in the health care setting. In: Mandell GL, Douglas RG, Bennett JE, eds. *Principles and Practices of Infectious Diseases*. Third edition, New York: Churchill Livingstone; 1989: 2233.
14. Liebes L, Mendoza S, Wilson D, et al. Transfer of zidovudine

(AZT) by human placenta. *J Infect Dis* 1990; 161: 203-207.

15. Lange JMA, Boucher CAB, Hollak CEM, et al. Failure of zidovudine prophylaxis after accidental exposure to HIV-1. *N Eng J Med* 1990; 322: 1375-1377.

16. Sacks HS, Rose DN. Zidovudine prophylaxis for needlestick exposure to human immunodeficiency virus: A decision analysis. *J Gen Intern Med* 1990; 5: 132-137.

17. Mishu B, Schaffner W, Horan JM, et al. A surgeon with AIDS: Lack of evidence of transmission to patients. *JAMA* 1990; 264: 467-470.

18. Rhame FS. The HIV-infected surgeon (editorial). *JAMA* 1990; 264: 507-508.

19. Gramelspacher GP, Miles SH, Cassel, CK. When the doctor has AIDS. *J Infect Dis* 1990; 162: 534-537.

Editorial Note written 17 years later: Wags back then suggested that HIV/AIDS actually comprised three epidemics: an epidemic of disease, an epidemic of fear, and an epidemic of meetings (see editorial note on page 285). After 1990 my editorials on HIV/AIDS became increasingly technical or scientific. The advent of the protease inhibitors in 1995/1996 made HIV/AIDS a highly treatable condition. The protease inhibitors also allowed us to use potent combination regimens for post-exposure prophylaxis, thereby taming much of the anxiety reflected about "HIV, surgeons ... and all of us." Those of us who were caught up in the HIV/AIDS epidemic from the beginning were privileged to live through what amounted to a short history of medicine, truncated between 1981 and 1996. We journeyed from the Dark Ages during which we were clueless to the age of molecular biology with its incredibly powerful diagnostic and therapeutic tools. (See Bryan CS. Theodore E. Woodward Award. HIV/AIDS, ethics, and professionalism: Where went the debate? *Trans Am Clin Climatol Assoc* 2003; 114: 353-367).

Fort Host

J *SC Med Assoc* 1991; 87: 151-155

"Ain't gonna study war no more."
—From "Down by the Riverside"

It was the dean's introductory address on our first day of medical school. "And now ... I'm going to let you in on a well-kept professional secret." He paused as if to make sure that nobody from the outside world might be listening, or perhaps to suggest that we weren't to share the forthcoming secret with the laity. Then he let it fly: "Most of the time, patients get better on their own."

That our bodies usually win without outside help is remarkable, but it's even more remarkable that we never even hear about most of the battles fought in our behalf. Untold hordes of microbes, chemicals and would-be cancers assault the towers of our inner recesses on a daily basis. We nearly always turn them back. We win because of superior weaponry. Host defenses.

Certain writers of national prominence object to society's frequent use of military metaphors when speaking of disease. Why must we *fight* heart disease, *crusade* against cancer, or form *task forces* against AIDS? Why not take a more benign and wholistic posture: there are no friends or enemies, only ecosystems? Why the incessant attack and kill?

As this issue of *The Journal* approaches deadline (February 1, 1991), our national conscience wrestles with war in the Persian Gulf. Fascinated yet troubled, apprehensive yet optimistic, we share with trepidation our President's vision of a new world order. Perhaps someday we will disprove historian Barbara Tuchman's judgment that our species "makes a poorer performance of government than of almost any other human activity."[1] In the meantime we learn once more that military preparedness seems to be the upfront price for security.

I therefore defend the use of the military metaphor — at least when speaking of host defenses against foreign invaders. The

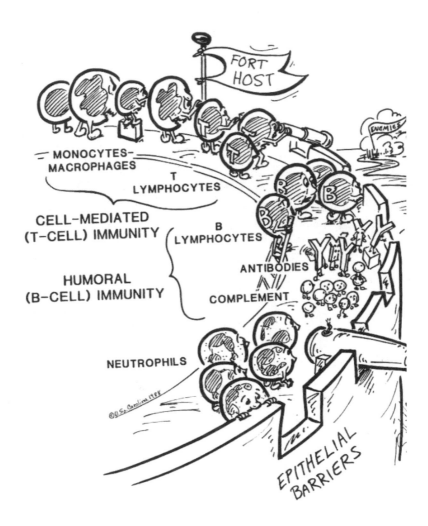

Figure 1. *Fort Host braces for approaching enemies, shown here as a cloud on the horizon (upper right). Sensitized T-lymphocytes, caricatured here with a telescope, spend their entire lifetimes looking for one or another foreign antigen.*

HIV/AIDS epidemic bears grim witness to what happens with-without them. For several reasons, the time seems appropriate to display some drawings done for me several years ago by Sue Hilfer, a medical illustrator, of what I choose to call Fort Host (Figure 1). Let us review briefly this most remarkable bastion.

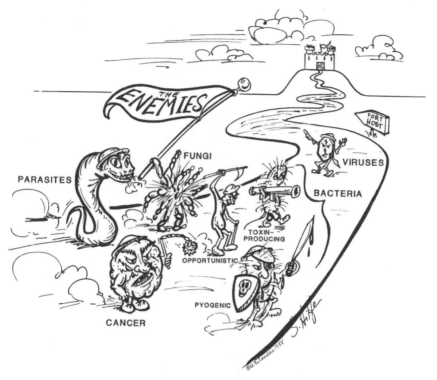

Figure 2. *The approaching enemies often hunt in packs, counter to the classic version of the germ theory (one pathogen:one disease).*

Tough epithelial barriers form the first walls of defense. Pathogens that manage to break through these walls encounter three systems that, much like the army, navy, and air force of a twentieth-century nation, compete but more often cooperate. These are the neutrophils (polymorphonuclear leukocytes); humoral immunity (B lymphocytes, antibody, and complement); and cell-mediated immunity (T lymphocytes, monocytes, and macrophages). We'll examine these in turn, but let's begin by focusing on the potential enemies, which often attack in packs (Figure 2).

In this battle scenario, viruses lead the attack. Their plan is to soften Fort Host for the swarms of bacteria behind them. Pyogenic bacteria (such as the streptococci and staphylococci) carry tough shields to resist phagocytosis. Toxin-producing bacteria (such as the bacilli of tetanus and botulism) use chemical warfare. Opportunistic bacteria lurk around to take advantage of whatever footholds we will give them. Assorted fungi parasites, and would-be cancers bring up the rear.

When the Enemies reach Fort Host (Figure 3), each defending brigade responds according to assignment. Clockwise from the upper right, we find B lymphocytes shooting cannons of antibodies to neutralize viruses, activate bacterial toxins, and opsonize the more virulent bacteria and parasites to facilitate the work of the professional phagocytes neutrophils and macrophages. We find T lmphocytes and activated macrophages assuming primary responsibility for intracellular bacteria, fungi, parasites, and tumors. We find the ubiquitous complement components plugging the gaps and rallying the troops wherever they can. In most cases, the enemies are quickly routed.

Now ... after a deep breath, let's go back to our analysis of Fort Host.

If it is astonishing that we know so much already about the molecular biology of HIV infection,[2] it also astonishes that in the two decades prior to AIDS we learned so much about B and T lymphocyte function. Dr. Robert Gallo of the National Institutes of Health observed: "Had AIDS struck during the 1960s, we would have been in a black box ... we didn't even know what lymphocytes do." Our knowledge came just in the nick of time.

As a sophomore medical student in 1964 I was asked by a pathology instructor: "What do lymphocytes do?" "Sir," I responded, "they're implicated in antibody synthesis." This answer satisfied him enough to pass on to the next student. The whole subject of immunology seemed abstruse. We knew that lymphocytes were involved in both humoral and cell mediated immunity. But all small lymphocytes look pretty much alike, and we had no clues as to which ones did what.

It was around 1970 that medical schools were abuzz with talk about B and T lymphocytes. The concept was that although lymphocytes—like neutrophils and monocytes—originate in the bone marrow, they must go to school for further training

300

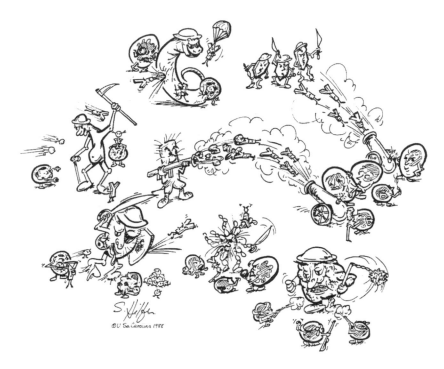

Figure 3. *When the enemies reach Fort Host, each defending component of the immune and phagocytic systems responds according to its specific assignment.*

(Figure 4). B lymphocytes go to school in the human equivalent of the chicken's bursa of Fabricius. T lymphocytes go to school in the thymus. This simple dichotomy brought coherence to what had previously been a morass of disjointed observations. Immunology suddenly made sense. Its laboratories now attracted streams of bright young investigators. All of this happened just in time for us to recognize what the HIV/AIDS.

Let us digress briefly into how the key observations were made, for the story makes a strong case for adequate funding of basic biomedical research. It is perhaps no surprise that the key observation about T lymphocytes was made by an established researcher studying the potential role of the thymus in leukemia.[3] Removal of the thymus from newborn mice impaired cell-

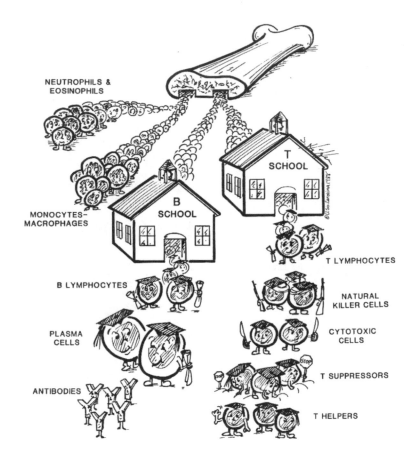

Figure 4. *Schools for lymphocytes. Emerging from the bone marrow, lymphocytes attend either "B School" (the human equivalent of the chicken's bursa of Fabricius), now thought to be the bone marrow itself) or "T School" (the thymus gland). Upon graduation they become either B lymphocytes responsible for humoral immunity or T lymphocytes responsibile for cell-mediated immunity.*

mediated immunity. However, the discovery of how the bursa of Fabricius affects antibody synthesis offers a classic lesson in serendipitous spin-off from basic research. Bruce Glick, a graduate student at Ohio State University, chose for his doctoral thesis the effect of removing the bursa of Fabricius from newborn chicks. Nothing much did. Glick therefore gave his bursectomized birds to a researcher down the hall who needed more chickens to make antibodies against *Salmonella* for his experiments. Glick's Rhode Island Reds and White Leghorns failed to produce antibodies and the rest is history.[4]

The elegant complexity of how lymphocytes seek out and destroy foreign invaders makes Patriot missiles seem like child's play. To make this point, I would ask any skeptical reader to consider just two passages from recent review articles. Having taken these passages from their contexts, I suggest that one make no attempt to follow the meaning—just appreciate the authors' enthusiasm and the systems' complexity.

First, consider this account of the antigen-binding sites in the antibodies formed by the B lymphocyte system:

> To understand how antibodies can differ without violating the rules of the genetic code, we must look at genes coding for the immunoglobulin V regions ... *Amazingly enough*, the heavy-chain V region is coded by three separate genes—V, D and J—and the light-chain V region by two genes—V and J. There are 500 to 1,000 different V heavy-chain genes ... (and) at least 200 different light-chain genes ... It is immediately apparent that an antibody combining site consisting of randomly chosen gene products from no fewer than five genes, each of which permits multiple choices, can present quite enormous variability—i.e., $10^3 \times 10 \times 4 \times 200 \times 6$ (or 5×10^7) to a first approximation (*emphasis added*).[5]

Next consider this account of how T cells respond to so many different antigens:

> T cell orchestration occurs as the result of a *precisely orchestrated* set of events involving the T3-Ti complex, the 15-kd sialoglycoprotein polypeptide growth factor interleukin-2 (formerly called T-cell growth factor), and the interleukin-2 receptor. Although resting T cells express no receptors for interleukin-2, they have a maximal number of surface antigen-MHC receptors (approximately 40,000 per cell). After the T-cell receptors are triggered by antigen and MHC gene products, the number of surface antigen receptors quickly diminishes,

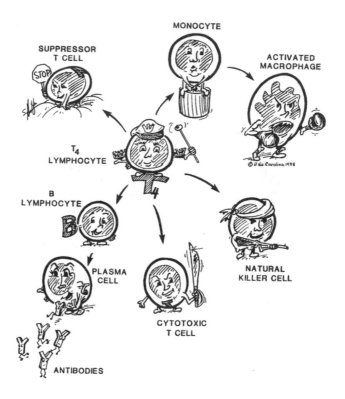

Figure 5. *The T4 lymphocyte (subsequently known as the CD4 lymphocyte) serves the immune system in much the same way as a conductor serves an orchestra or a general serves an army, directing the various components toward their respective functions. The human immunodeficiency virus (HIV) specifically targets the T4 lymphocyte, which explains why AIDS is such a devastating disease.*

and induction of surface interleukin-2 receptors occurs within hours (*emphasis added*).[6]

Let no one say that Fort Host's defenses are crude or primitive!

Let's now return to the military metaphor. Perhaps the day will come when we no longer need to study war, but it's likely that we'll always need to study defense. I cannot but think that the more we know about host defenses, the better off we'll be. The more we learn about Fort Host, the more we stand in awe.

Several years ago, I watched a prominent investigator show his latest movie of neutrophils engulfing bacteria. I cannot recall the details of the experiments, but I well remember his last sentence—applicable to all components of Fort Host.

"I'm just glad those guys are on our side!"

References

1. Tuchman B. *The March of Folly: from Troy to Vietnam.* New York: Alfred A. Knopf; 1994: 4.
2. Greene WC. The molecular biology of human immunodeficiency virus type I infection. *N Engl J Med* 1991; 324: 308-317.
3. Miller JFAP. Immunological function of the thymus. *Lancet* 1961; 2: 748-749.
4. Glick B, Chang TS, Japp RG: The bursa of Fabricius and antibody production. *Poult Sci* 1956; 35: 224- 225.
5. Nossal GJV: The basic components of the immune system. *N Engl J Med* 1987; 316: 1320-1325.
6. Royer HD, Reinherz EL: T-lymphocytes: ontogeny, function, and relevance to clinical disorders. *N Engl J Med* 1987; 317: 1136-1142.

Editorial Note: The principal motives for this editorial were (1) to provide practicing physicians with "talking points" for educating patients about the immune system, and (2) to publish the wonderful editorials prepared for me by Sue Hilfer, who was then the medical illustrator at the University of South Carolina School of Medicine. In the late 1980s, I entertained fantasies about writing a book on HIV/AIDS for a lay readership. Immunology is of course a fast-moving field; hence some of the terminology shown here may have changed. The overarching point is the incredible sophistication of the human immune system, and I sought in this editorial to convey yet another reason for awe and wonder about the intricacies of the human body.

"The Rights of the Child" Revisited

J SC Med Assoc 1994; 90: 613-614

Why bother with organized medicine? Why waste time going to meetings of the county medical society?

Recently, I pondered William Osler's answers to these questions while driving to my county society's meeting. Grabbing
his hat and coat one evening, Osler asked a younger colleague,
"Aren't you going to the medical society?" "No," the young
man replied, "I think it's a waste of my time." "Do you think
I don't!" exclaimed Osler, and off he went. Osler knew that
it's important to attend if for no other reasons than to promote
good will and to participate in the issues-of-the-day. And he
also knew he might actually learn something!

Still, I doubted that I would learn anything of a useful nature that evening. The announced topic was: "Violence in Our
Society: Prevention and Intervention." True, the subject is extremely important and affects us all. But as physicians—individually or collectively—can we really make a difference? The
speaker recited familiar facts. Each year, the 200 million guns in
the United States account for the deaths of some 25,000 people,
of whom 85 percent knew their killers in one way or another.
Battery is now the leading cause of injury to women in the United States, and more than one in three women are abused during their pregnancies. Nearly two million elderly persons are
abused each year. Well, what did I expect? After all, this was
the medical society—not the Optimist Club!

Then the speaker took a different tack. The basic problem,
he opined, is that more and more children are being raised in
homes without love. This is largely because illegitimacy has become almost the norm. In the speaker's home state, somewhere
north of the Mason-Dixon Line, 20 percent of white children, 64
percent of Hispanic children, and 77 percent of African-Ameri-
can children are born out of wedlock. The speaker suggested
that children raised without love become adults filled with
hate. He challenged organized medicine to do something about

it. He suggested that we, as physicians have the duty to teach people how to raise their children and fill their lives with love.

Quixotic? Perhaps. But driving home that night I had two thoughts. First, one should definitely try to attend the county medical society's meetings, for you never know what you'll learn or re-learn. Second, I formed the opinion that the speaker's basic message was hardly new. Indeed, I recalled in 1920 a lead article in *The Journal of the American Medical Association* was entitled "The Rights of the Child." Its author, by no coincidence, was our own state health officer and a former SCMA president — Dr. James Adams Hayne.[1]

After reviewing the evolution of our ideas about "the rights of man" and "the rights of woman," the eloquent (if often bombastic) Dr. Hayne asked:

> What of the child? Who has championed its right? Summoned against its will and without its consent into this world of trouble, pain, sickness, and finally death, what Rousseau or Voltaire shall sound the tocsin and call on the infant "mewling and puking in the nurse's arms," to demand that its own mother shall give it the lactic fluid that is its primal right ... Who shall demand for them the right to believe in fairies, the right to sunshine and to flowers, to the fresh air, and to green fields, to all that makes up the paradise of childhood. Who shall lead another Children's Crusade for these, their ancient rights?

He elaborated on the following rights in order of priority:

- The right to be conceived.
- The right to be born after conception.
- The right to have healthy parents.
- The right that "its mother shall be so cared for by the state that neither through poverty nor ignorance shall she bring it into the world in unhygienic surroundings ... "
- The right to "have its own mother's milk until it is old enough to be weaned."
- The right, "guaranteed by the state, that every baby born shall have an equal chance with other babies to develop into the normal healthy child."
- The right that, when it reaches school age, it shall have the

best that the resources of any government can command."
Hayne, it seems, was in some respects well ahead of his time.

More recently, the American Academy of Pediatrics has formulated a similar list of desiderata for children. Some refinements to Hayne's list of rights include the following:
• The right to immunizations.
• The right to good nutrition.
• The right to education about health and the health care system.
• The right to a safe environment.
• The right to adequate assistance for any handicaps.
• The right to live in a family setting "with an adequate income to provide basic needs to insure physical and intellectual health."
• The right to be free of environmental contamination.
• The right to live in a society that recognizes the special needs of young people.
And to this list, one might easily add the right to be wanted and the right to be loved.

Why bother with organized medicine? Perhaps the most basic reason is that it takes collective action not only to preserve and strengthen our own traditions but also to improve society. It should not escape our notice that medicine is being redefined. It has even been suggested that primary care medicine is almost an anachronism—that most functions of the front line physician can in fact be filled by others.[2] But let us not forget that the word "doctor" means "teacher" and that we do, indeed, have the right and the duty, the responsibility and the privilege, to teach our patients how to live, learn, and love. And let us not forget the enthusiasm with which Dr. Hayne ended his address: "If the rights I have tried to indicate are given the child, the future of the race is assured."

References

1. Hayne JA: The rights of the child. *JAMA* 1920; 75: 143-145.
2. Starfield B: Is primary care essential? *Lancet* 1994; 344: 1129-1133.

The Politics of Medicine

Physician's Assistants

J SC Med Assoc 1977; 73: 122-123

A telephone shatters the night stillness. Silence follows. A voice then strides forth: "Give him 40 milligrams of Lasix right away, and I'll be over."

What thought processes underlie this confident imperative?

At one extreme is the clinician-scientist. The pathophysiology of heart failure provides his daily fare, garnished last night by perusal of the latest research on sodium metabolism. He knows the patient through and through, and as he sheds his pajamas and buttons his shirt he estimates what the right atrial filling pressure will be when he gets there.

At the average, there is the concerned and capable clinician. Understanding basic principles, seasoned by experience, and practical in his decisions, he judges the database to indicate volume overload on the left ventricle. He knows the patient well, indeed the patient is his friend, and he can't wait to get there in order to be of help.

At the bottom, sadly, there is the individual for whom the order to "give him 40 milligrams of Lasix" lacks any scientific rationale. He knows little about the drug and less about the patient. His voice projects confidence but is the voice of a charlatan. The clinical problem may be volume depletion rather than excess, but he reaches for the loop diuretic just as his ancestor reached for the pocket lancet. Worse still, he may care less about the patient's welfare than about his own wallet.

That the mannerisms of a doctor are rather easily assumed explains in part the success of the occasional imposter, who successfully fools most of the people some of the time before his inevitable discovery. The fear is sometimes expressed that the trained physician's assistant might be tempted to assume such a role. Especially in rural areas, the people might demand such a role of him if, for instance, their only doctor were to cease his practice. Lacking a thorough grounding in basic sciences and unable to keep abreast of developments, he would ultimately do more harm than good.

I believe this fear to be unreasonable.

There is increased interest by both government and by organizations such as the SCMA to assure adequate licensing and regulation of all persons in the health care delivery system. Further, the network of health care extension into rural areas (see data in this issue provided by Mr. Hardy Wickwar) will make it increasingly difficult for the potential imposter to "go it alone," unwatched.

We should look instead at other aspects of the physician's assistant concept, and we should encourage the growth of this concept within well-regulated bounds.

In this issue, Dr. Kenneth J. Buhmeyer comments on the current status of physician's assistants in South Carolina. His analysis of their use of algorithmic protocols is of interest. His concluding paragraph carries a message which should be read and remembered. Of further interest is the article by Dr. Lawrence Jowers on the medicolegal problems posed by the physician's assistant concept.

It has been shown that patients managed by supervised physician's assistants in a rural setting "fare about as well as those seen by a physician."[1] Such studies have, however, used physician's assistants who were fresh from the academic environment. Hopefully, there will be long-term evaluations. We should be sensitive to the problems of identity which these young people will experience:

> The self-image of the paramedical professionals themselves will be an important factor in determining the future of this field. On the whole, their acceptance of this new role has been good, but they are anxious about career mobility, limitations of responsibilities, exploitation by physicians, and achievement of a salary level commensurate with their productivity and responsibility.[2]

Physician's assistants need the approval not only of patients and physicians but also of non-physician members of the health care team. Recent years have seen enormous subspecialization within the nursing profession. In South Carolina, for example, the new laws governing nursing define the scope of practice for eleven nurse categories. These will be summarized in a future issue of *The Journal*. Quantitatively, the problem of defining more clearly the role of nurse practitioners far exceeds the problem of defining the role of physician's assistants. The new regulations, for instance, refer to the "extended role of the licensed practical nurse" and to the "expanded role of the registered nurse." The scope of practice of the new breeds of nurse subspecialists is considerable, and it is not surprising that some nursing educators have opposed the physician's assistant concept.[2]

Such regulations are tedious but necessary. We should give them our attention. And we should wish these young people well, while maintaining our concern to protect the public interest.

References

1. Kane, RL, Olsen DM, Castle CH. Medex and their physician preceptors: quality of care. *JAMA* 1976; 36: 2509-2513.
2. Murray RH. Acceptance of paramedical professionals. *Ann Intern Med* 1972; 77: 467-468.

Editorial Note: In 1977, controversy surrounded both physician's assistants and nurse practitioners (see the following editorial). In hindsight, this proved to be much ado about relatively little. Many tasks now formerly carried out by physicians are now performed by physician's assistants and nurse practitioners and, as best I can tell, the relationships are almost uniformly felicitous.

The New Nurse and Territorial Rights

J SC Med Assoc 1977; 73: 337-338

It's three o'clock in the morning and your patient is in shock. You examine him carefully and think through the steps necessary to correct lactic acidemia and to restore patency to the microvasculature. As the last of your detailed orders flows from your ballpoint pen, you look around to see who will carry them out. The ward seems empty. Only vaguely aware of the perspiration on your forehead, and ignoring the gnawing epigastric (or substernal) discomfort, you are seized with an urge to run down the corridor paraphrasing Shakespeare: "A nurse! A nurse! My kingdom for a nurse!"

We need more nurses—few would question this desideratum. Not infrequently, one hears a further stipulation that "we need more *good old-fashioned nurses*." Nursing educators agree that we need more nurses, but do not necessarily agree that we need more of the good old-fashioned kind.[1] Rather, the nurse whom you need at 3 A.M. can do *much more* than her (or his) predecessor—she can measure the pulmonary capillary wedge pressure, interpret the arterial blood gas analysis, add positive end expiratory pressure to the mechanical respirator, adjust the constant-rate infusion pump for anticoagulant or vasopressor drug therapy, and evaluate the simultaneous urine and serum osmolalities. She will not only help you; she will, in part, replace you.

In this issue of *The Journal* appears a synopsis of the 1975 amendment to the Laws Governing Nursing in South Carolina. These laws and their implications have been the subject of an ongoing, productive dialogue by members of the Joint Practice Commission of the South Carolina Medical Association and the South Carolina Nurses Association, chaired by Dr. Michael C. Watson of Bamberg. It is clear, as the commission points out,[2] that the "day of the physician being almost solely responsible for the delivery of health care is long since past." There are *extended* and *expanded* areas of nursing by which *additional* acts can be carried out; the definitions (outlined in the synopsis) are important.

Those interested in the implications of these laws might profit from the informative articles in this issue by non-physicians Vincent and Reeder. Describing the functions of the family planning nurse practitioner in a summer beach environment, they note with candor:

Medical doctors have been very protective of their profession and frequently rebel against anyone interfering in the health care arena. The unavailability of medical doctors, however, results in many individuals being deprived of health care. Professional protectiveness is not only confined to medical doctors. Nurses likewise have been concerned about other types of health professionals infringing upon their *territorial rights* (*emphasis added*).

At this moment, with perceived shortages of both physicians and nurses, the importance of these territorial rights seems small. But when the numbers of both groups increase — as they should — what confrontations might we expect?

Vincent and Reeder assume a shortage of physicians. Let us envision an increase in physicians so that their seaside community has a surplus of eager young physicians — family practitioners, internists, pediatricians, and gynecologists — offering their services to the same clientele. Imagine their attempts to compete with the family planning nurse practitioner: she not only has a lower overhead, but also profits from free advertisement provided by bartenders, streamer-pulling airplanes, posters, Frisbees, and a band! And her services (as mother points out) extend far beyond what used to be considered "family planning." Times change!

Below, Dr. William Weston of Greenville comments on the role of the new breed of nurse practitioners. Surely, the nursing profession is to be commended for its innovations. We should also applaud the Joint Practice Commission of our medical and nursing associations; hopefully, its activities will allow us to minimize conflicts over territorial riots. None could disagree with the commission's assessment: "It is a new day and there are new opportunities on the horizon for improving the quality of care patients receive from our health care system and we should be prepared to take advantage of them."[2]

References

1. Campbell CS: Where are the nurses of yesteryear? (editorial). *Am J Surg* 1977; 133: 143.
2. Joint Practice Commission of the South Carolina Nursing Association and the South Carolina Medical Association: Recent changes in the role and practice of the nurse (draft statement).

Handgun Control

J SC Med Assoc 1981: 245: 77

O wad some Power the giftie gie us
To see oursels as ithers see us!
                              —Robert Burns

As this issue goes to press, the President is recovering from a gunshot wound. The assassination attempt can be expected to heighten the arguments abroad whether America—where three of the last six Presidents have been fired at with one injury and one death—can continue to be entrusted with leadership of the Free World. The attempt can also be expected to heighten the arguments concerning handgun control.

Few issues evoke more controversy. Basic rights are in opposition — on the one hand, the Bill of Rights asserts the right to bear arms; on the other hand, the Declaration of Independence asserts the duty of governments to secure the rights to life, liberty, and the pursuit of happiness. Despite arguments to the contrary, the association between access to handguns and homicide seems clearcut, as was recently pointed out in one of our medical journals.[1] It seems paradoxic to hear individuals assert that "the President (or Michael Halberstam, or John Lennon, or ...) could just as easily have been injured with a knife as with a handgun," yet seldom if ever assert that "that child could have been killed just as easily on roller skates as on a moped."

It has become clear that the issue of handgun control, like the issue of nuclear disarmament,[2] is one that will not be resolved by easy formulas within the near future. A good case can be made that our profession, with its first-hand familiarity with the consequences of violence, should participate actively in the ongoing quest for solutions.

References

1. Rueben ER, Leeper JD: Homicide in five southern states: A firearms phenomenon. *Southern Med J* 1981; 74: 272-277.
2. Lown B, Chivian E, Muller J. et al: The nuclear-arms race and the physician. *N Engl J Med* 1981; 304:726-728.

Editorial Note: Like many Americans, I've been deeply concerned about the ready availability of handguns in our society and about its impact on our image abroad. However, South Carolina being a famously conservative state, I suspect that many readers of *The Journal* do not share my views. I therefore positioned this editorial after similarly short pieces on "Weight Control" and "Cost Control." As editor I've sought to minimize inserting my opinions on divisive issues, recognizing the potential for such opinions to be construed as positions of the South Carolina Medical Association.

The CT Scan and the Technological Imperative

J SC Med Assoc 1981; 77: 411-412.

It is to be regretted that, in the medical profession, as in many others, when a good thing is introduced often the pendulum swings too far, and discredit is thrown upon the thing or method before maturer experience causes it to swing in its proper arc, proving the old Latin axiom to be true, "In medias res tutissimus ibi."

— L. C. Stennis, M.D.

The *Journal* 76 years ago — in 1905. The title of Dr. Stennis's article was "Physiological saline solution: its uses and abuses"!

Leading the battery of newer tests is the computerized tomographic (CT) scanner, now available for searches beyond the cranial vault, where it first found wide application. It seems inevitable that if the future historian considers the most important medical instrument of the mid-twentieth century to have been the telephone, he or she will consider the most important instrument of late twentieth century medicine to have been the computer. Some of our prophets predict that computers will radically transform medicine as we know it. Some allege that computers can already replace physicians for recording the medical history. No less a sage than Dr. Lawrence Weed suggests that computer storage capacity makes traditional memorization of medical facts and habitual journal reading obsolete. It seems highly likely that computers will change the current cumbersome format of medical records. But the most dramatic application of computer technology to medicine to date has to be the invention, by enterprising Englishmen, of the CT scan.

In the preceding editorial, Dr. Frederick Greene reminds us of the overwhelming battery of new diagnostic tests that now find frequent application in clinical medicine. How future historians will judge our current diagnostic maze makes interesting food for thought, but we should remember that such confusion and second thoughts are almost inevitable after the introduction of a new procedure. The above quotation from Dr. Stennis of Greenville appeared in the inaugural issue of *The Journal*. I predict that within the foreseeable future the CT scan will seem as routine to medical practice as physiologic saline.

Although many of us will no doubt continue to protest wide and indiscriminate application of the CT scan, the method is clearly here to stay and will be used with ever-increasing frequency and accuracy. With nostalgic narcissism, we will wave the banners of the meticulous history, the unhurried physical examination, and the thoughtful bedside deliberation—and we will order the scan anyway. The imperative to use available technology for a patient's benefit is a powerful force, and a not altogether undesirable one.

Indeed, newer imaging methods such as radionuclide scans, diagnostic ultrasound, and now the CT scan rank among the most humane diagnostic tools ever devised. They will spare numerous patients the need for invasive procedures such as arteriograms, pneumoencephalograms, biopsies, and explorations. We in medicine should remember with humility that most of these advances were given to us by scientists in other fields, and we should strive to use these tests responsibly. We should try to reduce their costs and thus make them available to all who need them.

Editorial Note: In the intervening years, CT scans have indeed become "as routine to medical practice as physiologic saline." One seldom hears concerns such as those expressed above. Still, many of us worry about (1) a tendency to substitute CT scans and other imaging techniques (notably, ultrasound and magnetic resonance imaging) for careful history-taking and physical examination; (2) a tendency to delay the rest of the diagnostic workup until these studies have been completed; (3) the potential for unnecessary exposure to radiation; and (4) the impact of these technologies on the cost of medical care.

"Wellness" — New Catchword or Novel Concept?

J SC Med Assoc 1981; 77: 510-512

Our president, Dr. William Hunter, is a persuasive individual. I find it difficult to say no to Bill.

And so, when he asked me to give a keynote address at the first Statewide School Nurse Conference, I found myself sputtering, hemming and hawing over the proposed subject: "Wellness." Saying "Yes" despite the better judgment of my neocortex and the admonitions of my gastric parietal cells, I realized that I would feel more comfortable talking about just about anything — say, "African green monkey kidney disease" or "pseudopseudohypoparathyroidism" — other than "wellness."

Needing more information on the subject, I reached for the two dictionaries on my desk. Surprisingly, neither recognized "wellness" as a word. Clearly, I needed expert advice — but where might I find it?

A quick inquiry around the hospital settled the issue. Since June 8, 1981, the hospital, I learned had a new employee — a young woman bearing the title, "Wellness Coordinator." I called her immediately and asked whether she could inform me about the subject in the hospital cafeteria at noon the next day. She agreed to meet me at one o'clock, but not at noon — since that was when she did her daily exercises. Chuckling inwardly, I began to contemplate a tongue-in-cheek editorial in the finest Art Buchwald tradition ("Over a large bowl of organically-grown millet seeds and alfalfa sprouts, she went on to elaborate...."). But what I learned the next day was most informative.

A wellness movement now sweeps across the land. Like the weather, it started in California. That our hospital now boasts a wellness program in addition to a conventional employee health program typifies the trend. Such programs are now the pride of many major companies — Bank of America, Boeing, Exxon, Liberty Life, Mobil Oil, Weyerhauser, and Xerox, to name just a few. Employers may soon offer their employees not "sick days" but "well days," to reward health rather than illness. Some employers provide "exercise breaks," as the Japanese have been doing for years, rather than "coffee breaks" or "cigarette breaks." Persons bearing the title "wellness educator" now turn up in all sorts of places, from hospitals to health spas.

Still searching, I formulated several questions:
• How does the concept of "wellness" as used in this movement differ from the customary concept of "health"?
• What brought about the wellness movement — what perceived needs does it seek to fill?
• Where does the wellness movement stand *vis-a-vis* traditional medicine? Are there any actual or potential areas of conflict?
• Should organized medicine attempt to have input into the wellness movement and, if so, how?

I shall address each of these issues, continuing to acknowledge my ignorance.

The Concept

Central to the movement is the catchword "wellness." Although "health" and "wellness" might seem to be synonymous, the "wellness educators" seek to go beyond the traditional definition of health.

Health has usually been defined as the absence of disease. We pronounce people to be "healthy," for instance, if we find no disease after a comprehensive examination. This notion has stood the test of centuries, and was even given a ponderous affirmation by the great theologian Paul Tillich in one of his last addresses:

> Health is not health without the essential possibility and the existential reality of disease. In this sense, health is disease conquered, as eternally the positive is positive by conquering the negative.[1]

However, the apostles of the new wellness movement employ an expanded definition of health. They embrace the World Health Organization's recent definition of health as "a state of complete physical mental, and social well-being and not merely the absence of disease or infirmity." "Wellness," then, denotes optimum functioning of the individual, not just a normal physical examination combined with some reassuring laboratory studies.

A leading spokesman of the wellness movement defines "high level wellness" as a state of self-actualization:

> Wellness begins when an individual sees himself or herself as a growing, changing person. High level wellness means giving care to the physical self, using the mind constructively, channeling stress energies positively, expressing emotions effectively, becoming creatively involved with others, and staying in touch with the environment.[2]

It is argued that untold thousands of persons pass their physical examinations and are declared "healthy" yet "are in fact bored, depressed, tense, anxious, or generally unhappy with their lives." It is perceived that these individuals have a lifestyle detrimental to their health and that they can be helped.

Justifications

There appear to be three major justifications for the wellness movement.

First, it is perceived that we physicians have to some extent abdicated our roles as "wellness advisers." The wellness movement begins with the premise that about 80 percent of premature deaths attributed to heart disease, cancer, and stroke are preventable. It is perceived that a major way to prevent these deaths is to modify lifestyles. Traditional medical training does not prepare physicians to answer the innumerable nitty-gritty questions pertaining to lifestyle. Speaking as one physician, I can recall entering practice with the ability to recite the latest classifications of the hyperlipoproteinemias and the mucopolysaccharidoses but being completely unable to field a simple question such as "What do you think of the Scarsdale diet?" I had to "wing it" (that is, "fake it").

Second, it is suggested that the growing popularity of the wellness movement may reflect, in part, public hostility toward traditional medicine. Such hostility is, of course, as old as medicine and I have no further comment.

Finally, and probably most significantly, it is suggested that the popularity of the wellness movement reflects a growing dependency in our society for expertise. If one wishes to take any activity seriously nowadays, it seems necessary to join a club, pay an instructor, subscribe to a magazine, and/or buy a videotape. Why should "wellness" be an exception? One local wellness program, for instance, offers each participant a monthly newsletter, social events, a book, and a T-shirt. The program lasts a year and includes physical activities such as aerobic dancing, instruction in relaxation techniques, and workshops in nutrition and in stress control. One emerges with an altered lifestyle, designed both to reduce the risk of disease and also to enhance one's capacity for creative living.

Potential Conflicts

All of the aims of the wellness movement appear to be quite consistent with the aims of traditional medicine. For years, we have advocated lifestyle modification based on established cause-and-effect risk factors such as obesity, smoking, and dependence on alcohol and drugs. For years we have conducted research into other risk factors, such as stress, which might be modified. Seen as a supplement to traditional medical examinations, wellness programs appear to be quite admirable. However, three potential areas of conflict emerged from my cursory overview.

First, some of the leaders of the wellness movement seem to imply that traditional medicine may be anachronistic. The author of a leading book, for instance subtitled his work "an *alternative* to doctors, drugs and disease" (emphasis added). The argument states that traditional medicine deals only with the symptoms and signs of conditions leading to premature death, whereas "high level wellness" does much more.[2]

The second area of potential conflict concerns what is carried out in wellness programs. Are participants sufficiently informed about the trade-offs involved in this or that exercise program? We should remember that establishing the actual benefit from most "lifestyle modifications" can be extremely difficult.[3] Jogging provides an excellent example. One wonders, for instance, how today's avid joggers will view their benefits twenty to forty years hence as they nurse their osteoarthritic knees (*Editorial note written 26 years later*: I wish I'd heeded my own warning here!).

Finally, and most importantly, there is the question of qualification of persons identified as "wellness educators." The woman at our hospital has a master's degree in her field and clearly knows what she is talking about. She appreciates the significance of each of the baseline physiologic and laboratory tests which her participants undergo, and she considers physician input to be essential to her program. It is perceived, however, that a cadre of largely untrained persons may proclaim themselves to be "wellness educators," advising the public about this or that new diet or exercise program with little appreciation of the underlying issues. It does not require an Alvin Toffler to envision that such persons, equipped with a bookshelf of the latest manuals and some do-it-yourself laboratory tests, could replace physicians as the providers of the "annual check-up." I cringe to imagine that a cherished friend who recently underwent resection of an early colon carcinoma, found by her internist on a routine physical examination, might still be out there doing her jogging and relaxation exercises under the enthusiastic supervision of a poorly-qualified "wellness educator" blissfully unaware of a metastasizing malignancy.

Conclusions

A Mississippi physician wrote recently that "lifestyle is our generation's big medical fad" and argued against the trend toward lifestyle intervention.[4] An increasingly large segment of the public would disagree. So, I think, would many (perhaps most) of the leaders in our profession. One recalls especially the many exhortations of Dr. Harrison Peeples during his SCMA presidency that lifestyle education should begin early in the public schools. One recalls the excellent summary of lifestyle interventions expressed at the Governor's Conference on Health.[5]

We cannot ignore the basic thesis of the wellness movement; we should support it.

We should support these persons and their programs in two ways. First, we should insist on some standard of certification for wellness educators. We should recognize the potential for the public to be badly served by a new band of self-proclaimed paraprofessionals who are poorly prepared to comprehend the limitations of their methods. Second, we should work with qualified "wellness educators" toward sharper definition of those methods of intervention that have been shown to be beneficial. One long-term follow-up study, for instance, indicated that the patterns of psychological defense mechanisms provide an excellent prediction of illness[6] — but how can these be modified effectively? We should continue to emphasize that the data in many areas are simply too scanty to make dogmatic recommendations.

The wellness movement does not seem to be a novel concept. We have always known that health — in its broadest sense — means more than the absence of disease. I am reminded especially of the words of Freud who, pressed for a definition of health, responded that health is "the ability to work and to love."

References

1. Tillich P. The meaning of health. *Perspect Biol Med* 1961; 5:92-100.
2. Ardell DB. *High Level Wellness: An Alternative to Doctors, Drugs, and Disease*. Emmaus, Pennsylvania: Rodale Press; 1977.
3. Szlko M. The epidemiologic basis of prevention: how much data do we need? *Johns Hopkins Med J* 1981; 149: 64-70.
4. McGee RR. "Stop blaming the patient for being sick." *Medical Economics*, 10 August 1981: 57-59.
5. [South Carolina] Governor's Conference on Health: Prevention for the Eighties. December 5, 1980 [Prospectus].
6. Vaillant GE. *Adaptation to Life*. Boston: Little, Brown and Company; 1977.

Chiropractic Legislation: Two Broken Records

J SC Med Assoc 1982; 78: 170-172

*We feel that we are beginning to sound like a broken record,
but our chiropractic legislation remains far and away the most
prominent issue facing the legislature.*
— Legislative Update, *Journal of the South
Carolina Medical Association,* January, 1982

The nineteenth century witnessed many unifying theories
of disease, usually made by one individual on the basis of
one or several observations and usually discarded by the end
of that individual's lifetime. By the end of the century, what is
now called the scientific method had become well-established
and broad, sweeping theories of disease were no longer acceptable to qualified physicians. Curiously, such a sweeping theory
arose toward the end of the nineteenth century, took roots outside of orthodox medicine, and, while still without scientific
validation, again needs a response from our profession.

In September 1895, Daniel David Palmer, the proprietor
of a "magnetic healing" studio in Davenport, Iowa, allegedly
restored the hearing of a deaf janitor by adjusting one of the
vertebrae. Apparently unaware that the eighth cranial nerves
lie entirely within the skull, Palmer concluded that malalignments of vertebrae cause most if not all disease processes. His
theory obtained a following. For the next thirty years, qualified
physicians—perhaps because they had little to offer patients
with nagging backaches—permitted leeway to chiropractic.
Not surprisingly, many chiropractors promoted the notion that
malalignments of the vertebrae caused most disorders, not just
backache. And, not surprisingly, many chiropractors branched
out into modes of therapy other than spinal adjustment.

The many skirmishes between organized medicine and organized chiropractic will not be reviewed in detail here. Suffice
it to say that chiropractic made enormous strides during the
1970s:

• In 1973, chiropractors gained approval for reimbursement by both Medicare and Medicaid.

• Shortly thereafter, they received licensure in Mississippi and Louisiana, thereby attaining the right to practice in all fifty states.

• In 1974, an accrediting agency for their schools was recognized by the United States Commission of Education, which had previously listed chiropractic schools as "spurious."

Political pressure, made possible by sophisticated organization among the nation's chiropractors, was instrumental to all of these gains. These gains came paradoxically at a time when established medicine validated the scientific basis for its practices at an astonishing rate. Yet the unity and cohesiveness of established medicine paled by comparison to the unity and cohesiveness of chiropractic.

The American Medical Association, harassed by the Federal Trade Commission and sued for restraint of trade, eventually adopted a report by the Board of Trustees holding that chiropractic would no longer be viewed as an "unscientific cult" nor would it declare that voluntary association by physicians with chiropractors was unethical. Today, chiropractic flourishes. Some 23,000 chiropractors treat at least eight million Americans each year (estimates run as high as 35 million Americans). Each year, more than 2,000 new chiropractors graduate from their schools. It can be concluded safely that "chiropractors appear to be winning their struggle to survive."[1]

All of this seems quite remarkable when one reflects on the absence of scientific proof of the basis for chiropractic theory. No experimental evidence supports the thesis that minor malalignments of the vertebrae give rise to significant internal disease processes. The logical viewpoint that chiropractic should validate its claims was recently stated by one of our leading editors, Dr. Arnold Relman:

> It is up to the chiropractors to demonstrate that their theories are sound, their diagnostic techniques accurate and their treatments effective. They must do research and they must publish their evidence.... Medicine accepts these obligations. It recognizes its limitations, but

it uses methods of science to advance its understanding. Medicine supports its theories with evidence and submits its diagnostic and therapeutic claims to objective tests. Let chiropractic do the same.[2]

Chiropractors counter such arguments by stating that they need not submit to the same standards that physicians choose to impose upon themselves.

However poorly understood it might be, chiropractic manipulation as one method for treating musculoskeletal aches is not a current issue. The present SCMA position paper holds that "the majority of physicians in the medical community feel that most chiropractors are ethical within their range of training." We should perhaps remember that not all of our own remedies have been well-proven by either controlled observations in the laboratory or by prospective, randomized, double-blind clinical trials. One observer pointed out recently that "one is tempted to imagine that if it had been chiropractic rather than acupuncture that was brought out of China to a palpitating American public less than ten years ago, chiropractic might have fascinated and conquered the lay and professional community with its miraculous effects."[3] It is acknowledged that physicians, including orthopedists, sometimes refer patients to chiropractors for manipulation.

The principal issue is the tendency of some chiropractors to go well beyond their traditional boundaries. In 1975, *Consumer Reports* conducted an exhaustive survey of chiropractic.[4] Chiropractic educators and officials invariably told interviewers that "the chiropractor's role was that of the primary physician." Chiropractors felt that they should have the same rights as family physicians to serve as "portals of entry" to the health care delivery system. The report mentioned one institution within our own state:

At the Sherman College of Chiropractic in Spartanburg, S.C., for example, the criteria for accepting a patient are liberal indeed. According to an Editorial by ... a Dean of the College, requirements for a "chiropractic case" are threefold: "Does the patient have a spinal column? Does the patient have a nervous system? Is the patient alive?"[4]

The Consumer's Union concluded that Palmer's theory of disease belongs to the dusty pages of nineteenth century history, "along with bleeding, purging, and other blind alleys of medicine," and pointed out the potential for chiropractic to cause harm. It provided clear-cut guidelines for persons desiring to use a chiropractor, and recommended that "licensing laws and Federal health insurance should limit chiropractic treatment to appropriate musculoskeletal complaints."

In South Carolina today, there is abundant evidence that some chiropractors go well beyond their traditional boundaries. One advertisement, for example, promotes "colonic therapy with oxygen," to prevent "build up of poisons by anaeriobic [sic] bacteria in the body." Such therapy might be beneficial for headache, constipation, diarrhea, abdominal pain, low back pain, flatulence, or unusual fatigue. Another advertisement indicated "only chiropractic can help" a number of illnesses including life-threatening infectious diseases such as pneumonia and spinal meningitis. The advertisement goes on to declare that "two facts should be clear ... first, that our profession is not limited in scope ... (and second) that the cause of much sickness is due to spinal nerve interference."

A thoughtful review of the current problem of chiropractic concluded with the recommendation that limitation of scope — along the lines of the SCMA-sponsored bills (S. 636 and H. 2606) — is the soundest policy.[1] The possibility was raised that chiropractic might evolve to the status of a recognized "limited" specialty analogous to podiatry, optometry, speech therapy, or audiology. It was felt that evolution of chiropractic into a "limited role" would be better for the public than either preserving the status quo or attempting to eliminate chiropractic altogether.

Two developments in medicine should have a bearing on the eventual role of chiropractic. First, an increasing number of specialists in areas such as neurology and orthopedics are bringing new sophistication to the diagnosis and management of nagging musculoskeletal pains. Secondly, an increasing number of physicians specializing in primary care should eliminate

329

the need for persons in smaller towns and rural communities to seek out chiropractors due to difficulty obtaining an appointment with a physician. We should not assume, however, that increasing numbers of physicians in those communities will necessarily mean fewer tendencies for patients to see chiropractors. In a study conducted in Iowa, it was found that a growth in the physician manpower pool was accompanied by a slight increase — rather than decrease — in the use of chiropractic services.[5]

The hazards of chiropractic manipulation are well-known, and the list continues to grow.[6] The number of services offered by chiropractors has also expanded. With increasing specialization in medicine and wider availability of medical services, there is no reason for chiropractors to be offering services such as ultrasound, "vascular analysis," and other procedures for which physicians are specifically trained and certified. Limiting laboratory tests to professionals trained to interpret them also makes sense.

As this editorial is being prepared for press, the House and Senate are considering the two SCMA-sponsored bills for limitation of the scope of chiropractic. Let us conclude with our second "broken record"... the repeated urgings that all physicians should support organized medicine. Those who don't are clearly receiving a "free ride." We should emphasize again that the enormous gains made by chiropractors during the 1970s were due almost entirely to their unity and organization.

References

1. Wardell WI. The future of chiropractic. *N Engl J Med* 1980; 302: 688-690.
2. Relman AS. Chiropractic: Recognized but unproved. *N Engl J Med* 1979; 301: 659-660.
3. Silver CA. Chiropractic: Professional controversy and public policy. *Am J Public Health* 1980; 70: 348-351.
4. Chiropractors: Healers or quacks? *Consumer Reports*, September and October 1975.
5. Yesalis CE III, Wallace RB, Fisher, WP, et al. Does chiropractic

utilization substitute for less available medical services? *Am J Public Health* 1980; 70: 415-417.

6. Kureger BR, Okazakai H. Vertebral basilar distribution infarction following chiropractic cervical manipulation. *Mayo Clinic Proc* 1980; 55: 322-332.

The New Economics of Health Care Delivery: A Time for Ideas and Input

J SC Med Assoc 1983; 79: 506-507

Cost control is coming and the implications are enormous. One need look no further than one's favorite source of business news. The economics of health care delivery are about to change radically and drastically. The Congressional decision to restructure Medicare reimbursements will precipitate a cascade of repercussions. These changes come at a bad time — a time of economic uncertainty and of possible physician surplus. Everyone predicts keen competition: hospital versus hospital, hospital versus physician, and — yes — physician versus physician.[1,2] And these changes are likely to tarnish the image of our profession, an image built up gradually over more than a century of steady scientific achievement.

Sounding the battle cry against mounting medical care costs are not only government and insurance carriers but also private industries. Recently, for instance, Joseph A. Califano outlined sweeping changes in the way by which Chrysler corporation would provide health care for its workers.[3] Pointing out that the corporation's total health care bill per car produced rose from $75 per car in 1970 to $600 per car in 1983, Mr. Califano concluded that the burden had become intolerable. Exhorting industry to "deal with the cost of health care — a cost that bears little relationship to the quality of care and none to the efficiency with which it is delivered," he urged a radical restructuring of health care financing.

How did these grave prognoses and radical remedies come about? Although we have persistently pointed out that much, perhaps most of the spiraling rise in health care costs owes to factors pervading our society and beyond our direct control, social critics often disagree. They argue that physician pressures, not patient demands, propelled American medicine from a small and divided enterprise into the nation's second largest employer (after education) and third largest burden for consumer spending (after food and housing). In a book published just before enactment of the recent congressional legislation, for instance, sociologist Paul Starr argues that sweeping changes were inevitable:[4]

• Physicians managed to dominate the American hospital during its reorganization between 1870 and 1930, thereby capping most of the bureaucratic control characteristic of our times.

• Physicians defined the boundaries of public health in America to suit their own interests. The denouncement by the Chicago Medical Society of a philanthropically-sponsored venereal disease clinic as "unfair competition" in 1919 presaged the relegation of public health to secondary status.

• Physicians kept corporations from intervening in their relationships with patients. They thwarted the attempts of various corporations such as the railroads to change to their liking certain aspects of health care delivery.

• Physicians headed off the development of government health insurance programs through the 1940s and 1950s. In 1947, no less a personage than Bernard Baruch suggested a national system of voluntary health insurance for high income Americans and of compulsory health insurance under Social Security for low income Americans. However, American physicians often equated "socialized medicine" with "communism." America became the only country in which anti-communism sentiment was "channeled into opposition of health insurance."

• Physicians won accommodation to their own existing forms of organization during the development of commercial health insurance plans, such as the Blues and Kaiser-Permanente. A system of financing arose by which an ever-increasing share of the gross national income was channeled into health care.

• Physicians derived enormous benefits from the liberal philosophies of the post-war years. Between 1950 and 1970, national health care expenditures rose from 12.7 to 71.6 billion dollars per year, or from 4.5 to 7.3 percent of the gross national product. Despite a great increase in the demand for medical care, however, there was little or no increase in the supply of physicians. A perceived physician shortage resulted.

• Physicians derived enormous benefits from government programs that infused monies into medical research, mental health, the Veterans Administration, and community hospital construction under the Hill-Burton program. During enactment of each of these programs, physicians managed to win respect for "the sovereignty of the medical profession and local medical institutions."

• Physicians likewise profited when the financing of Medicare came to be based within previously-organized insurance systems, designed to suit "provider interests" rather than "consumer interests." The government thereby surrendered direct control of Medicare and its costs. Enormous increases in health care expenditures ensued.

• Young physicians with no previous records of customary charges for their newly-minted procedures billed Medicare at unprecedented levels and — owing to the way by which the system had been organized — were reimbursed. Costs soared to new heights.

• Responding to runaway costs, three powerful forces came

to align against health care providers and to seek greater government intervention: the insurance industry, employers, and government itself.

Whether or not one agrees with Starr's interpretations of recent history, the challenges faced by organized medicine are obvious and twofold. First, we must cope with the new economics in ways serving the best interests of both society and the medical profession. Second, we must minimize the extent to which the sharp axes of social change will splinter our profession into an ever-increasing number of special interest groups working toward conflicting goals.

South Carolina physicians should know that the staffs of the SCMA and of the South Carolina Medical Care Foundation, aided by the firm of McManis Associates have completed a detailed survey of the current socioeconomic terrain and that the SCMA officers and council members are devoting large portions of their time to these problems. There are no ready answers. This is a time for input from SCMA members and for fresh ideas. Mr. Califano, in concluding his talk to the Economic Club of Detroit,[3] quoted G. K. Chesterton: "I do not believe in a fate that befalls people however they act. I do believe in a fate that befalls them unless they act." Can we not heed the same advice?

References

1. Hospitals and doctors compete for patients, with rising bitterness. *The Wall Street Journal*, 19 July 1983.
2. The upheaval in health care: Government cost controls will soon have hospitals under the knife. *Business Week*, 25 July 1983.
3. Califano JA Jr. Can we afford one trillion dollars for health care? Address given to the Economic Club of Detroit, 25 April 1983.
4. Starr P. *The Social Transformation of American Medicine*. New York: Basic Books, Inc.; 1982.

Diagnosis Related Groups (DRGs): Implications and Uncertainties

J SC Med Assoc 1984; 80: 78-79

D RGs, like Carl Sandburg's fog, came on little cat feet and covered the future of medical practice like a blanket before we knew what was upon us. Few bells of alarm were heard prior to the passage of the 1983 Amendments to the Social Security Act (P.L. 98-21). On October 1, 1983 — a date likely to be recalled time and time again by future social historians — the system of prospective Medicare payments to hospitals went into effect. A current editorial in *The Lancet* tells the story accurately: "October 1, 1983 marked a turning point in American health care ... the consequences for the practice of medicine and the delivery of health care could be far-reaching."[1]

So sweeping are the implications of DRGs that it remains striking, in retrospect, that passage of this legislation occasioned so little public debate. In future editorials in *The Journal*, physicians from various health care delivery sectors in South Carolina will examine some of these implications. First, however, let us review the brief history of DRGs and let us sample some of the prognoses that have been offered.

The concept of diagnosis related groups (DRGs) as a method for identifying patients who according to discharge diagnoses should have similar needs during hospitalization was developed by researchers at Yale University during the 1970s. Congress elected to apply this system to Medicare payments to hospitals over a three-year period, so that by October 1, 1986, Medicare payments will be 100% of the national DRG rate for each of 467 diagnostic categories. In 1985, the Department of Health and Human Services is to report "on the advisability and feasibility" of extending DRGs so that they would also include physician charges. Legislation would, if appropriate, be recommended to use the system for reimbursement of physicians as well as hospitals.

The accompanying tables (*Editorial note*: The tables, now of historical interest only, are omitted here for the sake of brevity) summarize some of the pros and cons of DRGs as they affect patients, physicians and hospitals. Conflict between and among these three groups seems inevitable.

All major health care insurance companies in the United States may adopt the concept of DRGs within the near future. Current estimates hold that as many as one-sixth of our hospitals will be forced to close their doors.[1] Bearing an especially large brunt of the burden will be tertiary care centers responsible for acutely ill patients.

Hospitals will bring pressure on physicians to limit use of diagnostic tests, expensive therapies, ancillary services, and prolonged hospital stays. Formerly, all of these utilizations brought revenues to the hospitals; now they will either reduce profits or add to debts. Physicians will find that expenses generated by their activities will be monitored by computers. Those who fail to cooperate with hospital administrators may find their admitting privileges denied. Such warnings have already been issued to physicians in New Jersey. Heretofore, it is often pointed out nowadays, those physicians who admitted the most patients, ordered the most diagnostic studies, and gave the latest therapies were the hospital's heroes; now, they will be viewed as enemies to the hospital's very existence.

The pace of medical progress will slow considerably. No longer, for instance, will hospitals compete with one another to provide the latest imaging devices. The old but cost-effective equipment will have to suffice. It has been suggested that DRGs "will mean good news for computer software makers and bad news for some new medical instrument technologies."[2] Most advances in medicine within recent memory have meant increased costs. Under the new system, most potential advances will be unaffordable.[3]

An epidemiologist at Yale, where DRGs originated, observes that this concept is but the latest of a series of acronymic attempts to control medical costs, following in the wake of UR (utilization review), PSRO (professional standards review organization), CON (certificate of need), and HSA (health systems agencies). He suggests that "these acronymic maneuvers will be unsuccessful even in containing costs, and they will do little to improve patient care, provide better access for the underserved, or secure more equity in medical care services generally."[4] Is such pessimism warranted? For the sake of our patients, our hospitals, and ourselves, let us hope not. It is obvious, however, that physicians and hospital administrators, perhaps as never before, will need to sit down and define their common interests. Government policy spawned the notion that health care, whatever the cost, is a basic American right. Now government taketh away, and it is up to us to walk the tightrope between fiscal responsibility and practicing our art and science according to the Golden Rule.

References

1. Payment by diagnosis (editorial). *Lancet* 1983; 2: 1403-1404.
2. "Medicine by the numbers." *Forbes*, 16 January 1984: 84-85.
3. Connolly NK. "DRGs": Their relationship to hospital practice. *South Med J* 1983; 76: 1082-1083.
4. Silver CA. Solution by acronym. *Lancet* 1983; 2: 1433-1434.

Medical Education and DRGs

J SC Med Assoc 1984; 80: 511-512.

In its search for more efficient ways to finance health care, the government must not lose sight of the fact that teaching hospitals reached their current position by responding to the demands society placed on them.[1]

As Dr. Allen Johnson points out in the preceding editorial, the network of American teaching hospitals offers the most comprehensive, sophisticated medical care in all of history. These hospitals built excellence upon four pillars of government support: state and local governments, Medicare, the National Institutes of Health, and the Veterans Administration. Somewhat paradoxically, however, none of these funding sources viewed teaching as their primary aim. The current climate of cutbacks in funding for both research and patient care will inevitably affect the funding of teaching hospitals and therefore of medical education.

Already palpable is the impact of DRGS. For a variety of reasons, well-outlined by Dr. Johnson, the prospective payment system places considerable pressures on teaching hospitals. Although still incompletely defined, these pressures seem destined to cause university hospitals to specialize, at least to some extent.[2] Competition will dictate that these hospitals can no longer offer the entire spectrum of medical and surgical care and remain solvent. The era of the all-providing "Mecca" may be drawing to a close.

Part of the solution to this quandary must be the teaching of cost-effective medical care to the current and coming generations of medical students and residents. Unfortunately, their teachers and role models learned medicine during an era in which young physicians were by and large given a *carte blanche* to do whatever they deemed best for the patient. Many of us can recall being told during our own training by residents just ahead of us that "the faculty will seldom criticize you for ordering too many tests—but they'll criticize you if you forgot something." Reputation thus came to those residents who seldom overlooked the 24-hour urine collection for 5-hydroxyindoleacetic acid or the three morning gastric aspirates for AFB culture. Failure of the faculty to insist on cost/benefit calculations prior to such diagnostic adventures helped spawn what critics might call, with at least a measure of justification, a generation of medical spendthrifts.

A recent editorialist in *The Lancet* states the problem succinctly. Pointing out that the luxury of modern medical care is made "possible only because our industries and agriculture produce sufficient excess wealth to provide for more than the bare necessities of life," the writer notes that it is high time for medical educators to raise the banner of cost containment. Unfortunately, he notes that "the authoritarian natures of medical practice and medical knowledge tend to stifle criticism ... (perhaps) it is time to encourage a more questioning outlook in medical undergraduates."[3] Students and residents should not only learn cost-containment from their mentors; they should challenge their mentors.

There is a definite need for more critical dialogue about the cost effectiveness of the things we do. Such dialogue should lead to rational policies or operational rules-of-thumb to guide decision-making.

For example, it is clear that untold thousands of dollars are spent to increase the level of confidence that something does not exist (i.e., the "rule out") from say, 95 percent to 99 percent. Let us consider a single situation: the alcoholic patient presenting to the emergency room of an urban teaching hospital with a seizure. Prevailing opinion holds that the patient deserves skull x-rays, an electroencephalogram, and a CT scan if these have not been done previously. These studies are expensive. Although most us can recall the occasional unsuspected subdural hematoma, the yield of such studies is admittedly small. In a recent study, only one of 94 alcoholic patients with seizures but without focal deficits on neurologic examination was found to have a potentially reversible lesion on CT scan.[4] Assuming that the scan costs $300, the cost of detecting that one patient would be $28,200. Arguably, that one instance of potentially reversible disease would have been detected by a policy of careful follow-up observation without CT scans for patients without focal neurologic deficits or signs of trauma. Also arguably, the real cost of a CT scan is not $300 but the cost of the technician's time and of the x-ray film. Similar data are needed in many areas of medical practice and dialogue is needed to convert such data into practical guidelines. There is nothing to prevent teaching hospitals from showing the way.

In the Northeast, many hospitals have developed prototypes for providing data for cost-effective medical practice. For the first time in recent memory, physicians are finding that frugality may be rewarded while spendthrift ways may be punished. Has the time not clearly come for physicians practicing in teaching hospitals to be role models for cost-effective practice and for residents to be rewarded on the basis of conscientious utilization of resources rather than on their test- and procedure-ordering ingenuity? The future of both medical education and of teaching hospitals may be at stake.

References

1. Inglehart JK. Moment of truth for teaching hospitals. *N Engl J Med* 1982; 307: 132-136.
2. Bergen SJ, Roth AS. Prospective payment and the university hospital. *N Engl J Med* 1984; 310: 316-318.
3. High technology medicine: A luxury we can afford? (editorial) *Lancet* 1984; 2: 77-78.
4. Feussner JR, Linfors EW, Blessing CL et al. Computer tomography brain scanning in alcohol withdrawal seizures: Value of neurologic examination. *Ann Intern Med* 1981; 94: 519-522.

Of Cost Containment and Cat-Bellers

J SC Med Assoc 1985; 81: 87-88

Reprove not a scorner, lest he hate thee: rebuke a wise man, and he will love thee.
— Proverbs 9:8

A prerequisite for worthwhile evaluation ... is for all doctors to cultivate a self-critical attitude to their practices. The authoritarian natures of medical practice and medical knowledge tend to stifle criticism ...[1]
— *Lancet* 1984; 2: 77-78

In this issue of *The Journal*, Dr. Conyers O'Bryan of Florence has both edited a symposium on cost-effective cardiovascular drug therapy and also written the preceding editorial on the implications of DRGs for office-based physicians. In next month's issue, Dr. Mims Mobley of Greenwood will provide the latest of our planned series of editorials on DRGS, conceived during 1983 and begun a year ago. We can anticipate that dialogue regarding these two topics — cost-effective therapy and the implication of DRGs — will continue to appear in these pages for years to come. In the meantime, Dr. O'Bryan points out that while DRGs perhaps cloud the immediate future of medicine, there may be at least one silver lining: an incentive for high-volume, cost-effective outpatient medical care.

The delivery of a greater proportion of medical care in outpatient settings will predictably promote efforts to extend the concept of DRGs to those settings. We have already been told that the Department of Health and Human Services plans to extend the DRG approach to ambulatory care.[2] Like it or not, the issue of cost-effectiveness in all we do is here to stay.

The percentage of our gross national product spent on health care more than doubled during the past 25 years. During this period, leaders of our profession frequently sounded the need for cost containment and for medicine to "maintain its own house." Why did these cries fail to bring about effective self-regulation long before the enactment PL 98-21 in October, 1983? Were our leaders ineffective?

I suggest that our failure to bring about cost control prior to the recent legislation was due not to lack of leadership but rather to the nature of the problem. Talented persons from many areas—organized medicine, academic medicine, practicing physicians, and the lay public, to name a few—addressed the issues both frequently and forcefully. However, the problem was analogous to that facing the mouse of the familiar fable who proposed placing a bell around the cat's neck. Who was to actually bell the cat?

At least two factors have stymied efforts to promote cost-effectiveness. First, society has yet to give us a suitable ethical and legal framework upon which to take cost-effectiveness into account when we make certain key decisions. As patient advocates, we understandably feel compelled to do "everything possible" even when the cost-potential benefit ratio seems exceedingly high. The second factor is human nature, which poses powerful barriers to truly effective peer review. Knowing that our fellow physicians—like most people including ourselves—sometimes tolerate criticism poorly, we are usually reluctant to give it. We therefore keep to ourselves our opinions that some of our colleagues could practice medicine in a much more cost-effective manner.

As individuals, we cannot bell this cat by ourselves. We need society's advice and consent regarding the extent to which we can base clinical decisions on estimates of cost-effectiveness. We need our profession's help to provide the data for making these estimates. As a recent editorialist puts it:

> It will be far better (compared to a complicated set of rules and regulations) if American doctors begin to build up a social ethic and behavioral practices that help them decide when medicine is bad medicine—not simply because it has absolutely no payoff or because it hurts the patient—but also because the costs are not justified by the marginal benefits.[3]

We must encourage the development, both on a national and

local basis, of effective guidelines on which to base such judgments. We must encourage the development of more effective quality assurance and peer review activities at our hospitals. We must become more self-critical and more willing to give criticism to others and accept their criticism in turn.

A new mind-set for medical practice (code name: cost-effective medicine) must support and supplement the old one (code name: scientific medicine). We must all become cat-bellers.

References

1. High technology medicine: A luxury we can afford? (editorial). *Lancet* 1984; 2: 77-78.
2. Omenn GS, Conrad DA. Implications of DRGs for clinicians. *N Engl J Med* 1984; 311: 1314-1317.
3. Thurow LC. Learning to say "no." *N Engl J Med* 1984; 311: 1569-1572.

Editorial Note written 22 years later. These three editorials about reimbursement according to diagnosis-related groups (DRGs) reflected a national debate that turned out to be much ado about relatively little. As it played out, DRGs were only another example of a well-intended scheme that failed to stem the rising costs of health care in the United States. Health care expenditures as a percentage of our gross domestic product steadily increased. Attempts by various physician groups to suggest ways for reducing health care costs likewise failed — largely because society didn't seem ready to hear the message. Especially innovative was the "Oregon Plan," whereby physicians in that state ranked various medical interventions in order of cost-effectiveness and then asked citizens to "draw a line" regarding what they were willing to assure for everyone. As I understand it, the Oregon Plan failed because a few patients and their attorneys prevailed in the courts. Perhaps the day will come when necessity will force the American public to invite our serious input.

Black Physicians, South Carolina Medicine, and the SCMA

J SC Med Assoc 1988; 84: 260-261.

Sullivan's Island evokes many memories, mostly pleasant. Summer breezes remind us July afternoons on the beach. The streets numbered after stations remind us of the old trolley line. The history-minded recall the fortifications that once guarded Charleston Harbor, while the literary turn to Edgar Allen Poe's "The Gold Bug." To black Americans, the memories are — or should be — less pleasant. It was on Sullivan's Island that untold thousands of slaves were quarantined before being carted off to the auctions. The historian Peter H. Wood suggests that this storied spit of land "might well be viewed as the Ellis Island of black Americans," since "the colonial ancestors of present-day Afro-Americans are more likely to have first confronted North America at Charlestown than at any other port of entry."[1] Alone among American immigrants, they did not come voluntarily, seeking a better way of life.

More than any other issue, race relations define the history of South Carolina. It is hard to imagine a competent historian, sociologist, or anthropologist starting elsewhere. First came the clash between Native Americans and white opportunists seeking slaves for their Caribbean colonies and, later, land. Then came black slavery to power the plantation economy. In Georgetown County, the most extreme example, slaves comprised 85 percent of the population at the outbreak of the Civil War. The theory that the war was not fought over slavery is no longer tenable. South Carolina's fervor to secede prompted a long and bitter Federal occupation. When the troops finally pulled out, white populists quelled whatever chances there might have been for peaceful cooperation within a participatory democracy. Finally and more recently, the relative ease with which desegregation came about in South Carolina won praise from many quarters. Race relations provide a litmus test for measuring how just about any generation of South Carolinians responded to just about any issue. One need not talk about it openly. The problem is there.

Given the primacy of race relations to our history, one would anticipate that many articles and editorials would have discussed this issue over the years. This does not seem to have been the case. As best I can tell, the special problems of black physicians had not been the subject of a single article or editorial before this issue, in which Dr. Burnett Gallman rectifies this situation with what he calls a "brief overview." He recognizes that much more remains to be done. Likewise, I recognize that I cannot do justice to the subject's complexities in one editorial. However, several aspects deserve emphasis.

Dr. Gallman notes with understatement that "the practice of medicine in South Carolina for Black physicians has been historically difficult at best." After the long years of college, medical school, and residency, blacks faced almost insurmountable barriers. Their denial to membership in county, state, and national medical associations was bad enough, but the worst blow was denial of hospital privileges. Well-qualified black physicians were forced to surrender their patients at the hospital door. White physicians frequently stole those who were able to pay, leaving their black counterparts to care for large numbers of indigents. Records document that many black physicians relocated to the North. Others continued in practice partly out of a sense of obligation. Many burned out early. A common expression of the weary black physician to a younger colleague entering practice was, "I've paid my dues."

The lives of South Carolina black physicians who endured these hardships deserve more adequate recognition. Consider, for example, Matilda Evans of Columbia. Three times between 1898 and 1916, she attempted to open hospitals against all odds. Consider L. W. Long of Union. In the early 1930s, he opened a community hospital, started an annual program of post-graduate clinics for black physicians, and at his own expense started a program of preventive health services for black school children. Edward H. Beardsley points out that this was ironically beneficial to white children also: "Realizing that black schools were

345

getting something that theirs were not, Union whites became very uncomfortable and began to press for a public health center (where formerly they had opposed it) so that they could enjoy similar services and reestablish their racial pre-eminence."[2]

Adding to black physicians' problems were their small numbers. In 1890 there was one black physician per 23,000 citizens in South Carolina (compared to one per 420 citizens for whites). By 1920 there was one per 10,200 citizens (compared to one per 651 citizens for whites). Blacks not only found it difficult to obtain medical education but also found it difficult to get started in practice. Todd L. Savitt identifies several problems: (1) black patients were distrustful of black physicians after years of conditioning by white physicians; (2) black patients would often take advantage of black physicians' good will when it came time to pay their bills; (3) occasional well-entrenched black physicians were perceived as incompetent and would undermine the standing of other black physicians; and (4) root doctors and other unorthodox practitioners would undermine black patients' trust in their own physicians.[3] Looking back, it is amazing that blacks went into medicine at all.

In theory, ours should be an era of rapid social change. Medical schools no longer discriminate. Hospital staffs are open. Medical societies welcome all comers. Overt prejudice has largely disappeared from polite conversation. However, it would be naïve to opine that all wounds are healed. We in South Carolina can take comfort only in the observation that the problems are now recognized to be national, not just local or regional. Many of the great expectations spawned by *Brown v. Board of Education* have simply not happened. Allan Bloom of the University of Chicago writes pessimistically of the college scene:

> White and black students do not in general become friends.... the gulf of difference has proved unbridgeable. The forgetting of race in the university, which was predicted and confidently expected when the barriers were let down, has not occurred.... The programmatic brotherhood of the sixties did not culminate in integration but veered off toward black separation.[4]

By necessity, blacks have long had their own medical societies (the National Medical Association and in South Carolina, the Palmetto Medical, Dental, and Pharmaceutical Association and others). I shall now pose two questions. First, why do black physicians need the SCMA? Second, why does the SCMA need black physicians?

The answer to the second question comes more readily. The SCMA needs *all* South Carolina physicians. To be credible and effective, we must serve the best interests of *all* South Carolinians. The answer to the first question is less straightforward. In the other traditional professions — the ministry and the law — blacks have achieved great prominence in our state. This has not been the case in organized medicine. The first black physician has yet to serve on the SCMA Board of Trustees. Given the competing priorities for their time, why should black physicians bother to become involved in the SCMA?

As individuals, we should and must remain ever-sensitive to the subtle damages wrought by years of injustice. As an organization, we should encourage not only participation but also leadership among all identifiable subgroups of physicians. We must do this if we are to be credible where it counts. That some differences may never completely disappear, at least not during our own lifetimes, is no reason not to try, no reason why the SCMA cannot be in the forefront of those who seek to make things better for future generations.

References

1. Wood PH. *Black Majority: Negroes in Colonial South Carolina From 1670 through the Stono Revolution*. New York: Alfred A Knopf; 1975: xiv.
2. Beardsley EH. Making separate, equal: Black physicians and the problems of medical segregation in the pre-World War II South. *Bull Hist Med* 1983; 57: 382-396.
3. Savitt TL. Entering a white profession: Black physicians in the new South, 1880-1920. *Bull Hist Med* 1987; 61: 507-540.
4. Bloom A. *The Closing of the American Mind*. New York: Simon and Schuster; 1987: 91.

Editorial Note: In 2005, 17 years after the above editorial was written, Gerald Wilson (right), a Columbia surgeon, was installed as president of the South Carolina Medical Association, the first African American to hold that office. Having chaired the nominating committee that previously put Gerald up for president of the Columbia Medical Society, I'm proud to have played a small role in his success but suspect he'd have made it to the top anyway — after all, cream rises.

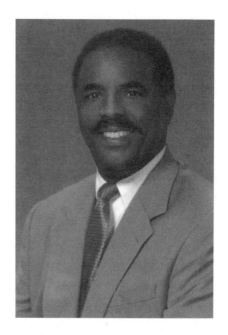

Appropriate Health Policy: A Larger View

J SC Med Assoc 1992; 88: 121-122

Frequently consider the connection of all things in the universe and their relation to one another.
— Marcus Aurelius

As Allan Bloom has pointed out, American society rewards performers, not thinkers.[1] We lionize movie stars, concert pianists, and quarterbacks but pay little heed to the lonely intellectuals who think seriously about the issues-of-the-day in their larger contexts. The current debate over healthcare policy provides yet another example: a shouting match mainly between performers, not thinkers.

This is a shame because we have so many fine thinkers in our society, and especially within the medical profession. In South Carolina, we are fortunate to have Dr. C. D. Bessinger of Greenville, who is interested in systems theory and not at all afraid of addressing the Big Questions, as in his first book, *Religion Confronting Science*.[2] In this issue of *The Journal*, Don Bessinger raises the possibility that systems theory may apply to the problem of appropriate and cost-effective healthcare delivery.

His basic message comes as a breath of fresh air especially during this election year when so many alternative solutions are being put forth in the public arena. Dr. Bessinger builds his recommendation on his earlier work, in which he interpreted Albert Schweitzer's concept of "reverence for life" within the framework of what we now know about homeostatic ecosystems. Dr. Bessinger's proposal for health care would require the physician to examine not only the needs of the patient before him but also the needs of society. We can no longer afford to expend our resources, unmonitored, for marginal patient benefit. There must be ongoing evaluation of "all component subsystems."

Is such thinking naïve and utopian? I think not. However, the concept will not work without a mandate from society as stipulated by government. As physicians, we must participate in the debate but must recognize that we are but one of many voices. Perhaps our most important input should be the definition of "appropriate care." We can and must inform the public about what really works, what is cost effective, what adds not merely to the length of life but also its quality. We can and must inform the public about which aspects of our technology should be considered luxury items rather than basic necessities. Data of the kind already generated by hospitals could be used to monitor such a system as proposed by Dr. Bessinger. Already, a new computer methodology known as "neural networks" is being used to provide feedback to physicians.[3] Cannot this methodology be applied to the system as a whole? In theory, yes indeed!

Some may consider Dr. Bessinger's plea for rethinking the two-tiered health system to be discriminatory. However, as Dr. Arnold Relman has opined: We cannot afford all the care a market-driven system is capable of giving."[4] Dr. Relman does say, however, that "we can afford all the care that is medically appropriate according to the best professional standards."

Our task is to define what represents "the best professional standards." We must be careful not to impose our version of the Golden Rule on others, for each person is entitled to decide how he or she would like to be treated. But we can educate the public, participate in the debate, and help government define more clearly what represents "appropriate care." No group of persons is better able to do so than physicians — and perhaps especially primary care physicians.

If we are to be a part of the solution, we must participate in the dialogue. Dr. Bessinger, with his global way of looking at things, has again suggested a conceptual framework. Can we make it work?

References

1. Bloom A. *The Closing of the American Mind*. New York: Simon and Schuster; 1987.
2. Bessinger D. *Religion Confronting Science*. Greenville, S.C.: Orchard Park Press; 1991.
3. Guerriere MRJ, Detsky AS. Neural networks: What are they? *Ann Intern Med* 1991; 115: 906-907.
4. Relman AS. The health care industry: Where is it taking us? *N Engl J Med* 1991; 325: 854-859.

When Democrats Last in the Dooryard Bloom'd

J SC Med Assoc 1993; 89: 220-221

Pardon the poor attempt at literary allusion. Also, please don't construe what follows as partisan politics. The issue at hand is how best to respond — individually and collectively — to the challenge of sweeping health care change (or, to use the popular parlance, "reform"). What can we learn from what one recent editorialist called "the ghosts of reforms past"?[1] How can we best provide input into the current political debate?

Let us consider what happened during the first administration (1933-1937) of President Franklin D. Roosevelt. Health care reform was proposed but didn't happen. Why? What were the long-range consequences?

The early FDR years resembled the current era in the following ways:

•Democrats controlled the White House and both branches of Congress.

•There was widespread uncertainty about the economy (to put it mildly).

•The public was preoccupied with domestic issues, not foreign affairs.

•There were a number of ongoing experiments in health care financing, including the nascent movements that produced to-day's Blue Cross and Blue Shield.

•There was a preference for solutions at both the state and the federal levels.

•There was uncertainty about whether the public was truly committed to a government solution to the problem of health care financing.

Soon after taking office, Roosevelt put together a blue ribbon Committee on Economic Security (again, does this sound familiar?). Membership included FDR's most intimate advisors, the Secretary of Labor, and some high-ranking academicians. Many of these advisers hoped that health insurance would be part and parcel of the Social Security package that was to be

put before Congress. Comprehensive health legislation would include the following:
•Improved access to health care, through sweeping reforms.
•A contributory insurance system to provide, in part, for the health care of otherwise uninsured patients.
•Improved quality of health care.
•Incentives for states for the development of innovative health insurance plans that met minimum standards for health insurance.

The American Medical Association vigorously opposed these changes and, assisted by such influential physicians as the great neurosurgeon Dr. Harvey Cushing, prevailed.[2] The AMA took the following positions:
•The medical profession should control all aspects of medical practice.
•Third party payors should not come between the patient and the physician.
•Any system for providing medical care for uninsured persons should be limited to people below a "comfort level" standard of income.
•There should be no restrictions on treatment or prescribing.
The Roosevelt administration was able to tinker with health care here and there, but was unable to bring about anything remotely suggestive of "reform." The time was not ripe.

It was not until three decades later, under Lyndon Johnson, that Medicare legislation was passed and much of what the Roosevelt administration had envisioned became reality. Third party payers became the norm. Physician reimbursement actually improved, at least for a time. But greater government involvement brought layers of bureaucracy and regulations, just as earlier prophets had predicted.

Today, organized medicine's successful opposition to the FDR proposals would seem to have been a Pyrrhic victory, at best. As this issue goes to press, the lead story in *American Medical News* contains the following observation:

Organized medicine has come a long way fast [toward addressing the issue of access to health care].... But ardent reformers have forgotten that for most of the

352

century the AMA led the fight against national health insurance. Medicine's past opposition to reform and its current reticence to say what it's willing to sacrifice, make it a suspect convert.[3]

Thus, to return to the original question: How can we best contribute to the debate?

The obvious answer: we must be involved both individually and collectively. Nobody has all of the answers, and any proposed solution is likely to be flawed. Yet, here and there, as we look around us, we find glimmers of hope that it might just be possible to develop what has been notably lacking from American health care policy: a shared vision based on shared values. People are beginning to ask the serious questions: in an era of limited resources, what price and should we pay for health care delivery — and when and for whom and how? In the absence of shared societal values, our ability to do so much (but at great cost) inevitably makes up part of the problem. Only by participating in the public dialogue — whenever, wherever, and however we can — will it be possible for us to be part of the solution. We must have the courage to trust that, in the long run, what is good and right for society is also good and right for us.

References

1. Dans PE. Perverse incentives, statesmanship and the ghosts of reforms past (editorial). *Ann Intern Med* 1993; 118: 227-229.
2. Goldfield N. The AMA faces down FDR and wins. *Physician Executive* 1993; 19(1): 3-8. 1993.
3. *American Medical News*, 22 February 1993.

"The Character and Usefulness of This Calling": Thoughts on the Coming Sesquicentennial

J SC Med Assoc 1997; 93: 162-163

Bill Mahon and Audria Belton reminded me that next year—1998—will be the South Carolina Medical Association's (SCMA) sesquicentennial. How should we celebrate? Should we change the letterhead design of *The Journal*? Should we plan a special symposium issue? Should there be a 150th Anniversary Ball at the Annual Meeting? The editorial board of *The Journal* joins the officers, trustees, and staff of the SCMA in welcoming your ideas!

However we choose to celebrate in public, we would do well to reflect privately on the significance of the SCMA. Such reflection should prompt us to rededicate ourselves to the ideals of our profession. But what exactly are our ideals, and what is a profession? These questions are always worthy of open-ended debate, for the answers are not entirely clear-cut. One thing is clear: No profession exists unless it is organized. It was in that spirit that, on February 14, 1848, an organizational meeting took place in Charleston at which Dr. Elias Horlbeck of Charleston offered a Preamble and Resolutions that began:

> Whereas, the members of the Medical Profession of the State of South Carolina are assembled on this occasion for the general purpose of advancing the character and usefulness of this calling ...

In 1848, medicine in South Carolina as elsewhere lacked sharp definition, regulation, and cohesiveness. Dr. Horlbeck and his colleagues resolved to do something about it.

They did not operate in a vacuum. Indeed, the notion of a state society had been incubating in Charleston since 1789, when 14 physicians formed a committee "to consider of such matters as will tend to improving the Science of Medicine, promoting liberality in the Profession and Harmony amongst the Practitioners in this City." On December 24 of that year, 10 of the 14 physicians met at the home of Dr. Peter Fayssoux and agreed unanimously to form what became the Medical Society of South Carolina.[1] During the next half-century, similar county or state medical societies were begun throughout the United States with mixed success. By the 1840s, it was apparent that there were too many people claiming to be physicians, and that both medical education and medical practice needed standards. Thoughtful persons recognized that if such standards were to happen, medicine must be organized. In 1846, a National Medical Convention was proposed at a meeting in New York. In 1847, representatives from many societies met in Philadelphia and resolved to found what we now know as the AMA.[2]

South Carolina was represented at the AMA's historic Philadelphia meeting 150 years ago by Drs. James Moultrie, Jr. William T. Wragg, and J. P. Jervey. Moultrie was elected vice-president. Dr. Samuel Henry Dickson of Charleston, a brilliant professor who had been unable to attend the organizational meeting, was made chairman of the Committee on Medical Sciences, members of which included Jervey and Wragg. It was in this context that the SCMA was born. To their enormous credit, the members of the Medical Society of South Carolina—proud Charlestonians though they were—recognized that they could not speak for the entire state. They therefore published the following discussion:

> The Committee are decidedly of the opinion that, with the exception of such as relate more immediately to incorporated Medical Schools, the objects contemplated in the proceedings of the Convention, will be more likely to be fulfilled by a special movement in this Society, than by leaving them to be severally considered by the different corporations and individuals to whom they are referred. The Society, however, having but little influence beyond the limits and suburbs of this city [Charleston], it appears to the Committee both expedient and proper that it should proceed in consecutive order, attempting that which is practicable now, and leaving the rest to be pursued as events or occasions may hereafter determine.

In accordance with these views, the Committee begs
leave to recommend, as a preliminary and essential
move, the incorporation of a state society.[3]

These sentiments led quickly to an organizational meeting for
such a true state society. Were they able to join us 149 years
later, what would these gentlemen say to us?

The founding fathers would no doubt take enormous pride
in the rapid growth and expanded mission of the SCMA in recent years. They would take enormous pride in the quality of
the educational programs at the Annual Meeting. They would
take enormous pride in the diligence displayed in our Reference Committees and in the House of Delegates. They would
take enormous pride in that what they started has continued
almost without interruption.

The founding fathers would hardly recognize, of course,
most of the tools, drugs, and facilities that we enjoy. They
would hardly recognize the way medicine is financed and they
would shudder at the amount of paperwork that is now necessary, computers notwithstanding. But they would have little
difficulty recognizing many, perhaps most, of the issues bearing on our relationships to our fellow humans and to each other. The Latin root of "celebrate" means "to frequent, go in great
numbers, honor." They would be pleased to have us honor our
heritage, but they would be more pleased to see us go forth in
great numbers, in unison, to promote what—in their words—
are indeed "the character and usefulness of this calling."

References

1. Davidson CG. *Friend of the People: The Life of Dr. Peter Fayssoux, of
Charleston, South Carolina*. Columbia: Medical Association of South
Carolina; 1950: 104-105.
2. King LS. American Medicine Comes of Age, 1840-1920. The Founding of the American Medical Association. *JAMA* 1982; 248: 1749-
1752.
3. Waring JL. *A Brief History of the South Carolina Medical Association*.
Charleston, South Carolina: South Carolina Medical Association;
1948: 24-25.

Of Hegel and Health Care Financing

J SC Med Assoc 1997; 93: 227-228

Our country's experiment with managed care evokes protests from many quarters. Patients protest that services — and especially the high technology to which they have become accustomed — are frequently denied. Physicians protest that the "hassle factor" of medical practice has never been greater. Academics protest that erosion of the financing of our great teaching hospitals threatens the fabric of medical education. Managed care also threatens the idea of professional solidarity, not only by lumping us with other health care providers, but also by pitting practice against practice, system against system. A recent article in *Time* proclaims: "Doctors, patients, unions, legislators are fed up and say they won't take it anymore."[1] What next?

We should take heart for at least two reasons. First, managed care as we now know it is unlikely to last without serious modifications. Second, we have by no means forfeited the right to work with everyone else toward better solutions for health care financing.

The concept of managed care or capitation was of course an inevitable reaction to the shortcomings of the fee-for-service system. The public largely shared our perception that American medicine was secondary to none, but became increasingly skeptical of its ability to pay for a system that consumed $1 out of every $6 of the gross domestic product. There was also the dilemma of some 45 million citizens being without any plan for regular health care. The fee-for-service system gave physicians little or no incentive to hold down costs despite the many exhortations to do so. Put simply, the fee-for-service system encourages overuse of services while managed care encourages underuse. Is it possible to strike a healthy mean?

The answer is yes, with the caveat that no solution is permanent. Changes in health care financing are likely to come about not so much by the replacement of older concepts with newer,

better ones (revolution) but rather by the ongoing tension between one idea and another (evolution).[2] Georg Wilhelm Friedrich Hegel (1770-1831), the great German idealist philosopher,
stated this famously as the dialectical method. With apologies to
serious Hegelians (whose ranks include Dr. William H. Hunter
of Clemson, S.C.), Hegel's method consists of dialectical triads
of thesis, antithesis, and synthesis. The inevitable flaws in any
idea or structure (thesis) generate the need for its opposite (antithesis), but neither the thesis nor the antithesis survives intact.
A synthesis emerges containing elements of both. This becomes
the new thesis, and the cycle repeats itself.

From the Hegelian viewpoint, we now witness a struggle
between one thesis (fee-for-service) and its antithesis (managed
care or capitation). As a thesis, fee-for-service was not all bad.
As an antithesis, managed care is not all good. Compromises
will inevitably emerge that contain elements of both the old and
the new systems. One can imagine, for example that Americans will eventually accept the notion that access to health care
should be a graded phenomenon in which nobody is denied
life-saving measures but in which many "luxury" services are
predicated on the ability to pay (for years, I've been puzzled
why we're so comfortable with the dentist's offering us a menu
of materials for our fillings, yet uncomfortable with applying
this concept to medical practice). The new synthesis will prevail
for a while, but cracks will prompt the search for something
even better.

Hegel was able to express his ideas with unusual clarity in
part because the German *aufheben* literally means "to lift up"
but also means both "to cancel" and "to preserve." In working with others in search of better ways to finance health care
delivery, we should acknowledge the limitations of the old fee-
for-service system while seeking to preserve its better aspects.
Through participation in organized medicine, we should network in ways that promote dialogue and goodwill among our
ranks, especially because managed care systems promote a "divide and conquer" mentality common to the marketplace.

Hegel died during a cholera epidemic. In a fee-for-service,
he would now be admitted to the hospital and given liter after

liter of IV fluids until he recovered. In a capitated system—well, let's just hope he'd get the right case reviewer!

References

1. Church GJ. Backlash against HMOs. *Time,* 14 April 1997: 32-39.
2. Washburn ER. Health care evolution? Or is it? *Physician Executive,* March 1997:14-16.

Editorial Note: Widespread use of managed care did not work out because, as I understand it, primary care physicians to their credit were reluctant to put the system's interests ahead of their patients' interests. Health care costs continue to spiral and, at the time of this writing, we're in yet another cycle of thesis/antithesis/synthesis.

Rightsizing the Healthcare Workforce

J SC Med Assoc 1998; 94: 231-233

The late Joseph I. Waring, MD, longtime editor of *The Journal*, had a wonderful flair for the English language and was quick to defend it against transgressions. He protested the common practice he called "verbing a noun." I suspect he would also protest today's widespread penchant for making one word out of two. It is therefore with tongue in cheek (or elbow on keyboard) that I've used "rightsizing," "healthcare," and "workforce" in the title of this editorial to suggest a point: Namely, this subject is far from straightforward despite the proclamations of various policymakers (here we go again!). In this issue of *The Journal,* Drs. Larry R. Faulkner and R. Layton McCurdy, deans at South Carolina's two medical schools, draw some reassuring conclusions.

Drs. Faulkner and McCurdy conclude that South Carolina has fewer medical students, residents, and physicians in relation to the population than is average for the Southeastern states or the United States as a whole. Moreover, 52 percent of residents now training in South Carolina are in primary care specialties, which meets the expressed national desideratum that one-half of graduating medical students should enter primary care (the so-called "50 percent solution"). Also, the number of first-year residency positions (PGY-1) offered in South Carolina in relation to the total number of graduating students seems about right. Nationally the number of PGY-1 positions is 140 percent of the number of graduating medical students, but South Carolina's ratio (118 percent) is close to the proposed "110 percent solution" designed to correct this disparity. Drs. Faulkner and McCurdy also review physician distribution in the Palmetto State and conclude that "available data suggest that South Carolina does not have the same degree of problems with its medical workforce as is present in many other areas of the country."

Still, this subject will continue to be contentious (as it has indeed been throughout recorded history). Here we stall pose three rhetorical questions: (1) Should the solutions be national or regional? (2) Are the solutions to be found in primary care or specialty training? (3) How will the solutions be impacted by the growing supply of nonphysician healthcare providers?

Should the solutions be national or regional? On the surface, recommendations of various national committees make a great deal of sense. If the number of PGY-1 positions offered in the United States were only 110 percent of the number of graduating medical students, then we would approximate a steady-state between physician supply and demand. If 50 percent of graduating medical students could be enticed toward primary care, then the overemphasis on expensive technology might be curbed. For reasons that are largely political, implementing these recommendations will be akin to belling the cat.

Yet the solutions must ultimately be national because doctors, like everyone else in our mobile society, go where the jobs are.

The solutions must remain national unless there are radical changes in the way healthcare and medical education are financed. The Canadian experience is often cited since their healthcare financing is delegated to the provinces. The Canadian provinces developed policies to limit medical school enrollments, adjust specialty mix to better accord with needs, and establish incentives for physicians to practice in underserved areas.[1] However, the surge of physician emigration from Canada may actually cause a shortfall of physicians by the early decades of the 21st century.[2] The Canadian experience may become relevant for the United States since it is widely predicted that federal funding for graduate medical education will be reduced. Still, national solutions should be sought if only to reduce the possibility (already predicted) that physicians will wander the country like nomads, alone or in groups, seeking opportunities to utilize their long and expensive training.

Are the solutions to be found in primary care or specialty training? Drs. Faulkner and McCurdy properly emphasize the role of primary care and observe somewhat cryptically that there should be downsizing and/or consolidation of "certain subspecialty programs in South Carolina." The oversupply of physicians in certain specialties and subspecialties is, however, again a national problem. Various specialties and subspecialties are already addressing these issues through their councils, residency review committees, and certifying boards. In some specialties — head and neck surgery is a good example — it seems that there will be a steady-state between supply and demand.[3] In other areas — gastroenterology is a good example — voluntary downsizing by prospective trainees is in full force even while national councils urge reductions.[4] Young physicians are unlikely to keep on training for jobs that aren't there; at least to some extent "the morrow will take care of itself."[5]

The second and larger issue concerns the extent to which twenty-first century Americans will prefer primary care versus specialty and subspecialty care. Eloquent spokespersons for both views can be found within medicine. Thus Eric Cassel, in

Doctoring, argues that the primary care movement "represents a shift away from the idea that has occupied twentieth-century medicine: that it is impersonal objective medical science that knows the disease and effects the treatment."[6] On the other hand, John D. Lantos, in *Do We Still Need Doctors?*, observes that when his father (an internist) gets sick, "he chooses the best specialist, and when the problem is fixed, he never goes back. Perhaps that's how the informed patient of the future will behave."[7] Medicine is one of the few areas in society in which today's policymakers stress generalism over specialism. In most other areas, the workforces are becoming more specialized in response to an information-rich, knowledge-based environment. Americans' appetites for technology are likely to shape their expectations of the healthcare system.[8] Reduction of medicine to technology delivered by strangers offends most of us, but it could well be that this is what most people will not only accept but even demand.

How will the solutions be impacted by the growing supply of nonphysician healthcare providers? Cooper's projection of current data to the year 2020 led to the conclusion that there is no major impending national surplus of physicians. However, the number of "nonphysician clinicians" is likely to double by the year 2010, equaling 60 percent of the number of physicians in patient care. It was concluded that the key determinant of whether we will have physician surpluses will be the extent to which patients utilize physicians for services that are also offered by nonphysician clinicians.[9] It is no secret that nonphysician clinicians are seeking and often getting their independence.[10] Also, on the horizon is an abundance of alternative medicine practitioners such as chiropractors, naturopaths, and acupuncturists. By one prediction, the per capita supply of these latter persons will grow by 88 percent by the year 2010, while the physician supply will grow by only 16 percent.[11] Can there be any doubt about the importance of organized medicine?

There are of course many other issues. Suboptimal distribution of physicians is an issue in South Carolina as elsewhere; physicians gravitate toward the larger metropolitan areas.[12] Affirmative action is an issue in South Carolina as elsewhere;

minority and women physicians are much more likely to serve minority, poor, and Medicaid populations.[13] My main point is that this subject will remain controversial, as perhaps it should given the ever-changing complexion of our calling. In the meantime, we can be grateful to Drs. Faulkner and McCurdy for analyzing the data in South Carolina and for reassuring us that, all in all, we are "about right" in relation to our peers.

References

1. Sullivan RB, Watanabe M, Whitcomb ME, et al. The evolution of divergence in physician supply policy in Canada and the United States. *JAMA* 1996; 276: 704-709.

2. Dauphinee WD. Medical workforce policy making in Canada: Are we creating more problems for the future? *Clin Invest Med* 1996; 19: 286-291.

3. Close LG, Miller RH. Head and neck surgery workforce in the year 2014. *Laryngoscope* 1995; 105: 1081-1085.

4. Meyer GS, Jacoby I, Krakauer H, et al. Gastroenterology workforce modeling. *JAMA* 1996; 276: 689-694.

5. Miller S, Dunn MR, Whitcomb ME. Initial employment status of resident physicians completing training in 1995. *JAMA* 1994: 277: 1699-1704.

6. Cassell EJ. *Doctoring: The Nature of Primary Care Medicine.* New York: Oxford University Press; 1997: 7.

7. Lantos JD. *Do We Still Need Doctors?* New York: Routledge; 1997: 27.

8. Sheldon GF. The health work force, generalism, and the social contract. *Ann Surg* 1995; 222: 215-228.

9. Cooper RA. Perspectives on the physician workforce to the Year 2020. *JAMA* 1995; 274: 1534-1543.

10. Cooper RA. The growing independence of non-physician clinicians in clinical practice. *JAMA* 1997; 277: 1092-1093

11. Cooper RA. Stoflet SJ. Trends in the education and practice of alternative medicine clinicians. *Health Affairs* 1996; 15: 226-238.

12. Guckian JC, Zetzman MR, Mullins CB. Physician work force in Texas: planning for the future. *Texas Medicine* 1995; 91: 50-57.

13. Cantor JC, Miles EL, Baker LC, et al. Physician service to the underserved: Implications for affirmative action in medical education. *Inquiry* 1966; 33:167-180.

Race and Health Care

J SC Med Assoc 1999; 95: 116-118

Here's the case, an all-too-familiar scenario. A 57-year-old African American man comes to the emergency room with shortness of breath and is found to have urgent hypertension, left ventricular failure, and pulmonary edema.

Here's the dialogue. "Have you ever been told you had high blood pressure?" "Yes." "Have you been treated?" "Yes." "Are you taking your medicines now?" "No. I stopped six months ago because I couldn't afford them."

Now, here's the question. Is his failure to take his medication (a) a socioeconomic problem?; (b) a healthcare delivery systems problem?; (c) his own problem, or a physician-patient relationship problem?; (d) a reflection of racism in our society?; or (e) all of the above?

My answer, at least for today: (e) all of the above.

The question is distressingly common and complex. Let's review the possible answers.

We can blame socioeconomics (or sociodemographics). Extensive studies in many cultures document the effect of socioeconomic status on health. As one writer puts it, "Top people live longer."[1] This effect may even be a biologic phenomenon. Some evidence suggests that social hierarchy correlates with health even in non-human primates. Researchers at the University of South Carolina recently found that a socioeconomic gradient extends even to pets. The pets of the better-educated and better-off live longer![2] Our patient could not afford his pills because he did not have a good job.

We can blame our healthcare delivery system. Our healthcare system allows many people to fall through the cracks of adequate insurance coverage. Why not make blood pressure monitoring and antihypertensive drugs available and convenient to everyone who needs them? Would this not cost society far less than the cost of managing hypertensive emergencies and end-organ failure? Our patient could not obtain good care because the system made it too difficult.

We can blame the individual patient and/or his doctor. Physicians and patients of different backgrounds often communicate poorly. Was adequate rapport established? Were the implications of hypertension sufficiently stressed? Were ethnic differences appreciated? According to one study, African Americans are more likely to perceive physicians' behavior as undesirable and are more likely to turn to God for control of personal destiny.[3] They may be more inclined to suffer stoically rather than seek handouts. Our patient and his doctor were on different wavelengths.

We can blame racism. Racism might have caused or contributed to his hypertension in the first place. Data suggest that among Blacks, blood pressure is related to the extent of racial discrimination, unfair treatment, inadequate social support, and stress.[5] One provocative study suggests that racial disrespect correlates with mortality not only in Blacks but also in whites.[6] Data also suggest that African Americans receive fewer invasive cardiac procedures than do whites, although the differences tend to be eliminated when insurance coverage is equalized.[7] Subtle racial tensions caused or at least exacerbated our patient's hypertension and muddled its treatment.

I do not know the best answer. Clearly the problem is multifactorial but with the various forces pushing and pulling at different rates in different patients and different doctors.

The symposium in this issue of *The Journal* came from a retreat held in February 1997 by the SCMA' Ethics Committee. Kristy Maher McNamara begins by pointing out that "there is a clear and persistent racial gap in health in the United States." As is well known, the health of African Americans declines at a faster rate at all ages compared to their white counterparts.[8]

Dr. McNamara's observations on the *what* do not solve the *why*. Drs. Stuart Sprague and Albert Keller describe Community Oriented Primary Care, an approach to making care more equitable. Today's management gurus inform us that most problems are actually systems problems, and Community Oriented Primary Care takes a systems approach to these issues. Finally, Dr. Robert Sade points out the dilemmas faced by African Americans in getting access to transplantation medicine.

These laudable papers leave us wondering about the extent to which inequalities in American healthcare can be eliminated.

In principle we turn to the ideal of equality expressed by the authors of the Declaration of Independence, influenced as they were by the philosophy of John Locke (who happened to be a physician). In practice we acknowledge that equality in healthcare or in anything else for that matter proves to be an elusive grail. We nostalgically turn to the ancient Greeks for the ideal of a noble profession embracing "love of humanity and love of the art," but access to healthcare in ancient Greece was decidedly class-determined. We turn to later generations, such as the Romans influenced by Scribonius Largus and the Scots influenced by John Gregory, for the ideal of charity in medicine, but this, too, is often tenuous. Charity—call it paternalism or *noblesse oblige*, if you like—is a flickering light that dims when times get tight. In sum, it's doubtful that true equality in goods and services can ever be achieved, at least in a free society. But how might we more nearly achieve it? And how might we eliminate forever the barrier of race?

As Americans we pride ourselves as belonging to the land of opportunity formed by immigrants. It was Clare Booth Luce who pointed out that this ideal translates historically to "a nation of white immigrants." It was Robert F. Kennedy who pointed out that racial discrimination is not a uniquely Southern problem but rather a national problem. Still, the history of the Palmetto State dramatizes how persons of different ethnic backgrounds do not always mix well (to put it mildly).

It was here, somewhere near Winyah Bay, that in 1526 the Spaniard Lucas Váquez de Ayllón brought African American slaves in his attempt to establish the first European settlement in what is now the United States. It was here during the eighteenth century that English colonists from the Barbados—the original "Goose Creek men"—indulged in the Indian slave trade, scouring the coasts for unsuspecting Native Americans. It was here on Sullivan's Island, the Black equivalent of Ellis Island, that one-half of the ancestors of all African Americans were quarantined before meeting their destinies at the markets. It was here along the coast, most notoriously in Georgetown County, that African slaves reached their densest populations when rice replaced indigo after the Revolution. It was here that thousands of freed men were left to fend largely for themselves and often knew discrimination of the worst kind.

We have come a long, long, long way. But there is more to be done.

On matters pertaining to race relations, organized medicine has not always led the way.[9] Certainly we should. Collectively we should explore such approaches as the use of "report card" approaches to monitoring care systems.[10] Individually we should acknowledge that pride of race and racial prejudice are ubiquitous, perhaps present in everyone if we're honest about it. We should resolve to celebrate our common humanity. We should resolve to treat everyone alike.

The SCMA's Ethics Committee is to be congratulated for taking on this thorny topic. This is, I think, another example that organized medicine is working hard toward the dream that Americans can indeed resolve their differences and for the common good.

References

1. Evans RG. Introduction. In: Evans RC, Barer, ML Marmor TR, eds. *Why are Some People Healthy and Others Not?* New York: Walter de Gruyter; 1994: 3.
2. Moloo J, Jackson KL, Waller IL et al. Xenotransmission of the socioeconomic gradient in health. A population based study. *Brit Med J* 1998; 317: 1686.
3. Ferguson, JA, Weinberger M, Westmoreland GR, et al. Racial disparity in cardiac decision mining: Results from patient focus groups. *Arch Intern Med* 1998; 158: 1450-1453.
4. Krieger N, Sidney S. Racial discrimination and blood pressure: The CARDIA study of young black and white adults. *Am J Public Health* 1996; 86: 1370-1378.
5. Strogatz DS, Croft JB, James SA. Social support, stress, and high blood pressure in black adults. *Epidemiology* 1997; 8: 482-487.

6. Kennedy BP, Kawachi L, Lochner K, et al. (Dis)respect and black mortality. *Ethnicity &. Disease* 1997; 7: 207-214.

7. Daumit GL, Hermann JA, Coresh J, et al. Use of cardiovascular procedures among black persons and white persons: A 7-year nationwide study in patients with renal disease. *Ann Intern Med* 1999; 130: 173-182.

8. Ferraro KF, Farmer MM. Double jeopardy to health hypothesis for African Americans: Analysis and critique. *J Health Social Behavior* 1996; 37: 27-43.

9. Nickens HW. A case of professional exclusion in 1870: The formation of the first Black medical society. *JAMA* 1985; 253: 2549-2552.

10. Smith DB. Addressing racial inequities in health care: Civil rights monitoring and report cards. *J Health Politics, Policy & Law* 1998; 23: 75-105.

Y2K.7. Myth, Magic, and Muggles: Harry Potter and the Future of Medicine

J SC Med Assoc 2000; 96: 514-515

It is our choices, Harry, that show what we really are, far more than our abilities.

— Albus Dumbledore to Harry Potter

The patient reader who has endured these musings on the new millennium will recall our convictions that while the future of medicine is bright indeed, that of the medical profession is unclear. Medicine is perhaps indeed *The Greatest Gift to Mankind* as declared by the title of Roy Porter's new popular history. However, the medical profession, having finally attained credibility based on science introduced in the nineteenth and twentieth centuries, faces a new reality: much, perhaps most of what we do can probably be done equally well by people who do not have the hard-won *Medicinae Doctor* degree. Where can we find the inspiration to take us forward? I found a measure of inspiration in an unlikely source: the Harry Potter novels by the brilliant British author J. K. Rowling.

Medicine, if it is to remain a profession and not just another way to earn a living, needs heroes. It needs not so much the heroes of great discoveries—the Harveys, the Jenners, the Pasteurs, the Listers, the Flemings—as it does the heroes of everyday life, physicians who treat their calling as a sacred trust, who willingly subjugate their egos and personal best-interests in lives of service to their fellow humans. And so what *is* a hero? What Joseph Campbell called the monomyth of the universal hero goes, in brief, like this. An ordinary person, residing in his or her hut or castle, is called to adventure by a mysterious person. Leaving behind the familiar, he or she enters an unknown realm and finds a series of tests and helpers in the context of a struggle between good and evil. The challenges culminate in a supreme ordeal. If our hero prevails—as invariably happens in fiction—he returns to the world with a boon to humankind, an elixir that restores to society something it had lost. Campbell taught that the monomyth should apply to us all. And why not?

Enter Harry Potter. Harry suffers tragedy as an infant when the evil Lord Voldemort kills his parents and tries to kill him, too. Left with a scar in the shape of a lightening bolt on his forehead, Harry is raised by his only relatives, the Dursleys. Being Muggles (that is, ordinary people), the Dursleys fear magic and try to suppress Harry, making him live in a cupboard beneath the staircase. Harry gradually comes to realize that he has unusual powers. Still pre-adolescent, he is called to enter Hogwarts School of Witchcraft and Wizardry by a gentle giant named Rubeus Hagrid. The school's motto, *Drago Dormiens Nunquam Titillandus* ("never tickle a sleeping dragon") is apt, for danger lurks everywhere. Harry encounters numerous obstacles, finds friends and helpers, overcomes adversity, and in each of the four novels to date accomplishes something that makes his world a better place. The immense popularity of the Harry Potter novels attests to the basic human need for myth and the recognition that a latent archetypal hero lies within each of us.

If the monomyth of the universal hero gives Rowling's novels their instructive value, it is her use of magic that makes them fun. Basing her principal characters on classical mythology and literature, Rowling writes with a zany humor that has enabled her to make millions of readers out of a generation habituated to television and video games. Just about everything that happens at Hogwarts involves magic including the school's key sport, quidditch, an aerial game played on broomsticks. But on reflection, I am struck by how much of what we take for granted in medicine would have seemed magical to our ancestors. Surgery without pain … antibiotics … computer-based imaging studies … gene mapping … and the list goes on. However, and as we began these essays, our magic involves a knowledge of good and evil; it can be used for better and for worse. At Hogwarts, the Dark Arts are ever present. Lord Voldemort, whose name is French for "flight of death," destroys people to obtain more power for himself. Will magic be used for personal power or public good? This is the tension at Hogwarts, and so it is for us.

And then there are the Muggles, the ordinary people who lack the heritage and/or training to become wizards or witches. Often they cannot even see the magic because of special charms used against them. Some of the students at Hogwarts are pedigreed witches or wizards, while others have Muggles for parents. A few students, notably Harry's arch rival Draco Malfoy, would like to banish anyone with Muggle ancestry. We find out, however, that Muggles can be quite useful—for example, there is Hermione Granger, one of Harry's best friends, an indefatigable problem solver. In medicine we have our Muggle equivalents—the legions of health care providers who lack the hard-earned M.D. degree. Yet we must remember that it is not we who own the magic. The magic belongs to society; we are merely its caretakers. We must have the faith that what is good for society will also be good for us.

In the fourth and most recent Harry Potter novel, the evil Lord Voldemort is restored to his former self, setting the stage for an inevitable showdown that will be Harry's supreme ordeal. Albus Dumbledore, the wise headmaster of Hogwarts, tells the students: "We are only as strong as we are united, as weak as we are divided." Is this not the message also for the medical profession? If we can just remember this one maxim, the third millennium surely holds greatness for our profession that we cannot even begin to imagine!

Health Care Reform: The Case for Communitarianism

J SC Med Assoc 2007; 103: 197-198

United States Senator Lindsay Graham addressed at the annual SCMA meeting in May the compelling need for health care access for the 45 Americans who lack insurance. SCMA president Gerald Harmon declared at the Board of Trustees meeting in July his main goal to be access of currently uninsured South Carolinians to decent health care. The current issue of *Consumer Reports* avers that 43% of Americans fortunate enough to have health insurance nevertheless feel "somewhat" to "completely" unprepared to cope with a costly medical emergency.[1] What's the root cause?

Political gadfly Michael Moore in his new documentary film *Sicko* lambastes our system (or non-system) for forcing millions of uninsured or inadequately insured Americans to choose between no health care and bankruptcy. He tacitly acknowledges that health care in the United States is second to none for those who can afford it. But with example after colorful example, Moore suggests that Americans' access to quality health care at an affordable price lags far behind that of all the other Western democracies and even (or especially) that of Cuba even though we spend more on health care than anyone else. This thesis is hardly new. For decades now, we've heard this refrain from far less controversial figures than Michael Moore. What's the root cause?

The root cause in my perhaps naïve opinion is that we Americans lack a shared communitarian vision of what constitutes an adequate and equitable health care delivery system.

We traditionally classify ourselves as "liberals" or "conservatives" based on our ideas of distributive justice and specifically of government entitlements — that is, "positive rights" to such goods as health care. Liberals tend to be generous with the public till; conservatives stress self-reliance. I've never been entirely comfortable with these labels and am beginning to understand why. Conservatives nowadays, by one only slightly tongue-in-cheek account, include at least 10 species: Austriocons, Buchanocons, Neocons, Aquinacons, Radiocons, Sociocons, Theocons, Republicons, Catocons, and Platocons.[2] Some conservatives, most notably certain talk show hosts, attack liberals at every turn even though, according to two recent surveys, only 18% to 20% of American adults identify themselves as "liberals" when asked. Over the past two decades we've seen both liberals and conservatives in the political driver's seat; health care costs have continued to spiral out of control and the plight of the uninsured and underinsured has only grown worse.

Libertarianism, a political perspective sometimes known as "classic liberalism," focuses mainly on "negative rights" such as the right to privacy and the right to freedom from government interference. Libertarians tend to judge actions by the extent to which they respect individuals' rights even when this means compromising society's overall well-being. Libertarians tend to oppose government forces that interfere with the free market. Many would hold this sentiment responsible, at least in part, for out-of-control health care costs. Thus, Dr. David

Blumenthal, director of the Institute for Health Policy at Massachusetts General Hospital, is quoted in *Consumer Reports* as saying: "We have very high prices because people can get away with charging them. In our decentralized, pluralistic system no single purchaser has the market power or political authority to impose cost controls."[1] Emerging in part as a reaction to libertarianism is an ethical and political philosophy known as communitarianism whereby stakeholders seek a shared vision of the optimum society.[3,4] Communitarians tend to favor government activities that promote equality and that impose social order, even if this might mean restricting certain individual liberties. Consider, for example, the lively debates about whether motorcyclists should be required to wear helmets. Libertarians, who currently prevail in South Carolina on this issue, hold that such a requirement impinges on their freedom from outside interference ("Nobody's gonna tell me what I can and cannot do, as long as I don't harm anybody else"). Communitarians would counter that the cyclists should wear helmets because survivors of closed head injuries impose substantial financial burdens on the rest of us. Communitarianism is best viewed as a way of thinking that honors the ability of people to seek mutually satisfactory solutions to their common problems.

I claim no special expertise in political theory. But what seems to be lacking in our health care system as in other aspects of our life together is a truly participatory (as opposed to representative) democracy in which well-informed people of different political stripes and self-interests seek compromise for the sake of a shared vision of what constitutes, as John Rawls famously put it, "justice as fairness."[5] And, speaking at least for myself, we're not even well informed about the issues.

Recently, a highly knowledgeable and thoughtful former hospital administrator asked me in casual conversation, "What do you think is the variance in the hospital charge for a chest x-ray — that is, what the hospital charges a patient exclusive of the radiologist's fee?" I waffled. "Come on, take a guess." "Well, I'd say anywhere between $50 and $200. He chuckled before informing me that in seven California hospitals the charge for a chest x-ray ranges from $120 to $1,519 — a variance of 1,266 percent! How is it that I'm reasonably well-informed about variances in, say, the price of gasoline, but am almost entirely ignorant about the things I order as a physician?

"Read on," suggested my friend. Researchers at the Dartmouth Center for the Evaluative Clinical Sciences estimate that up to one-third of the more than $2 trillion spent annually on health care in the United States is squandered on unnecessary hospitalizations, unproven treatments, over-priced drugs and devices, and end-of-life care that result in neither comfort nor cure for the recipients.[6] Several studies suggest that up to 50% of the health care delivered in the United States is not clinically justified. Patients with chronic illnesses who reside in "high-cost" areas such as Manhattan or Miami, Florida, receive much more aggressive and costly care yet often do worse than similar patients who reside in "low-cost" areas such as Salt Lake City, Utah. And whether one undergoes this or that procedure and whether one survives the surgery may be highly dependent on where one happens to live or chooses to be hospitalized. We have, to use the current lingo, a systems problem that calls for root-cause analysis and systems-based solutions.

Gerald Harmon emphasized that his interest in obtaining access to health care for all South Carolinians—that is, universal access—did not necessarily imply a commitment to a single-payer system. And that's a good thing. For a society as diverse as ours, I vote for pluralism. I vote for making basic health care for clearly-defined needs freely available to everyone. I vote for something akin to the failed Oregon Plan: Let us physicians rank what's cost-effective, then let society review and edit our conclusions and decide what it's willing to make available to everyone irrespective of ability to pay. I vote for transparency in what things cost. I also vote for setting reasonable limits on what constitutes "ordinary care" or "the standard of care" for everyone irrespective of ability to pay. Nobody in my opinion should bear financial hardship to have their streptococcal sore throat treated, their fracture set, their tumor resected, their coronary artery opened up, or their arthritic hip replaced. But nobody should be entitled to free and unlimited access to all that technology has to offer. Communitarianism requires setting limits on individual rights—both positive and negative—and on individual autonomy for the sake of fairness to all. Could it actually work here? I honestly don't know.

Approaching an election year, we brace for numerous proposals for health care reform by the various candidates. We brace for efforts by the prevailing presidential candidate and his/her party to enact legislation of proportions that rival the Medicare/Medicaid legislation of the 1960s. But, again in my perhaps naïve opinion, what's needed is not platitudinous political platforms but rather informed public participation. We don't need pat solutions so much as we need honest and open dialogue between and among ourselves (as will happen at the coming SCMA leadership retreat) and between and among representatives of all segments of American society. It's comforting to know that involved physicians such as our SCMA president continue to make equitable access to health care a top priority.

References

1. Are you really covered? Why 4 in 10 Americans can't depend on their health insurance. *Consumer Reports*; 2007 (September): 16-20.
2. Dean JW. *Conservatives Without Conscience*. New York: Viking; 2006: 20-21.
3. Daly M, ed. *Communitarianism: A New Public Ethics*. Belmont, California; Wadsworth Publishing Company; 1994.
4. Callahan D. Individual good and common good: A communitarian approach to bioethics. *Perspect Biol Med* 2003; 46: 496-507.
5. Rawls J. *A Theory of Justice*. Revised edition, Cambridge, Massachusetts: The Belknap Press of Harvard University Press; 1999.
6. Mahar M. The state of the nation's health. *Dartmouth Medicine* 2007 (Spring): 26-35.

Medical Journalism

The Case Report as Medical Scholarship

J SC Med Assoc 1976; 72: 184-185

*The countless interviews which make up the general practi-
tioner's everyday work are rarely chronicled, and even if they
were it would often be difficult to say whether the doctor's
skill or the patient's constitution deserved the credit. The artist, the poet and the research scientist record their work for the
benefit or scorn of posterity; but the doctor – like the school-
teacher, the barrister and the mother of a family – responds
to transient stimuli, and his skill (or perhaps genius), even if
recognized, usually goes unrecorded. His masterpieces – patients who recover – cannot defy time ...*

The above is from Desmond King-Hele's biography of Erasmus Darwin, a small town practitioner who authored a
theory of evolution that was later embellished and made famous by his grandson. Dr. Darwin's clinical reputation was un-
surpassed in eighteenth century rural England but has nearly
vanished because of his refusal to publish. Posterity's judgment
hinges largely on the written word, not hearsay.

Elsewhere in this issue, the skill (or perhaps genius) of one
country practitioner, Dr. William Markley Lee of Indian Town,
South Carolina, survives for our scrutiny. His five case reports
which appeared in the *Southern Medical and Surgical Journal* in
1836 describe a technique for acupuncture remarkably similar
to those circulating at the present time. His published experience, then allows our evaluation "for the benefit or scorn of posterity."

The case report is the traditional medium by which the practicing physician can make original contributions to the stream
of medical thought. Its historical base is old and substantial.
The Hippocratic writings contain 42 detailed case reports, 25
of them having a fatal outcome. Amid the present concern over
the medicolegal impact of a case report, it is worth recalling
that Hippocrates wrote: "I have written this down deliberately

believing it valuable to learn of unsuccessful experiments and to know the causes of their failure." Through the Renaissance and the seventeenth, eighteenth, and nineteenth centuries, the case report continued to be a major format for the published observations of master clinicians. Many of these observations remain indelibly stamped upon our collective memory. Nevertheless, the importance of case reports as scholarship has been questioned.

Questions regarding the value of a case report owe to the present emphasis on rigorous scientific methodology. It has become axiomatic in the Flexnerian era that basic medical discoveries are made, nearly always, only under controlled laboratory conditions. Further, clinical advances are made in large measure by rigorously controlled, preferably double-blind trials. But it should be noted that skepticism has now arisen over the actual benefit of much of basic research. Even more disturbing to clinicians has been the failure of controlled trials to resolve key therapeutic issues, such as the value of long-term anticoagulant therapy in cardiovascular disorders or of oral hypoglycemic agents in diabetes mellitus. Meanwhile, surveys of national and state journals reveals that the case report is as healthy as ever. This reflects the continued value of a single, if uncontrolled, observation.

A distinguished British investigator who has devoted most of his life to the study of atherosclerosis continues to hold the optimism that "the secret may be unlocked by observations in a single case." Not coincidentally, to the same physician is attributed the aphorism that one can judge a doctor by the strength of the batteries in his opthalmoscope.

The preparation of a succinct, informative case report is difficult and time-consuming. Evident in nearly all journals is a trend toward brevity. Some journals now publish case reports mainly as extended letters to the editor, as "brief recordings," or as short "clinical notes." The separate components of a case report merit review.

First, the INTRODUCTION should answer, in a single, straightforward sentence, the question, "Why do you consider this case to be worthy of reporting?" If such a statement cannot be written, the effort should be abandoned.

The BODY of a case report should be of length commensurate with the scientific content and importance. The content should depend upon the author's purpose. In general, data that relate to this purpose should be included: other information should be edited carefully. As Andrew Wyeth once said of his painting, the skill is not so much in choosing what to depict, but rather in choosing what to omit. Nonetheless, the likeness to reality must be sufficiently faithful that all facts that might reasonably have been expected to bear on the outcome should be included. One or more illustrations should be included, if possible, since these make the report more palatable for the reader.

The DISCUSSION should also focus upon the reason for reporting the case. Only rarely should an attempt to review the literature in exhaustive detail be made. A brief summary of the syndrome, disease, finding, treatment, or complication that is the major focus of the report should be included, but a lengthy "text book discussion" should usually be avoided. Previous experience, as gleaned from the literature, can sometimes be summarized most effectively by means of a table.

A SUMMARY is unnecessary in brief reports in which the discussion is limited to one or several paragraphs. In longer reports, a summary should be included. Finally, REFERENCES should be well-chosen, should be as few as possible, and should always reflect a perusal of the most recent volumes of the Index Medicus.

The succinctly-presented observations of Dr. William Markley Lee of Indian Town provided the impetus for this editorial. Some years ago, it was this editor's pleasure to receive a guided tour of the old graveyard at the Indian Town Presbyterian Church, courtesy of my friend William J. Cooper, Jr., a Kingstree native who is now Professor of History at Louisiana State University in Baton Rouge. Lovers of Thomas Gray's "Elegy Written in A Country Churchyard" could hope for no prettier spot. An attempt to verify Dr. Lee's presence in the Indian Town graveyard was therefore made, with the expectation that readers of *The Journal* could be assured that there "Dr. Lee sleeps on, surrounded no doubt by his therapeutic successes and failures alike."

But it was not to be. Bill Cooper, whose family planted in the environs of Indian Town for many generations, tells me that no record can be found there of a Dr. Lee. No history of Williamsburg County mentions a Dr. Lee, nor is there any record that he ever purchased or sold property, acquired debt, married, died, or left any other trace in the county's records. Perhaps his presence there was transient; alternately, he might have lived in another locale known unofficially as an "Indian town." It is clear that the definitive history of acupuncture in South Carolina remains to be written.

That Dr. Lee survives through his published experience is, however, indisputable. The purpose of this editorial is to exhort South Carolina physicians to emulate his efforts and to submit their observations for publication for the scrutiny of future generations.

Editorial Note: The purpose of this editorial, my first after being appointed assistant editor of *The Journal* under Ed Kimbrough, was to encourage practicing physicians to write. When in 1979 the Thomas A. Roe Foundation accepted Dr. William H. Hunter's proposal to fund an award for "the best article in *The Journal*," I suggested immediately that we should give the award on alternate years to a practicing physician or to an academic physician; competition should be within one's own reference group. Encouraging practicing physicians to write has been a constant theme of my tenure as editor and is reflected in *The Journal*'s Information for Authors.

The Journal — Expectations

J SC Med Assoc 1977; 73: 21-22

Why a state medical journal? As Ed Kimbrough's legacy of manuscripts and correspondence settled into a distant corner of my cluttered desk, I pondered this oft-raised question. The next morning's mail did little to mollify these doubts. The pile contained more than a dozen periodicals, of which some were scholarly subscription journals but the rest were those sleek, unrefereed publications commonly referred to as "throwaways." I visualized this scene recurring in physicians' offices and studies around the country, every day—an incredible bombardment of senses already numbed by the day's circuit of stubborn problems, fretful faces, chief complaints, anxious relatives, office paperwork, and the constant perturbations of Mr. Bell's invention. Surely, there are more than enough medical periodicals to fill the time available for their perusal.

Why, then, a state medical journal?

My own justification sprung from Jacob Bronowski's essay, *Science and Human Values.* Bronowski argues that "the society of scientists is more important than their discoveries." The attitude outweighs the specifics. It is the existence of the attitude that matters.

In this vein, I suggest that the existence of the state medical journal far outweighs the sum of its articles. *The Journal* benefits even the physician who for one reason or another seldom opens its cover. It arrives as a monthly reminder that the South Carolina Medical Association possesses a scientific identity, that the association serves the scientific interests of its members as well as their other interests. It arrives as a monthly reminder there exists a place for the practitioner to submit his or her observations for publication, should he or she choose to do so, and to an editor who is likely to be sympathetic. And no matter what his field, he should find an article title on the cover of at least potential interest. Although she may postpone its reading, it is there, among the pile of postponements accumulating on her desk, available if needed, and, even if remaining unread, serving to support her attitude that she would like to remain well-informed.

To follow Edward E. Kimbrough and Joseph I. Waring, the immediate past editors, challenges one's abilities to say the least. We should pause a moment and reflect on what they and others have accomplished.

Begun as the *Transactions of the South Carolina Medical Association* in 1869, ours ranks among the oldest state medical journals in continuous publication. We believe that its quality is competitive with the journals of all but the largest states. The library of the new SCMA building displays the aggregate of the journal's bound volumes, an impressive sight. From them one can glean a great deal of the medical history of the Palmetto State. One is also impressed by the array of substantive articles which have appeared in *The Journal* over the years. In recent years, special supplements and symposia published in *The Journal* have won national recognition.

"I'm amazed how many request for reprints I've received for that article I wrote for the *Journal of the South Carolina Medical Association*," a colleague from Boston remarked recently. To publish one's article in our journal is not to relegate it to obscurity; for this I can vouch. For an article published this year, requests for reprints continue to come in, many from foreign countries and bearing colorful stamps that made me regret I'd given up philately, one of my boyhood hobbies.

But *The Journal* exists primarily for the readers, not the authors. Therefore, a readership survey was conducted at the 1976 SCMA convention. We thank the respondents and aim to heed their suggestions.

Most respondents indicated that they would like to continue to see original scientific articles and commentary on social or economic issues. They also indicated their desire to receive association news, but the majority did not want to see the SCMA newsletter incorporated into *The Journal*. Fewer respondents wished to see case reports, but the lowest priority was given to historical and philosophical essays. This response may come as a disappointment to some of our readers, given the rich historical traditions of our state and of our medical association, but we respect it.

And the respondents provided practical, specific suggestions. One sought "more and better (more practical) articles on cardiology, diabetes, and arthritis." Another indicated that "*The Journal* should reflect the needs and experiences of practitioners" and not be a "research or history reporting journal." Rather, it should "relate to everyday needs and experiences." Clearly, the readership desires information relevant to patient care.

Information about the climate in which we practice was also sought. One respondent desired "access to conservative and liberal and consumer opinion without judgments made." Another wanted to be kept informed on "current legislative proposals that affect the practice of medicine." Input from the state agencies was also desired. One reader wanted "to know more about what the state can do ... that would be of use to my patients."

Based on these responses, we have set priorities. These are indicated in the revised "Information for Authors," to be found elsewhere in issue. There may be some readers and contributors who will dispute these priorities, and we welcome their thoughts. To the contributors, we feel a special obligation. We will seek to give all manuscripts a prompt review, to offer constructive criticism when revision is deemed appropriate, and to indicate with candor why some manuscripts might be considered unacceptable for publication. We continue to welcome comments from readers, both as criticisms of *The Journal* and as "Letters to the Editor" for possible publication.

Why a state medical journal? For the reader!

From the Report of the Editor of The Journal *to the House of Delegates of the South Carolina Medical Association, 2007:*

The year 2007 marks my 31st year as editor of *The Journal* and my 32nd year in office at the South Carolina Medical Association.... This almost surely constitutes a record for continuous service to the SCMA in an official capacity. With John Thomison's retirement several years ago from *Tennessee Medicine*, I suspect I'm now the longest-tenured medical journal editor in the United States. Through 2006, I've served as editor for 336 hard-copy issues of *The Journal*, containing by my count 1,085 articles of which 508 were by full-time faculty, 368 by physicians in private practice, and 209 by "other persons" including medical students, residents, physicians in state agencies, and non-physicians....

Please indulge me for a few reminiscences. One morning in 1975 I expressed an interest in *The Journal* to Ed Kimbrough as we walked into Richland Memorial Hospital from the physicians' parking lot. Ed called me a month or two later and asked if I'd like to become assistant editor. I gladly accepted, and became editor after Ed stepped down a year later....

Ed Kimbrough and I wrote two summary articles about *The Journal* in 2005 (citation numbers 283 and 284 in the bibliography that follows), and I shall therefore make only a few observations about my tenure. We removed the pharmaceutical advertisement from the cover. We revised the Information for Authors, set clear priorities for publication, and discouraged scientific articles by full-time faculty members that had previously "made the rounds" in the editorial boards of national journals. We encouraged symposium issues and established for them a model that would encourage active participation by physicians, both academic and practicing, throughout South Carolina.... We periodically reviewed our purpose and mission statement....

It has been a privilege to serve as editor these many years. I thank the 33 presidents (living and deceased), numerous members of the Council and Board of Trustees, three executive directors, five managing editors, and more than 1,100 authors with whom I've had the privilege of working.

Bibliography

Editorials in *The Journal of the South Carolina Medical Association*, 1976-2007

Editorial Note: This bibliography lists only my editorials. My policy has been to welcome and indeed often solicit guest editorials, and a complete listing of editorials can be obtained through MEDLINE, the *Index Medicus*, or archived collections of *The Journal*.

1. Bryan CS. The case report as medical scholarship. *Journal of the South Carolina Medical Association* 1976; 72: 184-185.
2. Bryan CS. Over-prescribing of antibiotics: Why, where, which, and by whom? *Ibid* 1976; 72: 285-286.
3. Bryan CS. Immunization against swine influenza: A major challenge for South Carolina physicians. *Ibid* 1976; 72: 303-304.
4. Bryan CS. On consumerism. *Ibid* 1976; 72: 323-324.
5. Bryan CS. The journal — expectations. *Ibid* 1977; 73: 21-22.
6. Bryan CS. The mission of a medical school. *Ibid* 1977; 73: 75-76.
7. Bryan CS. Impressions of council. *Ibid* 1977; 73: 121.
8. Bryan CS. Physicians' assistants. *Ibid* 1977; 73: 122-123.
9. Bryan CS. Stroke and hypertension in South Carolina. *Ibid* 1977; 73: 123-124.
10. Bryan CS. More on stamps and philatelists. *Ibid* 1977; 73: 124.
11. Bryan CS. Who should treat breast cancer? *Ibid* 1977; 73: 161.
12. Bryan CS. State of *The Journal*. *Ibid* 1977; 73: 161.
13. Bryan CS. Professional responsibility. *Ibid* 1977; 73: 232-234.
14. Bryan CS. The new nurse and territorial rights. *Ibid* 1977; 73: 337-338.
15. Bryan CS. Swine flu revisited: The beer factor. *Ibid* 1977; 73: 385.
16. Bryan CS. Waring Library Society. *Ibid* 1977; 73: 434.
17. Bryan CS. Alcohol and pregnancy. *Ibid* 1977; 73: 434-435.
18. Bryan CS. On committees and editorials. *Ibid* 1977; 73: 496-497.
19. Bryan CS. "For the millions who should not take aspirin . . ." *Ibid* 1977; 73: 497-498.
20. Bryan CS: Emergency rooms and cost containment. *Ibid* 1977; 73: 532-533.
21. Bryan CS: Hypertension: The night thief. *Ibid* 1977; 73: 534.
22. Bryan CS: Physicians and the environment. *Ibid* 74: 35-36, 1978.
23. Bryan CS. Reporting of diseases. *Ibid* 1978; 74: 36.

24. Bryan CS: In memoriam [Joseph Ioor Waring]. *Ibid* 1978; 74: 80-81.
25. Bryan CS: Joseph Ioor Waring: An appreciation. *Ibid* 1978; 74: 105-106.
26. Bryan CS. The medical education community orientation project. *Ibid* 1978; 74: 159.
27. Bryan CS. Death certificates. *Ibid* 1978; 74: 159.
28. Bryan CS: Parasites remain a problem. *Ibid* 1978; 74: 160.
29. Bryan CS: New trends in medical ethics. *Ibid* 1978; 74: 191-192.
30. Bryan CS: Personality and medical students. *Ibid* 1978; 74: 260-261.
31. Bryan CS: The JCAH and organized medicine. *Ibid* 1978; 74: 262.
32. Bryan CS. The limits of altruism. *Ibid* 1978; 74: 337.
33. Bryan CS: The new editorial board. *Ibid* 1978; 74: 377-378.
34. Bryan CS: Vasodilators versus digitalis. *Ibid* 1978; 74: 461-462.
35. Bryan CS: Heart disease, risk factors, stress, and physicians. *Ibid* 1978; 74: 462-463.
36. Bryan CS: Tuberculosis in community hospitals: Lessons from another year. *Ibid* 1978; 774: 464-465.
37. Bryan CS: Cost containment and laboratory tests. *Ibid* 1978; 74: 462-463.
38. Bryan CS. Robert Edward Jackson, M.D. *Ibid* 1978; 74: 511-512.
39. Bryan CS. J. Howard Stokes, M.D. *Ibid* 1978; 74: 512.
40. Bryan CS. Reviewing the utilization of utilization review. *Ibid* 1978; 74: 544-545.
41. Bryan CS. Library services for physicians: Collaboration between MUSC and USC. *Ibid* 1978; 74: 545.
42. Bryan CS. Cost containment and laboratory tests. *Ibid* 1978; 74: 545.
43. Bryan CS. To care and not to care. *Ibid* 1979; 75: 28-29.
44. Bryan CS. Beepers. *Ibid* 1979; 75: 83-84.
45. Bryan CS. Jim Clark. *Ibid* 1979; 75: 125.
46. Bryan CS. Sunset on the age of Keflin. *Ibid* 1979; 75: 187-188.
47. Bryan CS. Malpractice: The value of data. *Ibid* 1979; 75: 238.
48. Bryan CS. Doing good well. *Ibid* 1979; 75: 341-342.
49. Bryan CS. On symposia, case reports, the energy crisis, and "throwaway" periodicals. *Ibid* 1979; 75: 423.
50. Bryan CS. Are state medical journals obsolete? A rebuttal. *Ibid* 1979; 75: 473.
51. Bryan CS: Cost containment and physicians' fees: The St. Peters Parish solution. *Ibid* 1979; 75: 474.
52. Bryan CS. Thomas A. Roe Foundation announces award for scientific

articles written by practicing physicians. *Ibid* 1979; 75: 637.

53. Bryan CS. Requiem—"The ad on the cover." *Ibid* 1980; 76: 37-38.
54. Bryan CS. Prospectus: The eighties. *Ibid* 1980; 76: 37-38.
55. Bryan CS, Brenner EB. Drug-resistant bacteria: implications for community hospitals and practicing physicians. *Ibid* 1980; 76: 82-83.
56. Bryan CS: Bedside body language. *Ibid* 1980; 76: 144-145.
57. Bryan CS: The annual meeting: "Unity and concert of action." *Ibid* 1980; 76: 212-213.
58. Bryan CS: The second medical school—six years later. *Ibid* 76: 1980; 254-255.
59. Bryan CS: Reflections on the grievance committee. *Ibid* 1980; 76: 302.
60. Bryan CS: Disease reporting in South Carolina: Is there a need for new legislation? *Ibid* 76: 1980; 395-396.
61. Bryan CS. Hurrah for cooperation. *Ibid* 1980; 76: 395-396.
62. Bryan CS. Found: A point on the compass. *Ibid* 1980; 76: 442-443.
63. Bryan CS. Medicine in South Carolina is alive and well. *Ibid* 1980; 76: 487.
64. Bryan CS. Thomas A. Roe Foundation announces $5,000 award for scientific articles written by institution-based physicians. *Ibid* 1980; 76: 574-575.
65. Bryan CS. Medicine in Marlboro County. *Ibid* 1981; 77: 37.
66. Bryan CS. The hospital association survey. *Ibid* 1981; 77: 37.
67. Bryan CS. On the DDx of B & B. *Ibid* 1981; 77: 38.
68. Bryan CS. Should philosophy be required in the medical curriculum? *Ibid* 1981; 77: 94-95.
69. Bryan CS. Michael J. Halberstam, M.D.—a voice for our times. *Ibid* 1981; 77: 136-137.
70. Bryan CS. Weight control. *Ibid* 1981; 77: 244.
71. Bryan CS. Cost control. *Ibid* 1981; 77: 244.
72. Bryan CS. Handgun control. *Ibid* 1981; 77: 245.
73. Bryan CS. Sunset review of the medical licensing board. *Ibid* 1981; 77: 304.
74. Bryan CS. Publishing priorities for instiution-based physicians. *Ibid* 1981; 77: 305.
75. Bryan CS. The annual convention—perhaps the best ever. *Ibid* 1981; 77: 339.
76. Bryan CS. Eosinophils in sputum. *Ibid* 1981; 77: 339-340.
77. Bryan CS. New syndromes from staphylococci. *Ibid* 1981; 77: 340.
78. Bryan CS. What about coffee, doctor? *Ibid* 1981; 77: 341.
79. Bryan CS. Letters to the editor welcomed! *Ibid* 1981; 77: 341.
80. Bryan CS. The CT scan and the technological imperative. *Ibid* 1981;

77: 411-412.

81. Bryan CS. The nursing shortage: What can physicians do? *Ibid* 1981; 77: 455.

82. Bryan CS. Prevention of the congenital rubella syndrome: Physician participation needed! *Ibid* 1981; 77: 456.

83. Bryan CS. A new incentive for blood donors? *Ibid* 1981; 77: 456.

84. Bryan CS. Perplexing pulmonary problems. *Ibid* 1981; 77: 457.

85. Bryan CS. "Wellness" — new catchword or novel concept? *Ibid* 1981; 77: 510-512.

86. Bryan CS. The Pap smear — how many are enough? *Ibid* 1981; 77: 573.

87. Bryan CS. Malpractice liability — consultants and primary physicians. *Ibid* 1981; 77: 574.

88. Bryan CS. The non-tuberculous mycobacteria: neither "atypical" nor "anonymous." *Ibid* 1981; 77: 574.

89. Bryan CS. 535 North Dearborn Street. *Ibid* 1982; 78: 55-56.

90. Bryan CS. Hurrah for the men in orange! *Ibid* 1982; 78: 110-111.

91. Bryan CS. Chiropractic legislation: Two broken records. *Ibid* 1982; 78: 170-172.

92. Bryan CS. Children and chiropractic. *Ibid* 1982; 78: 240.

93. Bryan CS. The Lee report. *Ibid* 1982; 78: 285.

94. Bryan CS. Roe awards renewed. *Ibid* 1982; 78: 348-349.

95. Bryan CS. The annual meeting, 1982 — one person's perspective. *Ibid* 1982; 88: 349-350.

96. Bryan CS. Medicine and the male life cycle. *Ibid* 1982; 78: 400-401.

97. Bryan CS. What the polls tell us (and don't tell us). *Ibid* 1982; 78: 516-517.

98. Bryan CS. No medical schools or ten — does it make a difference? *Ibid* 1982; 78: 643.

98. Bryan CS. Hospitals for profit — No! *Ibid* 1983; 79: 39-40.

100. Bryan CS. On publishing, perishing, cherishing, and flukes. *Ibid* 1983; 79: 97-98.

101. Bryan CS. "Sunset on the age of Keflin" — revisited. *Ibid* 1983; 79: 97-98.

102. Bryan CS. A new high for medical advertising. *Ibid* 1983; 79: 179.

103. Bryan CS. Use of antibiotics in combination. *Ibid* 1983; 79: 296-297.

104. Bryan CS. Whither primary care? *Ibid* 1983; 79: 297-298.

105. Bryan CS. Medical information network becomes a reality. *Ibid* 1983; 79: 357.

106. Bryan CS. Preparation for medical school: What have we learned and what can we do differently? *Ibid* 1983; 79: 407-408.

107. Bryan CS. AIDS in South Carolina. *Ibid* 1983; 78: 452-453.

108. Bryan CS. The new economics of health care delivery: A time for ideas and input. *Ibid* 1983; 79: 506-507.

109. Bryan CS. Lewis W. Wannamaker, M.D. (1923-1983). *Ibid* 1983; 79: 648.

110. Bryan CS. Roe awards become perpetual. *Ibid* 1983; 79: 32.

111. Bryan CS. Diagnosis-related groups (DRGs): Implications and uncertainties. *Ibid* 1984; 80: 78-79.

112. Bryan CS. Second schools: Second thoughts. *Ibid* 1984; 80: 217-218.

113. Bryan CS. Bill's lesion. *Ibid* 1984; 80: 313-314.

114. Bryan CS. Medical education and DRGs. *Ibid* 1984; 80: 511-512.

115. Bryan CS. Antibiotics for hand infections. *Ibid* 1984; 80: 512-513.

116. Bryan CS. Acute bacterial meningitis: Current challenges. *Ibid* 1984; 80: 577-578.

117. Bryan CS. Hypertension in South Carolina: A small ray of optimism. *Ibid* 1984; 80: 633.

118. Bryan CS. Of cost-containment and cat-bellers. *Ibid* 1985; 81: 87-88.

119. Bryan CS. Fond memories of Emmett. *Ibid* 1985; 81: 145-146.

120. Bryan CS. Screening for HTLV-III antibodies: A government blunder? *Ibid* 1985; 81: 242-244.

121. Bryan CS. Fixed fees: A distant mirror. *Ibid* 1985; 81: 291.

122. Bryan CS. Philanthropia and philotechnia. *Ibid* 1985; 81: 292-293.

123. Bryan CS. The board affair: No cause for embarrassment. *Ibid* 1985; 81: 347-348.

124. Bryan CS. Our eightieth. *Ibid* 1985; 81: 348.

125. Bryan CS. A French connection. *Ibid* 1985; 81: 454.

126. Bryan CS. Hand emergencies: More data. *Ibid* 1985; 81: 455.

127. Bryan CS. The President's polyp. *Ibid* 1985; 81: 509-510.

128. Bryan CS. Leonard's legacy. *Ibid* 1985; 81: 659-660.

129. Bryan CS. Of motorcycles and helmets. *Ibid* 1986; 82: 92-93.

130. Bryan CS. What is "appropriate antimicrobial therapy?" *Ibid* 1986; 82: 249-251.

131. Bryan CS. Victims. *Ibid* 1986; 82: 313.

132. Bryan CS. Professional courtesy. *Ibid* 1986; 82: 653-655.

133. Bryan CS. Impressions of the second annual leadership conference. *Ibid* 1986; 92: 697-698.

134. Bryan CS. Crossroads. *Ibid* 1986; 92: 744.

135. Bryan CS. Real medicine. *Ibid* 1987; 83: 28-30.

136. Bryan CS. "Reverence for life": a unifying concept for ethical decision making? *Ibid* 1987; 83: 83-84.

137. Bryan CS. Young physicians and social change — A new challenge for organized medicine. *Ibid* 1987; 83: 131.

138. Bryan CS. Comprehensive health/lifestyle education in the secondary schools ... an idea whose time has come? *Ibid* 1987; 83: 229.

139. Bryan CS. AIDS policies. *Ibid* 1987; 83: 332.

140. Bryan CS: FLASH! *Ibid* 1987; 83: 447-449.

141. Bryan CS. Self expression welcomed! *Ibid* 1987; 88: 498.

142. Bryan CS: AIDS: Life on the new frontier. *Ibid* 1987; 88: 612-614.

143. Bryan CS: On the threshold of a golden age? *Ibid* 1988; 84: 38-39.

144. Bryan CS: Eulogy written in a country churchyard. *Ibid* 1988; 84: 94-95.

145. Bryan CS: AIDS and ethics — one year later. *Ibid* 1988; 84: 215-217.

146. Bryan CS: Black physicians, South Carolina medicine, and the SCMA. *Ibid* 1988; 84: 260-261.

147. Bryan CS: Waring Library Society celebrates tenth anniversary. *Ibid* 1988; 84: 418-419.

148. Bryan CS: "I've been there." *Ibid* 1988; 84: 511-512.

149. Bryan CS. Our Christmas gifts to South Carolina's children. *Ibid* 1988; 85: 595.

150. Bryan CS: Medicaid waiver for AIDS and ARC patients. *Ibid* 1988; 85: 596-597.

151. Bryan CS. Beliefs, attitudes, and health promotion. *Ibid* 1989; 85: 84-85.

152. Bryan CS. Slow poisons. *Ibid* 1989; 85: 86.

153. Bryan CS. Ciprofloxacin: Panacea or blunder drug? *Ibid* 1989; 85: 131-133.

154. Bryan CS. Peer review where it counts. *Ibid* 1989; 85: 209-211.

155. Bryan CS. True (Palmetto) blue. *Ibid* 1989; 85: 296-297.

156. Bryan CS. Ticks, tetracycline, and backyard terrorism. *Ibid* 1989; 85: 341-343.

157. Bryan CS. Of SCHIN and GRATEFUL MED (or computers to the rescue!). *Ibid* 1989; 85: 534-535.

158. Bryan CS. Peace and good will. *Ibid* 1989; 85: 580-581.

159. Bryan CS: High tech, high touch. *Ibid* 1990; 86: 114-115.

160. Bryan CS: The V-word and the Four C's. *Ibid* 1990; 86: 259-260.

161. Bryan CS: Pass the word! *Ibid* 1990; 86: 370-371.

162. Bryan CS: Gavin. *Ibid* 1990; 86: 411-412.

163. Bryan CS. Guidelines for symposium issues. *Ibid* 1990; 86: 417.

164. Bryan CS: First among the C's. *Ibid* 1990; 86: 461-463.

165. Bryan CS: "In this issue ..." *Ibid* 1990; 86: 464-465.

166. Bryan CS: HIV, surgeons, and ... all of us. *Ibid* 1990; 86: 513-517.

167. Bryan CS: Medical ethics: a promise fulfilled. *Ibid* 1990; 86: 636-639.

168. Bryan, CS. Sorry, Gavin. *Ibid* 1990; 86: 639.

169. Bryan, CS. Thanks, Art. *Ibid* 1990; 86; 640.

170. Bryan CS. Games played with balls. *Ibid* 1991; 87: 30-31.

171. Bryan CS. Fort Host. *Ibid* 1991; 87: 151-155.

172. Bryan CS. Good medicine. *Ibid* 1991; 87: 245-247.

173. Bryan CS. Well done! *Ibid* 1991; 87: 283.

174. Bryan CS. A tribute to Mike Jarrett. *Ibid* 1991; 87: 399.

175. Bryan CS. Practicing physicians and medical writing. *Ibid* 1991; 87: 400.

176. Bryan CS. A treacherous calm? *Ibid* 1991; 87: 401.

177. Bryan CS. Lyme disease: How common in South Carolina? *Ibid* 1991; 87: 438-439.

178. Bryan CS. Round three: HIV and public policy vs. health care workers and patients. *Ibid* 1991; 87: 479-482.

179. Bryan CS. Sinusitis: More than a headache. *Ibid* 1991; 87: 514-517.

180. Bryan CS. Thanksgiving. *Ibid* 1991; 88: 551-552.

181. Bryan CS. Seasons. *Ibid* 1992; 88: 27-31.

182. Bryan CS. Lyme, non-Lyme, and Lime. *Ibid* 1992; 88: 32.

183. Bryan CS. The chronic fatigue syndrome: *Caveat emptor. Ibid* 1992; 88: 79-81.

184. Bryan CS. Appropriate health policy: A larger view. *Ibid* 1992; 88: 121-122.

185. Bryan CS. Lipoprotein(a). *Ibid* 1922; 88: 122-123.

186. Bryan CS. L through Z (with apologies to Chris Hawk). *Ibid* 1992; 88: 199-201.

187. Bryan CS. William Osler and medical societies. *Ibid* 1992; 88: 447-449.

188. Bryan CS. Dear Mr. President. *Ibid* 1992; 88: 581-582.

189. Bryan CS. Flight 463. *Ibid* 1992; 88: 583.

190. Bryan CS. The white plague returneth. *Ibid* 1993; 89: 93-95.

191. Bryan CS. Tasteful advertising. *Ibid* 1993; 89: 148-149.

192. Bryan CS. The doctor-patient relationship. *Ibid* 1993; 89: 149.

193. Bryan CS. When Democrats last in the dooryard bloom'd. *Ibid* 1993; 89: 220-221.

194. Bryan CS. What is past is prologue. *Ibid* 1993; 90: 221.

195. Bryan CS. The courage to ration. *Ibid* 1993; 90: 307-308.

196. Bryan CS. Doctor Weston. *Ibid* 1993; 89: 349-350.

197. Bryan CS. The soul of medicine. *Ibid* 1993; 89: 598.

198. Bryan CS. A matter of time. *Ibid* 1994; 90: 74-77.

199. Bryan CS. Of ideals and heroes. *Ibid* 1994; 90: 193-194.
200. Bryan CS. Whither academic health centers? *Ibid* 1994; 90: 295-297.
201. Bryan CS. Deserving our remembrance. *Ibid* 1994; 90: 383-385.
202. Bryan CS. "The rights of the child" revisited. *Ibid* 1994; 90: 613-614.
203. Bryan CS. Toward a post-antibiotic era? *Ibid* 1995; 91: 35-37.
204. Bryan CS. Ehrlichiosis: more tick-borne terrorism? *Ibid* 1995; 91: 241-242.
205. Bryan CS. What is professionalism and can it be measured? *Ibid* 1995; 91: 243-244.
206. Bryan CS. Principle-centered change. *Ibid* 1995; 91: 276-277.
207. Bryan CS. *Aequanimitas* revisited. *Ibid* 1995; 91: 355-358.
208. Bryan CS. AIDS: Where do we stand? *Ibid* 1995; 91: 389-390.
209. Bryan CS. Managed caring (!) (?). *Ibid* 1995; 91: 507-508.
210. Bryan CS. Medical consultations: Ethics and etiquette. *Ibid* 1996; 92: 26-27.
211. Bryan CS. Family violence: Striking back. *Ibid* 1996; 92: 198-199.
212. Bryan CS. Kiva: making a difference. *Ibid* 1996; 92: 238-239.
213. Bryan CS. Just thinking. *Ibid*. 1996; 92: 280-282.
214. Bryan CS. Hit early, hit hard: New strategies for HIV. *Ibid* 1996; 92: 361-363.
215. Postic B, Bryan CS. Antiretroviral therapy in mid-1996. *Ibid*. 1996; 92: 400-403.
216. Bryan CS. Heart surgery in South Carolina comes of age. *Ibid* 1996; 92: 508.
217. Bryan CS. "The care of the patient" revisited. *Ibid* 1996; 92: 509-510.
218. Bryan CS. Thanks, Joy! *Ibid* 1996; 92: 507.
219. Bryan CS. "The character and usefulness of this calling:" Thoughts on the coming sesquicentennnial. *Ibid* 1997; 93: 162-163.
220. Bryan CS. Of Hegel and health care financing. *Ibid* 1997; 93: 227-228.
221. Bryan CS. Family physicians who write. *Ibid* 1997; 93: 259-261.
222. Bryan CS. Evidence-based medicine: Try it, you'll like it! *Ibid* 1997; 93: 352-354.
223. Bryan CS. Reflections on the SMA-1 (A.K.A., the medical history). *Ibid* 1997; 93: 387-389.
224. Bryan CS. Nothing could be finer. *Ibid* 1997; 93: 459-461.
225. Bryan CS. Humble origins. *Ibid* 1998; 94: 25-26.
226. Bryan CS. The duties of patients: A distant mirror. *Ibid* 1998; 94: 79-80.

227. Bryan CS. Primary prevention of myocardial infarction: A role for electron beam computed tomography? *Ibid* 1998; 94: 127-130.

228. Bryan CS. Sacred trust. *Ibid* 1998; 94: 190-191.

229. Bryan CS. Rightsizing the healthcare workforce. *Ibid* 1998; 94: 231-233.

230. Bryan CS. Only the good. *Ibid* 1998; 94: 327-328.

231. Bryan CS. Medicine's vocational rehabilitation. *Ibid* 1998; 94: 446-447.

232. Bryan CS. Jim Knight and the moral nature of medicine. *Ibid* 1999; 95: 37-39.

233. Bryan CS. Live as though seen. *Ibid* 1999; 95: 77-78.

234. Bryan CS. Race and health care. *Ibid* 1999; 95: 116-118.

235. Bryan CS. A very short history of the medical profession, as told to Patch Adams. *Ibid* 1999; 95: 168-170.

236. Bryan CS. John C. Hawk. *Ibid* 1999; 95: 203.

237. Bryan CS. Authors wanted! *Ibid* 1999; 95: 203.

238. Bryan CS. Heyward Gibbes, the Oslerian tradition, and the identity of internal medicine. *Ibid* 1999; 95: 204-206.

239. Bryan CS. Pew thoughts while listening to Pachelbel's canon in D. *Ibid* 1999; 95: 241-242.

240. Bryan CS. The coward's amygdala. *Ibid* 1999; 95: 275-276.

241. Bryan CS. Does infection cause atherosclerosis — and most other diseases? *Ibid* 1999; 95: 309-310.

242. Bryan CS. The English lesson. *Ibid* 1999; 431-432.

243. Bryan CS. Y2K.1. The tree of knowledge and the tree of life. *Ibid* 2000; 96: 34-35.

244. Bryan CS. Y2K.2. From rondelles to robots. *Ibid* 2000; 96: 131-132.

245. Bryan CS. Y2K.3. Hippocrates redux. *Ibid* 2000; 96: 192-193.

246. Bryan CS. Y2K.4. Virtues and values. *Ibid* 2000; 96: 276-279.

247. Bryan CS. Of Sims and Smoak. *Ibid* 2000; 96: 357-358.

248. Bryan CS. Y2K.5. *E. pluribus unum, Dum spiro spero, Esse quam videri. Ibid* 2000; 96: 390-391.

249. Bryan CS. Y2K.6. Town and gown. *Ibid* 2000; 96: 428-429.

250. Bryan CS. Y2K.7. Myth, magic, and muggles: Harry Potter and the future of medicine. *Ibid* 2000; 96: 514-515.

251. Osguthorpe JD, Bryan CS. Common respiratory infections: current treatment recommendations. *Ibid* 2001; 97: 37.

252. Bryan CS. Of compromise and incremental change. *Ibid* 2001; 97: 180-181.

253. Bryan CS. A journal for South Carolinians. *Ibid* 2001; 97: 254.

254. Bryan CS. Physical diagnosis and the technological imperative. *Ibid* 2001; 97: 259-261.

255. Bryan CS. Should religiosity be included in the medical history? *Ibid* 2001; 97: 353-354.

256. Bryan CS. September the eleventh—*ne cede malis*. *Ibid* 2001; 97: 483-484.

257. Bryan CS. Pres Darby—the man who met Massoud. *Ibid* 2001; 97: 527-528.

258. Bryan CS. *The Journal*—transitions. *Ibid* 2002; 98: 30.

259. Bryan CS. A hound dog in Anderson. *Ibid* 2002; 98: 30-31.

260. Bryan CS. Somatization: A disorder about "something." *Ibid* 2002; 98: 31-32.

261. Bryan CS. Electronic publishing: One small step for the SCMA. *Ibid* 2002; 98: 200.

262. Bryan CS. Palliative care for the terminally ill. *Ibid* 2002; 98: 200-202.

263. Bryan CS. What is a doctor? Reflections on the physician charter on professionalism. *Ibid* 2002; 98: 327-329.

264. Bryan CS. Tucker Weston and the SCMA Foundation. *Ibid* 2003; 98: 329.

265. Bryan CS. Pagination and enumeration. *Ibid* 2003; 98: 329.

266. Bryan CS. Christian Tucker Weston, Jr., M.D. (1919-2002). *Ibid* 2003; 98: 332.

267. Bryan CS. Dr. Pratt-Thomas: an appreciation. *Ibid* 2003; 99: 59.

268. Bryan CS. Yellow fever and the church. Ibid 2003; 99: 60-61.

269. Bryan CS. Thoughts on *The Doctor*. Ibid 2003; 99: 112-113.

270. Bryan CS. E. Carwile Leroy (1933-2002): *Lacrimae rerum*. *Ibid* 2003; 99: 114.

271. Bryan CS. Drug wars: Saying no. *Ibid* 2003; 99: 173-174.

272. Bryan CS. Pellagra in South Carolina: *Déjà vu*. *Ibid* 2003; 99: 249-250.

273. Bryan CS. Hiram Curry's vision and the future of primary care. *Ibid* 2003; 99: 251.

274. Bryan CS. Community service: Doing it willingly, wisely, and well. *Ibid* 2003; 99: 322-323.

275. Bryan CS. The South Carolina delegation: *macte virtue*! *Ibid* 2003; 99: 386.

276. Bryan CS. Advancing medical professionalism. I. Our public image. *Ibid* 2004; 100: 60-62.

277. Bryan CS. Advancing medical professionalism. II. One size does not fit all. *Ibid* 2004; 100: 123-125.

278. Bryan CS. One snake or two? Thoughts on the symbols of medicine. *Ibid* 2004; 100: 126-127.

279. Bryan CS. Advancing medical professionalism. III. Bearding the evils of specialization. *Ibid* 2004; 100: 205-207.

280. Bryan CS. Advancing medical professionalism. IV. Why higher professionalism hurts. *Ibid* 2004; 100: 265-267.

281. Bryan CS. Advancing medical professionalism. V. The social contract, and why tort reform is essential. *Ibid* 2005; 101: 47-49.

282. Bryan CS. Advancing medical professionalism. VI. Summing up. *Ibid* 2005; 101: 115-117

283. Bryan CS, Kimbrough EE. *The Journal of the South Carolina Medical Association* through the past century. *Ibid* 2005; 101: 172-174.

284. Bryan CS, Kimbrough EE. *The Journal of the South Carolina Medical Association* through the past century (Part II). *Ibid* 2005; 101: 280-284.

285. Bryan CS. The seven basic virtues in medicine. I. Introduction. *Ibid* 2005; 101: 327.

286. Bryan CS. The seven basic virtues in medicine. II. Prudence (practical wisdom). *Ibid* 2005; 101: 329-331.

287. Bryan CS. The seven basic virtues in medicine. III. Justice. *Ibid* 2005; 101: 388-390.

288. Bryan CS. Thank a doctor. *Ibid* 2006; 102: 21.

289. Bryan CS. The seven basic virtues in medicine. IV. Temperance. *Ibid* 2006; 102: 22-24.

290. Bryan CS. The seven basic virtues in medicine. V. Courage. *Ibid* 2006; 102: 134-135.

291. Bryan CS. Tomorrow's stethoscope: The hand-held ultrasound device? *Ibid* 2006; 102: 345.

292. Bryan CS. His blood runneth orange. *Ibid* 2006; 102: 346-347.

293. Bryan CS. The seven basic virtues in medicine. VI. Faith. *Ibid* 2006; 102: 348-249.

294. Bryan CS. The seven basic virtues in medicine. VII. Hope. *Ibid* 2007; 103: 21-22.

295. Bryan CS. The seven basic virtues in medicine. VIII. Love. *Ibid* 2007; 103: 74-75.

296. Bryan CS. The seven basic virtues in medicine. IX. Summing up. *Ibid* 2007; 103: 135-137.

297. Bryan CS. Health care reform: The case for communitarianism. *Ibid* 2007; 103: 197-198.

298. Bryan CS. The literature search: An essential skill. *Ibid* 2007; 103: 199.

299. Bryan CS. A polymath and a mathematical conundrum. *Ibid* 2007; 103: 201.

300. Bryan CS. "I'm not a missionary." *Ibid* 2007; 103: 273-275.

Index

Academic health centers, 249-253
Adams, Patch, 94-99
Adlerian psychology, 161
Accreditation Council for Graduate Medical Education, 138
Agramonte, Aristides, 135
AIDS. *See* HIV/AIDS
Altruism, 149-150, 170
See also Caring *and* Professionalism, as tiered construct
American Academy of Pediatrics, 308
American Association for the History of Medicine, 4
American Board of Internal Medicine, 89-90, 119-124
American Medical Association, 77, 82, 103, 126, 172, 327, 352
American Osler Society, 58, 59, 83
American Psychological Association, 184, 188
Anscombe, G.E.M. (Elizabeth), 178
Aristotle, 158, 159, 168, 177, 181, 188, 194, 199, 238
Association of American Medical Colleges, 98-99
Aurelius, Marcus, 348
Ayllón, Lucas Váquez de, 366

Bacon, Francis, 212, 254
Banov, Leon, Jr., 71
Baroody, Joe, 161, 163, 164, 167, 171
Baroody, N.B., 264
Barry, Daniel, 119
Beardsley, Edward H., 345-346
Beauchamp, Tom, 138, 194

Bell, Nora K., 156
Belton, Audria, 354
Bennett, William J., 184
Bentham, Jeremy, 283
Bessinger, C. Donovan, Jr., 45, 155-157, 349-350
Blachman, Morris, 17
Blalock, Alfred, 233, 234
Blank, Linda L., 119
Blair, Tony, 50
Bliss, Michael, 204
Bloom, Allen, 254, 346, 348-349
Blue Cross and Blue Shield, 351
Blumenthal, David, 372-373
Bonner, Walter, 204
Borg, Bjorn, 29
Brand, Paul, 66
Brand, Margaret, 66-67
Brieger, Gert H., 240-241
Bronowski, Jacob, 383
Brougham, Lord, 71-72
Brown v. Board of Education, 346
Browne, Sir Thomas, 41
Buchwald, Art, 320
Buhmeyer, Kenneth J., 312
Burton, Robert, 212

C's of medicine, 27, 138-139, 164-166, 167-171
Califano, Joseph A., 332
Campbell, Joseph, 86-87, 369
Caring, concepts of, 102, 139, 151-154, 171
Carroll, James, 135
Cassel, Eric J., 361-362
Chaplin, Charlie, 231
Character, 220-225

Children, rights of, 306-308
Childress, James, 138, 194
Chiropractic, legislation related to, 326-331
Churchill, Winston, 2, 25, 138, 204
Cleaveland, Clif, 56, 93
Cicero, 48, 194
Clemens, Samuel L., 187
Clinton, William Jefferson, 64, 87
Cohen, Jordan J., 98-99
Coleridge, Samuel Taylor, 212
Columbia Medical Society, 20
Communitarianism, 371-375
Competence, concept of, 138-139, 217
Compte-Sponville, André, 184, 204
Conroy, Pat, 37, 38
Coolidge, Calvin, 84
Cooper, Thomas, 243
Cooper, William J., Jr. 381-382
Cornwallis, Lord, 38
Courage, concept of, 137, 168-171
    as cardinal virtue, 204-207
Crosswell, Hal, 19, 67
Crump, Todd L., 65
Cushing, Harvey, 133, 204, 352

Darby, John T., 242
Darrow, Clarence, 194
Darwin, Erasmus, 379
Declaration of Independence, 317
Democritus, 158, 159
Depression, Great, 52-53
Dickson, Samuel Henry, 146, 243, 355
Doctor, The (painting), 54-57, 138, 141
Donato, Anne, 5
Drake, Daniel, 243
Duncan, Charles B., 282

Ebert, Robert, 239
Edelstein, Ludwig, 238
El Salvador, 16-20
Eliot, T.S., 154
Emerson, Ralph Waldo, 48
Englehardt, H. Tristram, 181
Enlightenment, the, 95-96, 97
Environmentalism, 273-275
Epictetus, 26, 106, 175
Epicurean philosophers, 238
Ethics, codes of, 172-173
Ethics, frameworks for, 127, 155-157, 185, 222, 282-285
Evans, Matilda, 345

Faith, as virtue, 208-211
Faulkner, Larry R., 104, 359-361, 363
Faulkner, William, 259
Fayssoux, Peter, 355
Felice, Gregory A., 125-126
Fildes, Luke, 54-57, 138, 141
Fitzgerald, Faith, 265
Fleming, Alexander, 369
Flexner Report, 96, 242, 251, 380
Franklin, Benjamin, 178, 244
Frankl, Viktor, 200
Franklin, Benjamin, 212
Freidson, Eliot, 107
French Revolution, 96-97
Freud, Sigmund, 325
Fye, W. Bruce, 267

Galen, 85, 133, 212
Galileo, 159
Gallman, Burnett, 345
Gallo, Robert, 300
Gazes, Peter C., 264-265
Gehrig, Henry Louis, 28
Gilman, Daniel Coit, 133
Glick, Bruce, 302-303

Goldberg, Arthur, 233
Golden Rule, 26, 175, 195, 337
Gracián, Baltasar, 41, 43
Graham, Lindsay, 371
Great Britain, 97
Greece, classical, 9, 97, 366
Greene, Frederick, 318
Gregory, John, 95-96, 366
Guarino, John, 235-236
Gulf War, 42

Halberstam, Michael, 317
Handgun control, 316-317
Harmon, Gerald, 371, 374
Harrison, Tinsley R., 220, 222
Harvey, William, 86, 133, 369
Hawkins, Alex, 15
Hayes, Helen, 33
Hayne, James Adams, 307-308
Hayne, Theodore Brevard, 21-23,
    135-136, 145, 169-171
Health care, disparities of. See Race,
    issues related to.
Health care, economics of. See
    Medicine, economics of.
Health care reform, 371-375
Health education, 247-249, 285-
    288, 320-325
Health Maintenance Organizations,
    32, 76
Hegel, George Wilhelm Friedrich,
    357-359
Hemingway, Ernest, 259
Henderson, Lawrence J., 110
Hero myth, universal, 85-87
Hill-Burton program, 333
Hillel the Elder, 218
Hippocrates, 79, 85, 95, 113, 133,
    379-380
Hippocratic Oath, 180, 237-238
Hobbes, Thomas, 126, 178, 284
Holmes, Oliver Wendell, 146

Homer, 177, 179
Hope, as virtue, 212-215
Horlbeck, Elias, 354
Hume, David, 95, 159
Humphries, J. O'Neal, 264-265
HIV/AIDS, 20, 23, 67, 111-114,
    127, 140, 158, 192-194, 206,
    275-279, 280-281, 282-285, 289-
    296, 297-305
Ethics and, 280-281, 282-285
Hunter, John, 14, 133
Hunter, William Harvey, 5, 60-63,
    237, 239, 320, 358, 382
Hurricane Hugo, 157, 158

Illich, Ivan, 107
Immune system, overviews, 276-
    277, 297-305
Influenza, 271-272
Iraq War, 115

Jefferson, Thomas, 28, 31
Jenner, Edward, 86, 133, 369
Jervey, J. P., 355
Jesus of Nazareth, 211
Johnson, Allen H., 249-250, 338
Johnson, Lyndon B., 233, 352
Johnson, Samuel, 204
Jones, Frederick, 27
Jonsen, Albert, 282
Jowers, Lawrence V., 167-168, 171,
    312
Justice, as cardinal virtue, 192-197

Kant, Immanuel, 127
Keller, Albert, 365
Kennedy, John F., 233
Kennedy, Robert F., 366
Kepler, Oliver, 151
Kilgore, Donald, 247
Kimbrough, Edward E., III, 4, 34,

382, 383, 384, 386
King, Lester, S., 76-77, 256
Koch, Robert, 133
Krause, Elliot A., 107, 220

LaGuardia, Fiorello, 233
Lombardi, Vince, 15
Lake, Kirsopp, 14, 208
Lancaster, Carol, 239-241
Lantos, John D., 92, 362
Lazear, Jesse, 135
Lee, William Markley, 379, 382
Lee Report on medical education,
    244-245
Lennon, John, 317
Leroy, E. Carwile, 58-59
Levinson, Daniel, 26
Lewis, C.S., 219
Lister, Joseph, 369
Livingston, Gordon, 60
Locke, John, 126, 366
Long, L.W., 345
Love, as virtue, 216-219
    importance to medical practice,
    171, 180
Lourie, Bernard, 271
Lowell, A. Lawrence, 240, 241
Luce, Clare Booth, 366
Lunceford, Emmett, M., Jr., 12-14
Lundberg, George L., 64, 75-76

Macaulay, Neill W.
Macaulay Museum of Dental His-
    tory, 3, 4
McCardle, Robert, 35
McCarthy, Eugene, 233
McCurdy, R. Layton, 359-361, 363
McEnroe, John, 29
McGovern, George, 233
MacIntyre, Alasdair, 164, 176, 179,
    195, 283, 284

McLendon, Baxter, 64-68
McNamara, Kristy Maher, 365
Machiavelli, 178, 180-181, 188
Mahon, William F., 354
Maker, William, 237, 239
Mangels, Jeannette, 186
Mann, Thomas, 105
Manners, 48-51
Marion, Francis, 38
Marx, Groucho, 166 n. 4
Maslow, Abraham, 142, 200-201,
    210, 219
Mayer, Orlando B., Jr., 7
Medicaid, 98, 107, 150, 251, 327,
    375
Medical education, 227-268
Medical history taking, 258-263
Medical journalism, 15, 379-386
Medical negligence, issues related
    to, 24-27, 124-129
Medical politics, 309-375
Medical professionalism
    See professionalism, medical
Medical societies, value of, 79-83
Medical Society of South Carolina,
    355
Medical University of South Caro-
    lina, 3, 7, 34, 40, 52, 58, 62, 63,
    66, 239-241, 243-246, 249, 250,
    264, 278, 290, 292
Medicare, 98, 107, 251, 327, 331,
    333, 335, 338, 352, 375
Medicine, economics of, 331-334,
    335-337, 338-340, 341-343, 351-
    353, 357-359
Medicine, as profession, 71-74, 75-
    78, 368-371
    See also Professionalism, medi-
    cal
Medicine, philosophy of, 371-375
Mencken, H.L., 85
Middle Ages, 97

Mildvan, Donna, 192
Miles, Stephen H., 101
Mobley, Mims, 341
Moseley, Vince, 235, 236
Moore, Michael, 371-372
Moultrie, James, Jr., 355
Musher, Jeremy, 280-281

Naisbitt, John, 162
Nation, Carrie, 198-199
Nation, Earl F., 198
National Institutes of Health, 251,
     338
National Medical Association, 347
Newton, Isaac, 159
Niebuhr, Reinhold, 219
Nursing, issues related to, 314-317

O'Bryan, Conyers, 341
O'Conner, Flannery, 113, 139
Optimism, 214-215
Oregon Plan, 343, 374
Organized medicine, value of, 30-
     31, 78, 79-83, 181-182, 196, 224,
     306, 353
Osler, William, 27, 41, 46, 86, 133,
     143, 160, 161, 208, 212, 233,
     235, 306

Pachelbel, Johann, 45, 47
Paget, Sir James, 229
Palmer, Daniel David, 326, 329
Palmetto Medical, Dental, and Phar-
     maceutical Association, 347
Paracelsus, 85
Paré, Ambrose, 85, 133, 214
Parker, Richard, 271
Pasteur, Louis, 133, 369
Patients, 8-11, 31-32, 45-47, 115-
     117, 149-150, 172-175, 221,
     224-225

Peabody, Francis Weld, 73-74, 151-
     154
Peck, M. Scott, 115
Peeples, Harrison, 248, 274, 324
Pellegrino, Edmund D., 175, 176,
     181-182, 206-207, 210, 217
Pepper, William, 56
Peterson, Christopher, 184
Pieper, Josef, 183
Percival, Thomas, 102-103
Philosophy, in premedical curricu-
     lum, 237-239
Physical diagnosis, 235-236, 264-
     268
Physician's assistants, 311-313
Physicians, supply of, 359-363
Platinum Rule, 195
Plato, 130, 137, 164, 177, 184, 186,
     187-188, 204, 238
Plutarch, 223
Poe, Edgar Allen, 344
Porter, Roy, 368
Pound, Roscoe, 71
Premedical curriculum, 237-239,
     239-242
Primum non nocere, 156
Profession, definition of, 88-89,
     91-92
Professional project, concept of, 88,
     95
Professionalism, medical, 54, 69-
     146, 181
Physician charter on, 100-104, 105
     As tiered construct, 109-114, 163
Project Professionalism. 89-90,
     119-124
Prudence (practical wisdom), as
     cardinal virtue, 186-191
Prudent Man Standard, 187
Public health, 269-308, 332
Pythagoras, 238

Race, issues related to, 344-348,
    364-368
Rand, Ayn, 178, 181
Rawls, John, 126, 373
Reade, Charles, 223
Reasoning, errors of, 190-191
Reed, Walter, 135
Relman, Arnold S., 32, 350
Renaissance, the, 97
Reverence for life, as concept, 155-
    157, 349
Reynolds, P. Preston, 117
Rockefeller Foundation, 22, 135-
    136
Rogers, George C., Jr., 7
Roosevelt, Franklin D., 233, 351
Rousseau, Jean-Jacques, 126, 307
Rowling, J.K., 55-56, 368-371

Sade, Robert M., 239-241, 365-366
St. Ambrose of Milan, 177
St. Augustine, 200
St. Paul, 137, 177, 179, 184, 217
St. Thomas Aquinas, 158-159, 168-
    169, 178, 180, 200, 204, 206, 284
Salvation Army, the, 17
Samaritan contract, 173, 218
SARS epidemic, 124-125, 206
Sandberg, Carl, 335
Sanders, Charles V., 183-184, 263
Sapira, Joseph, 265
Saunders, Donald E., Jr., 104
Savitt, Todd L., 346
Schweitzer, Albert, 155, 349
Scribonius Largus, 180, 366
Seligman, Martin E.P., 184, 215
Seven Deadly Sins, 199
Shaw, George Bernard, 207
Sheehy, Gail, 26
Shelley, William, 154
Sherman, William Tecumseh, 20
Sims, J. Marion, 133, 138, 169-171

Smith, Adam, 95-96
Social contract theory, 126
Social responsibility, of physicians,
    139
Socrates, 184, 191, 204, 238
Sophists (in Greek philosophy), 177
Soranus, 237
South Carolina, state of, attributes
    of, 36-40, 157
South Carolina Department of
    Health and Environmental Con-
    trol, 274, 276, 292
South Carolina Medical Association,
    xiii, 4-5, 13, 20, 33, 58, 63, 91,
    93, 149, 172, 317, 324, 334, 347,
    354-356, 365-367, 383, 386
South Caroliniana Library, 20, 40
Southgate, Therese, 64
Snyder, C.R., 213-214
Specialization, effects of, 115-118
Sprague, Stuart, 365
Starr, Paul, 332-334
Stevens, Rosemary A., 101, 105,
    107-108
Stevenson, Adlai, 233
Stevenson, Robert Louis, 105, 253,
    257
Stewart, Jimmy, 94
Stoic philosophers, 26, 126, 177,
    200, 238
Stokes, Hunter, 46
Stuckey, Melton R., 54
Sydenham, Thomas, 133

Tate, Sir Henry, 54
Taylor, Edmund R., 234
Technological imperative, 264-268,
    318-319
Temkin, Owsei, 4, 6
Temperance, as cardinal virtue,
    197-203
Thinking, critical, 253-257

Thomas, Lewis, 240, 241, 245, 256
Thomas L. and Shirley W. Roe Foundation, 66
Thomasma, David C., 175, 176, 181-182, 206-207, 210
Thompson, John, 29
Thomsonian movement, 96
Tillich, Paul, 208-209, 321
Toffler, Alvin, 324
Truman, Harry, 15
Tuchman, Barbara, 297
Tumulty, Philip A., 152-154

Unamuno, Miguel de, xiv
Updike, John, 36, 38
United States Public Health Service, 22
University of South Carolina School of Medicine, xiii, 104, 243-246, 250, 264-265
Urbani, Carlo, 124-125, 128, 132

Veatch, Robert M., 166, 181
Veterans Administration, 333, 338
Vietnam Conflict, 37
Virtue theory, 137, 140-141, 147-224
Virtues, cardinal, 180, 183-185
Virtues, theological, 180, 183-185
Voltaire, 307

Walton, Douglas N., 138, 168-169, 205-206

Waring, Ferdinanda Legaré, 6
Waring, Joseph Ioor, 3-7, 24, 243, 359, 384
Waring Historical Library, xiv, 5, 7, 40
Waring Library Society, 7, 34-35
Watson, Michael C., 314
Weed, Lawrence, 318
Welch, Claude Emerson, 72, 74
Wellcome Institute of the History of Medicine, 40
Weston, S. Nelson, 33, 91, 93
Weston, William, Jr., 7, 33-36
Weston, William, III, 33, 180, 315
Whetten, Kathryn, 193
Wickwar, Hardy, 312
Williams, Bernard, 179, 180
Williams, Robin, 94
Wilson, Gerald, 348
Wisdom, as virtue. *See* Prudence.
Withering, William, 133
Wood, Peter H., 344
World Health Organization, 124, 321
World War II, 251
Wragg, William T., 355

Yellow fever, 21-23, 135-136
Young, Foster, 16-17

Zuger, Abigail, 127